Frommer's Radiology for the Dental Professional

Frommer's Radiology for the Dental Professional

Tenth Edition

Jeanine J. Stabulas-Savage RDH, BS, MPH

Assistant Clinical Professor of Radiology
New York University
College of Dentistry
New York, New York

ELSEVIER

ELSEVIER

3251 Riverport Lane
St. Louis, Missouri 63043

FROMMER'S RADIOLOGY FOR THE DENTAL PROFESSIONAL,
TENTH EDITION

ISBN: 978-0-323-47933-2

Notices

Practitioners and researchers must always rely on their own experience and knowledge in evaluating and using any information, methods, compounds or experiments described herein. Because of rapid advances in the medical sciences, in particular, independent verification of diagnoses and drug dosages should be made. To the fullest extent of the law, no responsibility is assumed by Elsevier, authors, editors or contributors for any injury and/or damage to persons or property as a matter of products liability, negligence or otherwise, or from any use or operation of any methods, products, instructions, or ideas contained in the material herein.

Previous editions copyrighted 2011, 2005, 2001, 1996, 1992, 1987, 1983, 1978, and 1974.

International Standard Book Number: 978-0-323-47933-2

Director, Private Sector Education Content: Kristin Wilhelm
Senior Content Development Manager: Luke Held
Senior Content Development Specialist: Diane Chatman
Publishing Services Manager: Julie Eddy
Project Manager: Abigail Bradberry
Design Direction: Paula Catalano

Printed in India

Last digit is the print number: 9 8 7 6 5 4

Working together
to grow libraries in
developing countries

www.elsevier.com • www.bookaid.org

For my teacher, mentor, and friend,

Dr. Herbert H. Frommer

For his ever-present guidance and confidence.

And to my family,
For their love, support, and patience during this process.

Reviewers

Susan Bowen, CDA, BS
Dental Assisting Instructor
Perry Health Sciences Campus
Wake Technical Community College
Raleigh, North Carolina

Vicki Brett, RDH, CDA, BSDH
Dental Assisting Program Director
ECPI University
Chesapeake, Virginia

Joanna Campbell, RDH, MA, MA
Instructor, Dental Hygiene Department
Bergen Community College
Paramus, New Jersey

Charmaine Chappell, BS, MBA, CDA
Dental Assisting Program Coordinator
Centura College
North Chesterfield, Virginia

Lisa Childers, CDA, RDA
Associate Professor and Director
Dental Assisting Program
Arkansas Northeastern College
Blytheville, Arkansas

Leslie Koberna, RDH, BSDH, MPH/HSa, phD
Dental Hygiene Program Instructor
Texas Woman's University
Denton, Texas

Consulting Reviewer – 10ᵗʰ Edition
Alan Friedman, DDS
Dental Director
Joseph P. Addabbo Family Health Center, Inc.
Arverne, New York;
Private Practice Dentist
Brooklyn, New York;
Associate Clinical Professor (Retired)
NYU College of Dentistry
New York City, New York

Preface

As I planned the 10th Edition of this textbook, I seriously considered the dynamic changes in dental radiology since the first edition of this book was published. This textbook has grown from nine chapters and 160 pages to the present textbook of 25 chapters and more than 300 pages with an accompanying workbook. In addition, this text is currently augmented by the Evolve companion website with student practice materials and educator support. One has to be impressed with the changes that have taken place in the field of dental radiology. The 10th Edition now includes increased emphasis on utilization of rectangular collimation, cone beam computed tomography (CBCT), digital radiography, recognition by the American Dental Association of Dental Radiology as a specialty, the advent of established dental radiology private practice, implant placement, increased concern with radiation protection, and the universal use of the paralleling technique. I feel that we, as dental radiographic personnel, are a part of these monumental advancements and hope to reflect this in the current edition of this textbook.

This edition includes all the necessary content on dental radiology for the student of dental education and the dental professional. The textbook has been divided into three sections:

1. Foundation Knowledge of Dental Radiology
2. Foundation Knowledge of Radiographic Techniques
3. Foundation Knowledge of Radiographic Interpretation and Legal Aspects of Dental Radiology

The succession of the chapters has been changed as well to coincide with the addition of the previously mentioned three sections and to enable an improved flow of the dental radiographic educational concepts included in this edition. In addition, this 10th edition also includes the following **new features:**

- Full-color art program with new technique photos and modern illustrations
- Multiple-choice chapter review questions
- Critical thinking exercises
- Fully revised educational objectives
- Chapter introductions and summaries
- Additional helpful hints and notes within the chapters

The following **key features** remain, as they have resonated with students and instructors alike for the life of this product:

- Approachable writing style that simplifies complex concepts for improved understanding
- Step-by-step illustrated procedures for key skills and techniques
- *Common Errors* features to identify mistakes and ways to prevent and remedy them
- Advantages/Disadvantages boxes summarizing pros and cons of techniques
- Key terms highlighted in text and defined in a handy glossary

My intention is that the 10th Edition offering will improve the educational value of this textbook in contemporary dental radiology education and professional utilization.

Jeanine J. Stabulas-Savage, RDH, BS, MPH

Acknowledgments

I have some words of thanks for the colleagues and friends who have encouraged and helped me in preparing this tenth edition. I would like to especially thank Dr. Herbert H. Frommer for the confidence he has shown by entrusting me with this textbook that he originated back in 1974. The inspiration I employed while writing the tenth edition of this text emanates from his support and confidence in me to continue his work. I also could not have completed the manuscript without the help of my friend and colleague, Dr. Alan Friedman, whose knowledge of dental radiology and undying support was integral in the successful completion of this manuscript. I'd also like to acknowledge other colleagues and friends at the NYU College of Dentistry for their support with this project including Ms. Judith Cleary, Ms. Isabella Pellicciari, Ms. Letty Ponce, Dr. Debra Ferraiolo, Dr. Rajinder Jain, Dr. Lewis Lampert, Dr. Milton Palet, Ms. Cynthia Ruiz, Matthew Cardona, Dr. Denise A. Trochesset, Dr. Cheryl M. Westphal Theile, and my former chairperson, Dr. Joan A. Phelan. A special recognition goes to New York University's President, Dr. Andrew H. Hamilton; the Vice Dean for Academic Affairs and Research of New York University's College of Dentistry, Dr. Louis Terracio; and the Dean of New York University's College of Dentistry, Charles N. Bertolami for creating an academic environment that encourages and supports faculty scholarship.

Finally, I'd like to express my heartfelt appreciation to my husband, John Paul Savage; my daughters, Valerie and Vanessa Savage; and the Frommer family without whose encouragement, patience, and support this project could not have been completed.

Jeanine J. Stabulas-Savage

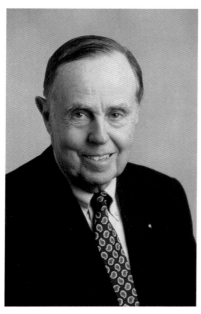

Herbert H. Frommer, DDS, was a Professor of Radiology at the New York University College of Dentistry, where he was a member of the faculty since 1971 (Emeritus since 2008). An internationally recognized expert in oral radiology, Dr. Frommer was the original author of Radiology for Dental Auxiliaries (currently titled Frommer's Radiology for the Dental Professional). Now in its 10th Edition, this textbook is used worldwide in educating dental professionals in oral radiology science and techniques. He was also author of the textbook Radiology in Dental Practice as well as 5 book chapters, 18 scholarly articles, and more than 100 lectures, including 4 at the prestigious International Congress of Maxillofacial Radiology. He was a founding member and former President of the American Academy of Oral and Maxillofacial Radiology.

Throughout his career as an educator, Dr. Frommer won tremendous acclaim from students and colleagues for his dedication to the craft of teaching. As the lead faculty member for one of the required first-year courses at the largest dental school in the country and as lead author of a popular textbook, Dr. Frommer had been involved in educating an entire generation of dental professionals. He served on the NYU Faculty Council and was President from 1993 to 1994 in addition to being a dedicated member of New York University's faculty senate. He was a past recipient of the College of Dentistry's Arnold and Marie Schwartz Outstanding Teacher Award and the NYU Distinguished Teacher Award.

In addition to his work in academic dentistry, Dr. Frommer was in private general dentistry practice for close to 50 years and had done consulting work reading CBCT scans for other practicing dentists.

Dr. Frommer received his AB degree from Columbia College and his DDS degree from the Columbia University School of Dental and Oral Surgery (now known as the College of Dental Medicine). He did his internship at Grasslands Hospital (now Westchester Medical Center) and has held multiple hospital appointments.

A member of the varsity crew team in college, Dr. Frommer served as faculty advisor and assistant coach of the NYU club crew team (where one of the shells is actually named after him). He was also a veteran of the United States Navy.

Dr. Herbert H. Frommer passed away peacefully on February 1, 2018. He is survived by his loving wife of 57 years, Eleanor Goldman Frommer and beloved sons, Ross and Daniel. He was the doting grandfather of Evan, Adam and Ariella; older brother of Paul and Alan, brother-in-law of Judith Goldman Frommer, Elizabeth Appell Frommer, and Jean Goldman; and father-in-law of Connie Dong and Jacqueline Frommer.

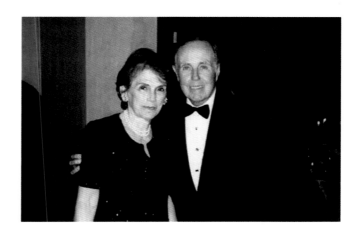

Contents

1

The History of Ionizing Radiation and Basic Principles of X-Ray Generation

EDUCATIONAL OBJECTIVES

Upon completing this chapter, the student will be able to:

1. Define the key terms listed at the beginning of the chapter.
2. Recognize the names, dates, and discoveries of the early pioneers affiliated with the discovery and the use of x-radiation in dentistry.
3. Define the term *radiation* and distinguish it from the term and definition of *radioactive*.
4. Discuss *electromagnetic radiation* and the significance of the *electromagnetic spectrum*.
5. List and describe the properties of x-rays.
6. Identify and describe the components of an atom and the process of ionization.
7. List and describe each of the components and respective functions of the x-ray tube, and explain the significance of heat production in the x-ray tube.
8. Describe the production of x-rays in the x-ray tube.
9. Describe the interactions that could occur at the target of the anode, including general radiation (bremsstrahlung radiation) and characteristic radiation.

KEY TERMS

anode
atom
atomic mass
atomic number
binding energy
bremsstrahlung (general) radiation
cathode
cathode ray
crest
duty cycle
duty rating
electromagnetic radiation

electromagnetic spectrum
electron
focal spot (area)
frequency
ionization
isotope
kilovoltage
milliamperage
molecule
neutron
nucleus
photons

proton
radiation
radioactive
radiographs
radionuclide
shell
target
thermionic emission effect
trough
tungsten filament
wavelength
x-rays

Introduction

We will begin our study of dental radiology by reviewing the history of x-rays, the basic terms and concepts associated with radiation, x-radiation, electromagnetic radiation, the electromagnetic spectrum, ionization, and x-ray production. This discussion will build the foundation of knowledge for the concepts to be discussed in the chapters to follow.

History of X-Rays

Names and Dates to Remember

- Wilhelm Conrad Roentgen, 1895
- Dr. Otto Walkhoff, 1896
- Walter Koenig, 1896
- Thomas Alva Edison, 1896
- Dr. C. Edmond Kells, 1896

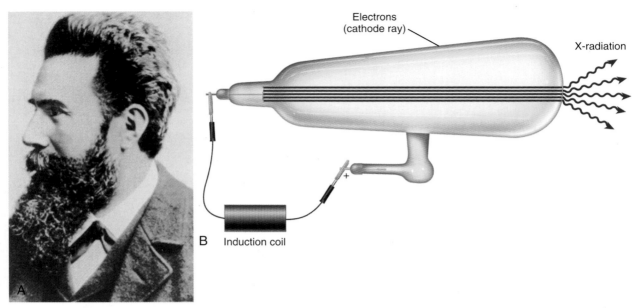

• **Figure 1.1 A,** Wilhelm Conrad Roentgen (1845–1923), discoverer of x-rays. **B,** Hittorf-Crookes tube, which Roentgen worked with at the time he discovered x-rays in 1895.

- William Rollins, 1896
- Dr. Frank Van Woert, 1913
- Dr. Howard Riley Raper, 1913
- William D. Coolidge, 1913
- Victor X-ray Corporation, 1923

It has been more than 120 years since the discovery of x-rays. Radiation can be best appreciated and understood by looking at the history of the development of the utilization of x-rays since the initial discovery. One can also learn about the hardships and injuries sustained by the early x-ray pioneers and how far science has come in reducing radiation exposure to patients and practitioners alike while improving diagnostic capabilities.

The x-ray was discovered on November 8, 1895, by **Wilhelm Conrad Roentgen**, a professor of physics at the University of Würzburg in Germany. He was working with a vacuum tube called a *Hittorf-Crookes tube,* through which an electric current from a battery was flowing (Fig. 1.1). Roentgen, like many of his colleagues, was interested in the cathode ray (a stream of electrons) and the type of light produced across a vacuum tube when an electric current was applied. Since he was concerned with light, he was working in a darkened room with black cardboard covering the Hittorf-Crookes tube. Coincidentally, there were many fluorescent plates in his laboratory at the time of his experiments with light. Thus, the stage was set for a discovery that would aid medical and dental science and has been ranked in importance with the discoveries of Pasteur (the principles of vaccination, microbial fermentation, and pasteurization) and Lister (pioneer of antiseptic surgery).

One evening, while working in his darkened laboratory, Roentgen noticed that one of the fluorescent plates at the far side of the room was glowing. He quickly realized that some form of energy coming from the Hittorf-Crookes tube was striking the fluorescent plate and causing it to glow. Because he did not know what it was, he called the phenomenon *x-ray,* "x" being the algebraic designation for the "unknown." He also noted that when he moved the plate closer to the tube, the glow grew stronger; and conversely, when the distance increased, the glow weakened. This specific observation demonstrated the inverse relationship between distance and intensity and is the basis of the "inverse square law," which is dealt with in later chapters. Roentgen also noticed that when placing various objects in the path of the x-ray beam, he could produce images of those objects on the screen. He inadvertently placed his hand between the tube and the screen and saw the faint outline of the bones of his hand. Roentgen went on to expose and produce images on photographic plates. Two of the first radiographs that Roentgen took were of his wife's hand, using a 15-minute exposure (Fig. 1.2), and of his shotgun. Thus, the first medical and industrial uses of x-radiation were demonstrated. It is interesting to note how closely the essential parts of Roentgen's tube and the modern x-ray tube resemble each other. They both are highly exhausted vacuum tubes with an anode and a cathode through which an electric current passes. Roentgen's tube had a fixed number of electrons available, in contrast to the present variable source (milliamperage), and the potential across his tube was fixed, whereas today it is variable (kilovoltage) as well.

Within a few weeks of his discovery, Roentgen presented a paper entitled "On a New Kind of Rays: A Preliminary Communication." In January 1896, **Dr. Otto Walkhoff**, a dentist in Braunschweig, Germany, made the first dental use of an x-ray, a radiograph of a lower premolar (Fig. 1.3).

Walkhoff used a small glass photographic plate wrapped in black paper and covered with rubber that he placed in his own mouth while lying on the floor. The exposure time was 25 minutes. Because of the plate's position in his mouth, the image showed parts of the upper and lower teeth, which actually resembled today's bitewing radiograph as opposed to just a lower premolar radiograph. This was followed in February 1896 by the work of physicist, **Walter Koenig**, who obtained a clearer image using only 9 minutes of exposure. Today, for a comparable image, these exposures would take fractions of a second (or impulses).

Interestingly, Roentgen's work was not greeted with universal acclaim, because the potential for diagnosis of disease was overshadowed by the public's concern about "something that could be used to see through people's clothing." His discovery was exploited by many who commercialized the use of x-rays. There were x-ray parlors in the United States in which individuals could have an image made of any part of their body made suitable for framing. These images were often referred to as *skiagraphs* (a photographic image produced on a radiosensitive surface by radiation

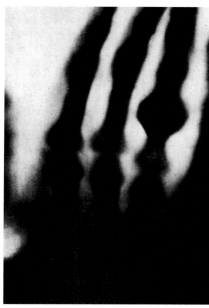

• **Figure 1.2** Radiograph taken of the hand of Mrs. Wilhelm Conrad Roentgen in 1895. (Reproduced with permission from Goaz PW, White SC: *Oral radiology and principles of interpretation*, ed 2, St Louis, MO, 1987, Mosby.)

other than visible light), from the Greek word meaning "shadow pictures." At the same time, in Victorian England, Roentgen was vilified for inventing a machine that could see through women's dresses.

For many years, the science of imaging using x-radiation was called *roentgenology*. His name is actually still used to express the amount of x-ray exposure, which is measured in "roentgens." For his work in the discovery of x-rays, Roentgen was awarded the first Nobel Prize in physics in 1901. Roentgen died in 1923.

The announcement of Roentgen's discovery was reported in the United States in 1896; within 2 days, **Thomas Alva Edison** and his staff at Menlo Park, New Jersey, had duplicated Roentgen's work. One of Edison's assistants was the first person to die as a result of repeated radiation experiments on himself and demonstrations on patients. Edison himself noted the development of redness around his own eyes. He discontinued his work with radiation and developed a fear of radiation that stayed with him for the rest of his life.

Dr. C. Edmund Kells, a New Orleans dentist, is credited with taking the first intraoral radiographs in the United States in April 1896. He had read about Roentgen's work and the new rays and immediately recognized its practical potential use in dentistry. Within a year, he set about acquiring the electrical equipment needed to produce the voltage necessary to charge the vacuum tubes available. He assembled all the equipment in Asheville, North Carolina, and gave the first demonstration of the use of x-rays before the Southern Dental Society. He used a variety of glass tubes—depending on the extent of the vacuum, age of the patient, and weather conditions—to make his choice. Because the handblown tubes were not standardized, the usual way for him to determine which tube was best for any procedure on a given day was to place his hand between the tube and a handheld fluoroscope and "set the tube" in that manner. This procedure could take a considerable amount of time; as a consequence, Kells developed radiation burns to the exposed areas that led to amputation of his fingers, then his hand, and, finally, his arm. These injuries are said to have led to his committing suicide.

Another early worker with intraoral radiographs was **William Rollins**, who developed the first dental x-ray unit in 1896. Many of the early pioneers working with dental x-rays suffered from effects of their work. Rollins also

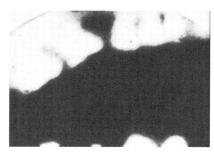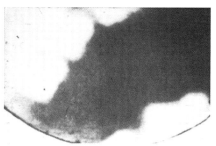

• **Figure 1.3** Early radiographs taken by Dr. Walkhoff.

reported burns to the skin on his hands and recommended lead shielding of both the tube and the patient.

It was not until 1913 that film was used instead of glass photographic plates to record dental images. **Dr. Frank Van Woert**, a New York dentist, was one of the first dentists to use and lecture about the new Kodak dental film.

Dr. Howard Riley Raper was the first to introduce radiology into the dental school curriculum at the University of Indiana and is credited with publishing the first dental radiology textbook.

The next great breakthrough was also in 1913, when **William D. Coolidge** invented the hot-cathode x-ray tube, which is the prototype of contemporary x-ray tubes. The hot filament provided a variable source of electrons in the tube and eliminated the need for residual gas as a source of ionization in the tube.

Additionally, in 1913, the first American dental x-ray machine was manufactured. In 1923, the **Victor X-ray Corporation**, which later became the General Electric X-ray Corporation and is now the Gendex Corporation, introduced a dental x-ray machine with a Coolidge tube in the head of the unit cooled by oil immersion.

The x-rays were produced in Roentgen's vacuum tube by the electric current applied to the tube, which caused ionization of the gas molecules in the tube; that is, the neutral molecules were broken into negative and positive ions. Because of the difference in electric potential, the negative particles (electrons) were attracted to the positive side of the tube, where they collided with the tube wall, and x-rays were produced. Modern dental x-ray tubes employ the same principle with some modifications, the most significant being a higher voltage, or difference in potential across the tube, and a variable source of electrons (hot filament). Today's tubes also have radiation safety features and cooling devices.

Radiation

The term radiation is defined as the emission and propagation of energy through space or a substance in the form of waves or particles. Particulate radiation consists of atoms or subatomic particles that have mass and travel at high speeds to transmit their kinetic energy. Some examples of particulate radiation are electrons (sometimes called *beta particles*), protons, neutrons, and alpha particles. These forms of particulate radiation most commonly are emitted from radioactive substances called radionuclides. However, the term *radiation* should not be confused with the term *radioactive*. The term radioactive refers to the process whereby certain unstable elements undergo spontaneous degeneration and produce high-energy waves called *gamma* and *particulate radiations*. Dental radiology specifically deals with x-radiations and not with radioactive materials. However, in the case in which dental patients are undergoing cancer therapy, they may receive radiation treatment from radioactive materials.

The use of x-rays is an intricate and essential part of dental diagnosis and is applied in many of the diagnostic imaging systems in both dentistry and medicine. X-rays are a type of radiation that are invisible waves or bundles of energy possessing certain properties that enable them to penetrate structures and record images that allow practitioners to see differences in densities in those structures. The images produced are viewed on either film or a digital display device and should be referred to as radiographs or images but not as x-rays. X-rays are the energy source that are waves with no mass and are part of a grouping called *electromagnetic radiation*.

Electromagnetic Spectrum

The electromagnetic spectrum is a grouping of energy waves known as electromagnetic radiation. What they all have in common is the weightlessness of the waves and the speed at which they travel (the speed of light—86,000 miles per second). The individual radiations of the electromagnetic spectrum differ in their wavelengths and frequencies and thus in many of their properties, including their ability to penetrate objects, also known as their "penetrating ability." Those radiations with shorter wavelengths and higher frequencies have more photon energy. Looking at Fig. 1.4, the reader can immediately recognize energy waves that are encountered every day, including radio waves, microwaves, and dental x-rays.

It is not known whether these electromagnetic radiations are actually waves of energy or the individual units of energy, called photons. Some phenomena can be best explained using the wave theory and others by considering the theory of discrete units of energy. If the radiation is considered a wave, its length is measured in angstrom units. If it is considered a bundle of photon energy, it can be measured in ergs. This text uses both forms, sometimes referring to waves of energy and at other times to photons of energy.

An energy wave travels in the same way that a ripple crosses a body of still water. The height of the wave is called the crest, and the depth of the wave is called the trough. The distance from the crest of one wave to the crest of another wave is called the wavelength and is usually abbreviated with the Greek letter lambda (λ). The frequency of a wave is the number of oscillations per unit of time (Fig. 1.5). The wavelength of x-rays is very short and is measured in angstrom units, which are 1/100,000,000 of a centimeter and can be expressed as 10–8 cm. The difference in the electromagnetic spectrum between visible light and x-rays is their wavelengths; x-rays have shorter wavelengths. The shorter the wavelength and the greater the frequency, the more energy it bears. This higher energy gives the x-ray the ability to penetrate matter—specifically, the teeth, bones, and gingiva of the dental patient—and cause ionization in tissue. Light waves, on the other hand, cannot penetrate teeth and bone because the wavelength is too long and does not have sufficient energy.

The effect of electromagnetic radiation on living organisms varies depending on the wavelength. Television and radio waves, which are ever present in the atmosphere, have no effect on human tissue. Microwaves, which are low-energy

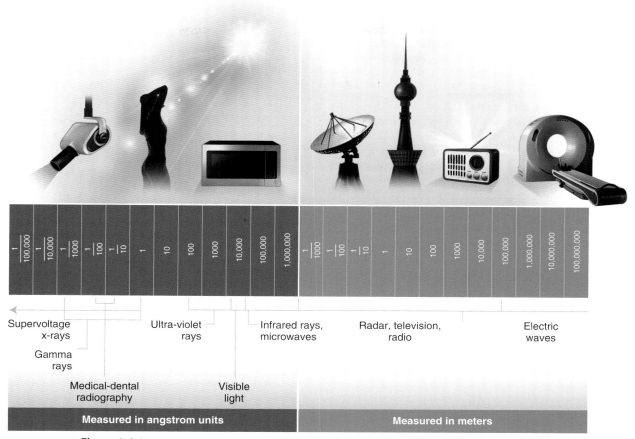

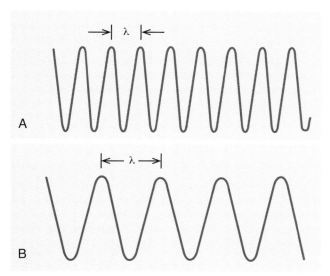

• **Figure 1.4** Electromagnetic spectrum. The shorter, more energized waves to the left are measured in angstrom units; the longer waves are measured in meters.

• **Figure 1.5** X-ray energy wave. The distance between the two crests is the wavelength lambda (λ) and the number of oscillations is the frequency. The wave in **A** has a shorter wavelength and a higher frequency than does the wave in **B**.

radiations, can produce heat within organic tissues and are thus employed in microwave ovens. However, microwaves do not have enough energy to be ionizing and therefore do not have the same effects on living tissue as x-rays, gamma rays, or particulate radiations. Electromagnetic radiations that do not contain sufficient energy to cause ionization are utilized in magnetic resonance imaging (MRI). MRI is used in medicine and dentistry for diagnostic purposes but does not possess the energy that x-rays have. These radiations are located in Fig. 1.4 near the radio waves on the electromagnetic spectrum.

Fig. 1.4 also shows that there is an overlap between gamma rays and the x-rays used for diagnostic purposes in medicine and dentistry because the two have identical wavelengths. Gamma rays and x-rays have identical properties if their wavelengths are the same; they differ only in their source. Dental and medical x-rays are the result of electron and atomic interactions within an x-ray tube, whereas gamma rays originate in the nuclei of radioactive materials.

Ultrasonic radiation, which is not part of the electro-magnetic spectrum, is another type of radiation used in medicine. Dental patients often question dentists about its use and relationship to dental x-rays. Ultrasound is a nonelectromagnetic, nonionizing radiation, with no effect on tissue that can be used to image internal structures. Because it is nonionizing, its use is acceptable in cases in which ionizing radiation might prove harmful (e.g., fetal imaging in pregnant women).

To explain the energy aspect of radiation, take the example of throwing a ball. Energy is imparted to the ball, which is expressed by the speed with which the ball travels. As this energy is lost, the ball falls, hits the ground, and rolls to a stop. The total energy is lost when the ball stops. This is also true of radiation. As x-rays travel over a distance, they lose their energy. For this reason, in the dental office, the operator stands a safe distance (6 feet) away from the patient having dental radiographs taken to avoid any personal exposure. If the ball is caught in midair, the energy can be felt by the impact on the hand catching the moving ball. The impact of the ball is in part a product of the weight of the ball and the speed with which it was thrown. X-rays and other radiations have no weight; they have only speed and energy, but their effect is as tangible as the sting of the ball on the hand. This effect is produced by interaction with the basic unit of matter, the **atom**, and the resultant ionization, which may adversely affect living tissue.

A preliminary understanding of x-rays and x-ray generation can be acquired simply by visualizing the everyday dental office procedure of taking a radiograph of a patient's tooth. The patient is seated in the dental chair. Because x-rays may produce harmful effects, the patient is draped with a lead apron (lead equivalent and lead-free aprons are also available for dental radiographic procedures). Following the infection control protocol (described in more detail in a later chapter), a film packet (or a digital sensor) in a holding device is positioned in the patient's mouth. The operator ensures that the activating switch is turned on and the dental x-ray machine is ready for the exposure procedure (Fig. 1.6). The open-ended, position-indicating device is then aimed at the film packet (or sensor) in the patient's mouth. The operator leaves the room or cubicle and makes sure to be standing at least 6 feet away from the source of radiation, which is also to avoid harmful effects. Radiation is produced for the appropriate length of time, and the film is exposed by pressing a button attached to an electric cord leading to the x-ray machine or mounted on the wall outside of the exposure room or cubicle. The film is then processed (when using conventional radiography) and interpreted.

From this description, some important observations can be made about the properties of x-rays. X-rays are produced by a machine whose source of energy is electricity; x-rays are produced by pushing a button that completes an electric circuit. Because no sign of x-ray production is apparent during the interval of exposure, x-rays must be invisible.

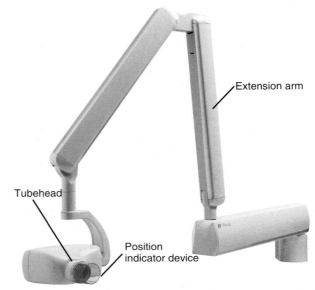

Extension arm

Tubehead

Position indicator device

• **Figure 1.6** Dental x-ray machine. (From KaVo Kerr, Orange, CA.)

The x-ray beam is directed at the film packet or sensor; thus, x-rays must travel in straight lines.

The ability of x-rays to produce an image on a film packet or digital sensor inside a patient's mouth by a machine positioned outside the mouth indicates that x-rays can penetrate opaque structures, such as skin, teeth, or bone.

After penetrating the dense tissue, x-rays can produce an effect on an imaging receptor, such as the dental film or sensor placed in the patient's mouth. This effect becomes visible by processing the film in the darkroom or by computer imaging so that an image of the penetrated structures appears on the film or computer monitor.

In summary, the following properties of x-rays are observed:

• X-rays are produced by the conversion of electrical energy into radiation.
• X-rays are invisible.
• X-rays travel in straight lines.
• X-rays can penetrate opaque tissues and structures.
• X-rays can affect a photographic emulsion, which, when processed, produces a visible image. X-rays can also affect a digital sensor to produce a digital image.
• X-rays can adversely affect human tissue.

Atomic and Molecular Structure

To understand both the concepts of x-ray production and the effect of x-radiation on tissue, the basic structure of matter (Fig. 1.7) must be understood. Matter is anything that has mass and occupies space. Matter is made of molecules. A **molecule** is the smallest particle of a substance that retains the property of that substance. Molecules are composed of atoms (Fig. 1.8). An atom contains a dense inner core, or **nucleus**, which possesses a positive electrical charge, and a number of light negatively charged subatomic particles called **electrons** that orbit around the nucleus. The nucleus

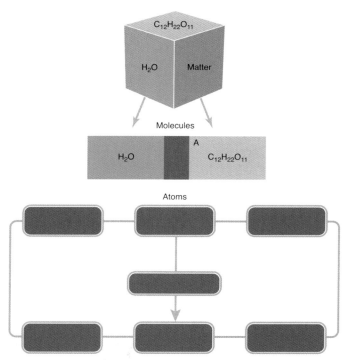

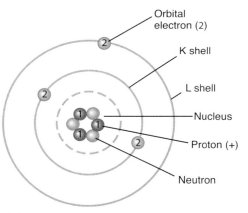

• **Figure 1.7** Components of matter.

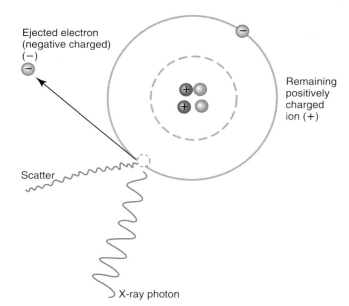

• **Figure 1.9** Ionization. The x-ray photon interacts with a neutral atom to form negatively and positively charged ions.

• **Figure 1.8** An atom. This is a lithium atom, whose atomic number (Z) is 3 and mass number (A) is 6.

of an atom is composed of positively charged subatomic particles, called **protons**, and particles that have no charge, called **neutrons**. The number of protons in the nucleus of an element is specific for each element and determines its **atomic number**. The number of protons, or atomic number, is designated by the symbol Z. The total number of protons and neutrons in the nucleus of an atom is the mass number and is designated by the letter A. An atom of an element that has the required number of protons for that specific element but a different number of neutrons in the nucleus is said to be an **isotope** of the element. Isotopes of an element have the same atomic number (number of protons) but a different **atomic mass** number (number of protons and neutrons) of the element (e.g., carbon-14). They may be stable or unstable, and the unstable isotopes may give off gamma rays, which are a component of the electromagnetic spectrum. Many isotopes are used as tracer elements in diagnosis or for the management of malignancies.

In the neutral or stable atom, the number of orbiting electrons (–) equals the number of protons (+) in the nucleus; thus, the atom is electrically neutral.

Electrons travel around the nucleus in definite orbits called **shells**. There is a maximum number of electrons that can occupy each shell and a definite energy level that binds the electrons in each shell to the nucleus. The shells farthest from the nucleus have less **binding energy** than the inner shells. The shell closest to the nucleus is called the *K shell*, the next outer shell the *L shell*, and then successively the *M*, *N*, and *O* shells. More energy is needed to remove an electron from the K shell than from the outer shells, because the binding energy is greater. This factor will come into play during the discussion of characteristic x-ray production.

Ionization

When an orbiting electron is ejected from its shell in an electrically stable or neutral atom, the process is called **ionization** (Fig. 1.9). The electrically neutral atom is then changed into two ions—one positively charged and one negatively charged. The remainder of the atom has a positive charge, and the ejected electron has a negative charge. Electrons can be removed from atoms by heating or interaction with x-ray photons. In all cases, however, the energy must be greater than the binding energy that holds the electron in orbit around the nucleus of the atom. Thus, the inner-shell electrons can be dislodged only by high-energy photons, such as x-rays, gamma rays, or particulate radiations, whereas the loosely bound electrons of the outer shell can be dislodged by low-energy photons, such as in ultraviolet light and heat. The new ions do not have the

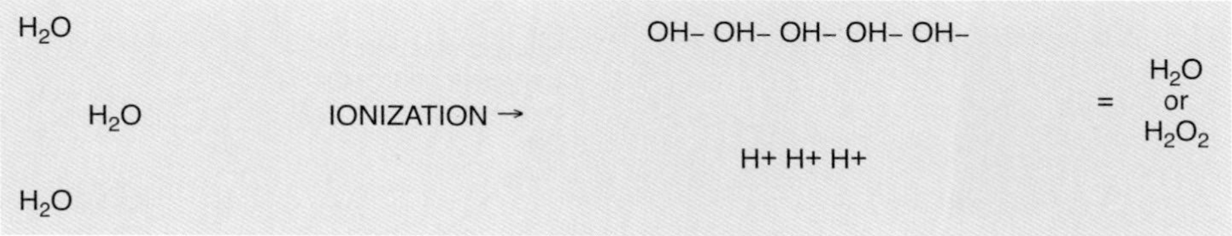

$$H_2O \qquad\qquad\qquad\qquad OH- \; OH- \; OH- \; OH- \; OH-$$

$$H_2O \qquad IONIZATION \rightarrow \qquad\qquad\qquad\qquad\qquad = \quad \begin{matrix} H_2O \\ or \\ H_2O_2 \end{matrix}$$

$$\qquad\qquad\qquad\qquad\qquad\qquad H+ \; H+ \; H+$$

$$H_2O$$

• **Figure 1.10** Ionization of a water molecule.

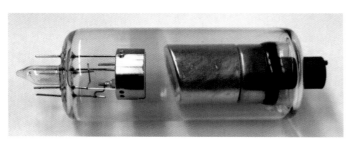

• **Figure 1.11** Dental x-ray tube. (From White SC, Pharoah MJ: *Oral radiology: principles and interpretation*, ed 7, St Louis, 2014, Mosby.)

same properties of the former neutral atom. Because x-rays, gamma rays, and some particulate radiation can cause this type of reaction, they are classified as ionizing radiations. The ionizing potential of certain radiations accounts for their harmful biologic effects. A simple illustration is the water molecule, H_2O. If it is ionized, as it can be by radiation, two hydroxyl ions are formed (free radicals). The two ions may recombine to form water or, in certain instances, they may recombine as H_2O_2, hydrogen peroxide (Fig. 1.10), which is used as an oxidizer, bleaching agent and disinfectant. Also, hydrogen peroxide is an oxidizing agent and is one of the primary tissue toxins produced by ionizing radiation.

X-Ray Tube

The dental x-ray tube (Fig. 1.11), although housed in the large tubehead of the dental x-ray unit, is quite small and is approximately only 6 inches long and 1½ inches in diameter. The three basic elements of an x-ray tube needed to produce x-rays are (1) high voltage to accelerate electrons across the tube, (2) a source of electrons within the tube, and (3) a target to stop the electrons.

High Voltage

As shown in Fig. 1.12, the x-ray tube has a positive electrode, called the **anode**, and a negative electrode, called the **cathode**. Electric current flows from a negative pole to a positive pole regardless of whether the cathode is positioned on the right or on the left of the x-ray tube. This voltage can be varied by adjusting the **kilovoltage** that controls the autotransformer, which then affects the step-up transformer and thus the kilovoltage across the tube. The greater the kilovoltage or potential across the tube, the faster the electrons will travel and the greater the energy that will be released when the electrons strike the target at the anode, thus the greater the penetrating capability.

Source of Electrons

The main source of electrons in the x-ray tube is the **tungsten filament** found at the cathode. This is a variable source of electrons, unlike Roentgen's tube, in which electrons were produced from the ionization of a fixed volume of gas. The tungsten filament is connected to the step-down transformer circuit. The hotter the resistant filament becomes, the more electrons are produced at the cathode. This production, or "boiling off," of electrons from the heated tungsten filament is called the **thermionic emission effect**. The **milliamperage** dial controls the amount of current in the filament circuit and thus the number of electrons that boil off. The tungsten filament is surrounded by a focusing cup made of molybdenum and directs electrons toward the anode that contains the target.

Target

The **target** in the x-ray tube also can be called the **focal spot** or **area**. At the anode side of the tube and when the circuit is complete, it has a positive (+) charge. It is made of tungsten and measures about 0.8×1.8 mm. This is the actual target. The effective target, or focal area, is smaller because of the tilting of the target that geometrically makes the target smaller when viewed from the opening in the tube. All modern dental x-ray machines have approximately the same size target. Tungsten is used as the target material, because it has a high melting point and a low vapor pressure at high temperatures and thus is not affected by the heat produced. The element tungsten is also desirable as a target material because of its high atomic number and thus its density and because, when it is bombarded by electrons, x-ray production is more efficient. However, tungsten does not have a high degree of thermal conductivity and must be embedded in a copper stem. The heat is dissipated into the head of the x-ray machine by the copper stem attached to the anode and cooled by air or oil immersion.

Heat Production

The dental x-ray machine is an extremely inefficient machine. Of the total energy produced at the anode by the collision of the electrons with the target, less than 1% is x-ray energy; the remaining 99% is in the form of heat. This is why the highly conductive copper sleeve and oil immersion tube surround the target. Although difficult to do, care must be taken not to overheat the tube.

Heat production at the target is the limiting factor of the milliampere (mA) setting of a dental x-ray machine. With a

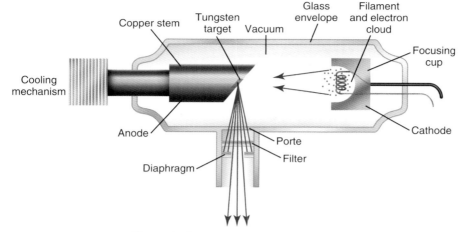

• **Figure 1.12** Components of a dental x-ray tube.

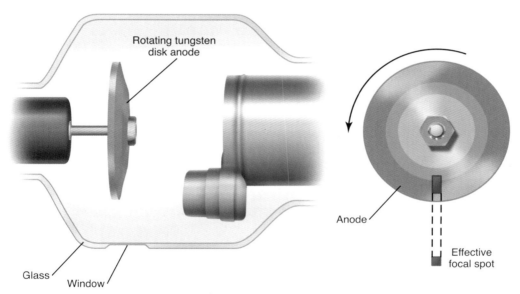

• **Figure 1.13** Rotating anode.

milliampere setting of more than 15, too many electrons hit the target and too much heat is produced. This overheating soon will destroy the target. Some panoramic and extraoral units have rotating anodes (Fig. 1.13) to dissipate the heat and thus can use higher milliampere settings. The standard dental x-ray machine has a fixed anode and a limit to the amount of milliamperage.

Overheating of a dental x-ray machine is not very likely under ordinary use. Each machine has a duty rating and a duty cycle. The duty rating refers to the number of consecutive seconds a machine can be operated before it overheats. The duty cycle refers to the portion of every minute that the dental machine can be used without overheating. To damage the x-ray tube, one would have to make about a 17-second exposure or work so fast that multiple exposures would be made per minute.

X-Ray Production

X-rays used in dentistry are produced in an x-ray tube and, as previously mentioned, with modifications the modern tube resembles the cathode ray tube used by Roentgen. The principles of high-speed electrons being attracted to and colliding with a positively charged target to produce x-rays and heat are still valid. Figs. 1.14 to 1.16 are schematic drawings of the production of x-rays in the dental x-ray tube.

When a dental x-ray machine is turned on and the indicator light is glowing, it is ready to produce x-rays. Turning on the machine closes the filament circuit and heats the tungsten filament, causing electrons to boil off by the thermionic emission effect. The electrons stay at the filament and are referred to as an *electron cloud* (see Fig. 1.14).

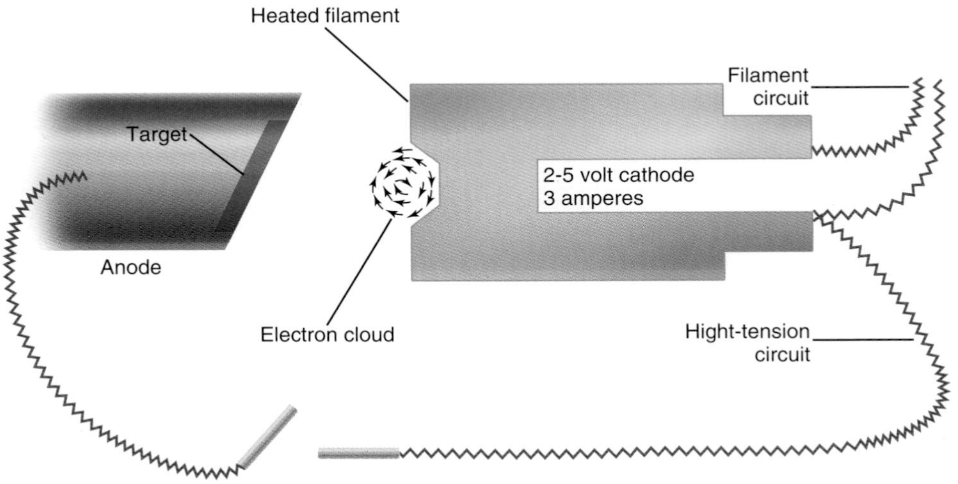

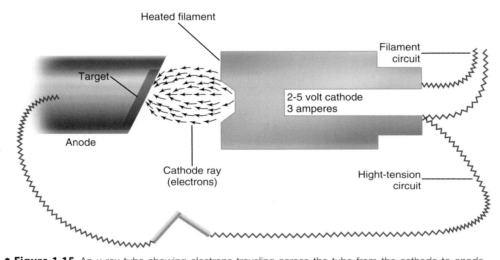

• **Figure 1.14** An x-ray tube illustrating formation of an electron cloud at the cathode as the filament circuit is activated. Note that the exposure switch is open.

• **Figure 1.15** An x-ray tube showing electrons traveling across the tube from the cathode to anode (target) as the high-tension circuit (exposure switch) is activated.

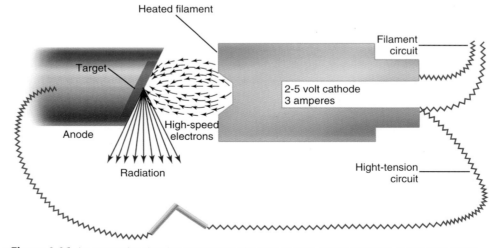

• **Figure 1.16** An x-ray tube showing production of x-rays as high-speed electrons collide with target.

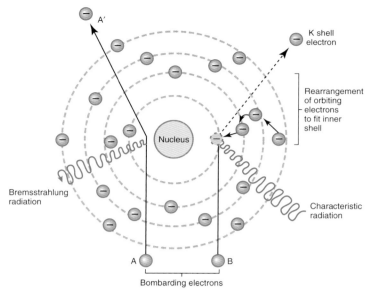

• **Figure 1.17** Electrons colliding with a simulated tungsten atom, forming bremsstrahlung radiation *(A)* and characteristic radiation *(B)*.

The electrons are attracted across the tube only when there is a difference in electric potential across the tube or, stated another way, when the high-voltage circuit is closed or completed. This high-voltage circuit is activated by the exposure switch and remains active for the length of time for which a timer is set as long as the operator maintains pressure on the switch.

With the high-voltage circuit completed by pressing the exposure switch, the electrons produced by the thermionic emission effect at the cathode are attracted to the positively charged anode, which contains a tungsten target (see Fig. 1.15). This stream of electrons crossing the tube is called the cathode ray. Federal regulations require that dental x-ray machines emit an audible signal when an exposure is being produced in addition to the signal light in the control panel.

X-rays and heat are produced in the tube when the high-speed electrons strike the tungsten target (see Fig. 1.16). This represents a transference of energy. The kinetic energy of the moving electron is converted to the energy-laden x-ray photon and heat energy. The faster the electrons travel across the tube, the more energized and penetrating are the x-rays produced. The speed of the electrons across the tube is determined by the kilovoltage.

As illustrated in Fig. 1.13, the tungsten target is angled and the x-rays produced are directed to an exit point (porte) in the tube. The rest of the x-ray tube is lead lined, and x-rays can leave the tube only through the porte. If x-rays leave the tube in any area other than the porte, the machine is said to have head leakage. This is a safety hazard to both patient and operator and is a violation of the radiation safety code. Consequently, during an x-ray inspection of the radiographic equipment in a dental facility, the inspector specifically checks the x-ray machines for head leakage.

Bremsstrahlung and Characteristic X-Rays

This section examines the formation of x-rays at the level of the atom; that is, the atomic mechanism of the formation of x-rays when the high-speed electrons strike the tungsten target.

The phenomenon of x-ray production can be best understood by considering the tungsten atom and the possibilities that arise when a high-speed electron enters its orbit, as it would by striking the target of a dental x-ray machine (Fig. 1.17). The tungsten target consists of an infinite number of tungsten atoms. Only one surface atom will serve as a representative example for the rest of the atoms in the tungsten target.

General Radiation or Braking (Bremsstrahlung) Radiation

General or braking radiation (bremsstrahlung) is produced when an electron hits the nucleus of the tungsten atom (which rarely occurs) or when the electron is attracted to the nucleus of the atom and comes close to it but does not hit it (represented by electron A in Fig. 1.17). This entering high-speed electron might hit the nucleus and give up all of its energy or may be slowed down and bent off its course by the positive pull of the nucleus. These possibilities represent a loss of energy that is given off as x-rays and heat and are the major sources of x-ray production in the dental x-ray tube. The sudden stopping or slowing down and veering off course of the entering high-speed electron with its loss of energy expressed in x-rays and heat is called bremsstrahlung, the German word for "braking radiation."

Because the tungsten target is not just one atom thick, this bremsstrahlung is repeated an infinite number of times.

The exiting electron A′ (see Fig. 1.17) will enter another tungsten atom; the reaction will be repeated with the production of more x-rays. A′ and the succeeding A″, A‴, and so forth, each will have less energy than the original entering electron A. Therefore, the x-rays produced at each succeeding bremsstrahlung will have less energy or longer wavelengths. Because of the multiple bremsstrahlung reactions, all of the x-rays produced do not have the same energy content (wavelength). Thus, a heterogeneous x-ray spectrum is produced. The later bremsstrahlung reactions produce x-rays whose energy is not sufficient to penetrate teeth and bone and, as will be seen, are removed by filtration.

Characteristic Radiation

Another possibility, represented by entering electron B in Fig. 1.17, is that the high-speed electron might hit and dislodge one of the orbiting inner-shell electrons of the tungsten atom. This can happen only when the entering electrons possess more energy than that binding the orbiting electrons to the nucleus. In the dental machine, this means it can happen only at settings of 70 kV (70,000 V) and above. If an orbiting electron is dislodged, a rearrangement or cascading of electrons inward fills up the electron vacancies in the inner shells. This rearrangement produces a loss of energy that is expressed in x-ray energy. The x-rays produced are called *characteristic x-rays* and account for a very small part of the x-rays produced in the dental machine. They occur only in those machines operating at 70 kV and above. Bremsstrahlung and characteristic radiation can be produced at the same time and are additive.

Chapter Summary

- X-rays were discovered by Wilhelm Conrad Roentgen in 1895.
- Dental radiography has progressed considerably since the work of the early x-ray pioneers, especially in reducing x-ray exposure to patients and practitioners while improving the diagnostic capabilities of radiographic images.
- The use of x-ray images is an integral part of dental diagnosis.
- X-rays are a type of electromagnetic radiation that have short wavelengths, high frequency, and greater penetrating ability.
- X-rays are related to ionization in two ways: (1) they are formed by the process of ionization, and (2) they can affect living tissue by the process of ionization.
- X-rays are produced in the dental x-ray tube when the dental professional presses the exposure button in a clinical setting.
- General, or bremsstrahlung, radiation and characteristic radiation are responsible for the x-ray energy that is produced at the target of the anode in the dental x-ray tube.

Chapter Review Questions

Multiple Choice

1. Which of the following pioneers is credited with the first dental usage of an x-ray?
   a. Walter Koenig
   b. Wilhelm Conrad Roentgen
   c. Thomas Alva Edison
   d. Otto Walkhoff
   e. William Rollins
2. Some examples of particulate radiation are:
   a. Electrons
   b. Alpha particles
   c. Beta particles
   d. Protons
   e. All of the above
3. The "frequency" of a wave is defined as:
   a. The distance from the crest of one wave to the trough of another wave
   b. The number of oscillations of a wave per unit of time
   c. The distance from the crest of one wave to the crest of another wave
   d. The penetrating ability of the wave
   e. The spectrum of the wavelength
4. The target of the anode:
   a. Is the positive side of the x-ray tube
   b. Is involved in x-ray production
   c. Is made out of aluminum
   d. Only answers a and b are correct
   e. Answers a, b, and c are correct
5. Which of the following components of the dental x-ray tube are considered part of the "cathode?" (Indicate all that apply.)
   a. Tungsten filament
   b. Molybdenum focusing cup
   c. Copper stem
   d. Aluminum filter
   e. Cooling mechanism

Critical Thinking Exercises

1. Explain how the properties of x-radiation can be understood simply by observing a dental radiographic procedure on a patient.
   a. Describe the steps of the procedure.
   b. Name the property of x-radiation related to each of those steps.

2. Explain x-ray production in the dental x-ray tube.
   a. Name each of the components of the x-ray tube and their functions as related to x-ray production.
   b. Name the three basic elements of an x-ray tube needed to produce x-rays and describe each element.

Bibliography

American Academy of Dental Radiology Quality Assurance Committee: Recommendations for quality assurance in dental radiology, *Oral Surg Oral Med Oral Pathol* 55:421–426, 1983.

American Dental Association Council on Scientific Affairs: An update on radiographic practices: information and recommendations, *J Am Dent Assoc* 132:234–238, 2001.

FDA Department of Health and Human Services, 21 C.F.R., Subchapter J Radiological Health, General § 1000.1 (1994).

Frommer HH: History of dental radiology, *Tex Dent J* 119:417–427, 2002.

Frommer HH, Fortier P: History of the American academy of oral and maxillofacial radiology, *Oral Surg Oral Med Oral Pathol Oral Radiol Endod* 80:511–516, 1995.

Iannucci JM, Howerton LJ: *Dental radiography: principles and techniques*, ed 5, St. Louis, MO, 2016, Elsevier Saunders.

Langland OE, Langlais RP: Early pioneers of oral and maxillofacial radiology, *Oral Surg Oral Med Oral Pathol Oral Radiol Endod* 80:496–511, 1995.

Langland OE, Langlais RP: *Principles of dental imaging*, Baltimore, MD, 1997, Williams & Wilkins.

National Council on Radiation Protection and Measurements: NCRP Report No. 145, Radiation in Dentistry. Washington, DC; 2004.

Thompson EM, Johnson ON: *Essentials of dental radiography for dental assistants and hygienists*, ed 9, Upper Saddle River, NJ, 2012, Pearson Education, Inc.

White SC, Pharoah MJ: *Oral radiology: principles and interpretation*, ed 7, St. Louis, MO, 2014, Mosby.

2

The Dental X-Ray Machine

EDUCATIONAL OBJECTIVES

Upon completing this chapter, the student will be able to:

1. Define the key terms listed at the beginning of the chapter.
2. Discuss the following related to electricity:
   - Differentiate between an alternating current (AC) and direct current (DC) and their uses in the dental x-ray machine.
   - Explain what is meant by *rectification* in older dental x-ray units.
   - Know how many impulses there are in a second and how they are related to the exposure time settings in dental radiography.
   - Define *voltage,* and differentiate between kilovolt (kV) and kilovoltage peak (kVp).
   - Define *amperage,* and explain what the milliamperage (mA) setting controls in the dental x-ray machine.
   - Discuss the function of a transformer, and name the three transformers used in dental radiography, as well as their respective purposes.
   - Discuss the process of x-ray production in the dental x-ray tube, including the components, their functions, and the electrical system utilized.
3. Discuss the two major circuits in the x-ray machine.
4. Differentiate between older and newer dental x-ray machines, and discuss timers.
5. Describe the following related to x-ray beams:
   - Discuss the process of collimation of the x-ray beam and the role of the position-indicating device (PID) in this process.
   - Summarize the three parameters of the dental x-ray machine (quality, quantity, and exposure time) and how kV and mA are related to these parameters.
   - Define and apply the concept of a *half-value layer (HVL)* in describing the x-ray beam quality and penetration.
   - Discuss the significance of the intensity of the x-ray beam and how it is related to the quality, quantity, exposure time, and target-receptor distance (or focal-film distance [FFD]).
   - Discuss the significance and regulation of filtration and collimation as they apply to the dental x-ray beam.
   - Explain why rectangular collimation is considered to be an important factor in reducing radiation exposure to the dental patient.

KEY TERMS

alternating current (AC)	direct current (DC)	position-indicating device (PID)
amperage	electric current	rectification
ampere	filter	scatter radiation
autotransformer	half-value layer (HVL)	self-rectified
central ray	half-wave rectified	step-down transformer
collimation	impulses	step-up transformer
collimator cutoff	intensity	transformer
cone	kilovolt (kV)	useful beam
cone cutting	kilovoltage peak (kVp)	voltage
cycle	milliampere (mA)	

Introduction

This chapter continues the discussion of x-ray production in the dental x-ray machine with a focus on its components, energy source, electrical circuits, control mechanisms, and characteristics of the x-ray beam.

Electricity

Because the primary source of energy for the x-ray machine is electricity, which is used to create x-rays, it is necessary to learn or review some basic concepts of electricity.

Electric current is the flow of an electrical charge. In electric circuits, this charge is often carried by moving electrons through a conductor. When the electrons flow in one direction, it is known as a direct current (DC), whereas in an alternating current (AC), electrons flow in one direction and then reverse and flow in the opposite direction in the circuit (Fig. 2.1).

Rectification

Most of the older dental x-ray machines operated on an AC wherein, for the x-ray tube itself, the polarity is reversed 60 times per second. When the direction of the current flow is reversed, the tungsten target becomes the negative pole and the tungsten filament becomes the positive pole. During the AC, when the current is reversed, few x-rays are produced, because there are few electrons available at the filament to travel across the tube and strike the target. Thus, the current is blocked from traveling across the tube. Also, because the tungsten target is negative during current reversal, electrons will not flow across the x-ray tube. This is due to the fact that negative charges repel each other. This blocking of the reversal is called rectification. Because the dental x-ray tube functioning on an AC is designed to produce this effect, it is said to be self- or half-wave rectified (Fig. 2.2).

In an AC, x-rays are not produced in a steady stream but rather in spurts or impulses. These impulses take place only during one half of the alternating current cycle. Most ACs are 60 cycles; thus, the dental x-ray machines express exposure units in impulses or sixtieths of a second. There are 60 impulses in a second; therefore, a ½-second exposure is equal to 30 impulses, ⅓-second of exposure is equal to 20 impulses, and ¼-second of exposure is equivalent to 15 impulses.

> ### HELPFUL HINT
> An easy way to remember how many impulses there are in a second is to recall that there are 60 impulses in a second, 60 seconds in a minute, and 60 minutes in an hour! These time intervals actually remain constant and are easy to remember!

Newer-model dental x-ray machines are designed to supply full-wave rectification (Fig. 2.3) by operating on a DC. In this circuitry, the negative portion of the AC cycle is reversed. If currents are then superimposed, there is less of a drop in voltage between cycles. These machines do not produce pulses of x-radiation but rather a constant stream of x-rays. Thus, exposure time can be reduced by one-half, because x-rays are being produced all of the time. Therefore, patient exposure is reduced in DC operated machines and, as a result, is an important consideration in patient protection. This is due to the fact that the mean energy produced by DC x-ray machines is higher than the mean energy from an AC machine operating at the same voltage. There are no dips in voltage in a DC machine, because you have a constant potential between the anode and the cathode. Thus, the x-rays are less heterogeneous, with a lot less x-rays with long wavelengths produced. However, both AC and DC units produce images that are diagnostic with conventional (film-based) and digital radiography. Voltage is the term used to describe the electric potential or force that drives an electric current through a circuit. The unit of measurement is the volt (V). The kilovolt (kV) is 1000 V. In an AC, in which the direction of the current is constantly changing, the voltage is also changing. The term kilovoltage peak (kVp) is used to denote the maximum or peak voltage that is described by the sine wave that plots the alternation of the current (see Fig. 2.1). A dental x-ray machine that is set for a potential of 90 kVp will reach 90 kVp only at the peak of the AC during exposure. As seen in the diagram of the exposure's sine wave (see Fig. 2.1), other voltage levels also occur during the exposure. This has great clinical significance, because these differences in voltage contribute to the heterogeneity of the x-ray beam

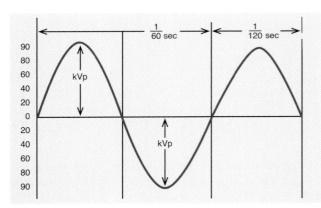

• **Figure 2.1** Sine wave of 60-cycle alternating electric current operating at 90,000 V (90 kVp).

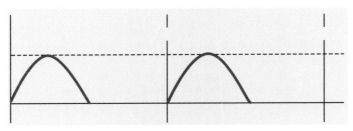

• **Figure 2.2** Half-wave rectification.

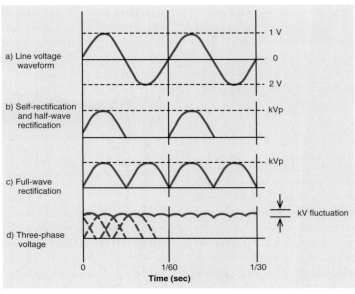

• **Figure 2.3** Full-wave rectification.

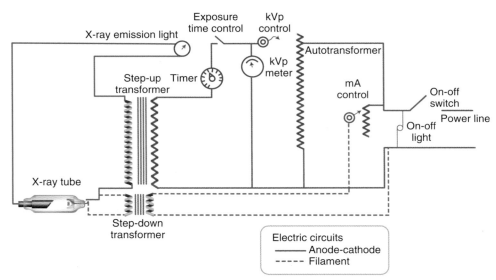

• **Figure 2.4** Basic electric circuits of dental x-ray machine.

and the need for proper filtration. It should be noted that the term *kilovolt (kV)* is used more often in contemporary dental radiography than the term *kilovoltage peak (kVp)*, which was formerly used.

Amperage is defined as the strength of an electric current measured in amperes. **Ampere** is the unit of measurement used to describe the amount of electric current flowing through a circuit. The **milliampere (mA)** is equal to 1/1000 of an ampere.

In dental radiography, both voltage and amperage can be adjusted by using the kV or mA control devices on the control panel if available. Some newer dental x-ray units have preset kV and mA settings. In either case, the mA setting will control the number of electrons at the cathode filament, and the kV setting will control the current passing from the cathode to the anode in x-ray production.

A **transformer** is a device that can either increase or decrease the voltage in an electric circuit. It is composed of two coils of electric wire insulated from one another. There are three transformers used in dental x-ray production (Fig. 2.4). The transformer that increases the voltage is referred to as the **step-up transformer**, and the transformer that decreases the voltage is referred to as the **step-down transformer**. The dental x-ray machine uses both of these in taking ordinary line or house voltage of 110- or 220-line voltage and stepping it up to a range of 65,000 to 100,000 V (65–100 kV) in the high-voltage circuit or stepping line voltage down to 3 to 5 V in the filament circuit—these being the two basic circuits in the dental x-ray machine. The dental x-ray machine also has an **autotransformer**, which uses only one coil and can be employed for making minor changes in voltage.

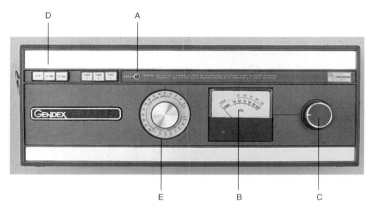

• **Figure 2.5** Control panel of an older-model dental x-ray machine. *A,* Exposure indicator. *B,* Kilovoltage peak (kVp) meter. *C,* kVp control. *D,* Milliampere (mA) control. *E,* Timer control. (Courtesy KaVo Dental/ GENDEX Imaging, Lake Zurich, IL.)

HELPFUL HINT

X-ray production can be easily understood by dividing the components and functions into two distinct phases:

Phase 1

The x-ray machine is turned on. The electricity travels from the wall outlet, through the arm of the x-ray unit to the tube head.

The current activates the filament circuit and the step-down transformer. 110 V (or 220 V) is reduced to 3 V to 5 V by the step-down transformer.

The filament circuit utilizes 3 V to 5 V to heat the tungsten filament at the cathode, causing the thermionic emission effect, which results in the formation of the electron cloud.

The milliampere (mA) controls the number of electrons that boil off the cathode filament and, thus, is responsible for the quantity of x-radiation produced.

Phase 2

Upon pressing the exposure button, the high-voltage circuit is activated, and the electrons produced at the cathode move across the tube as the cathode ray.

The step-up transformer increases the 110 V (or 220 V) to the 65,000 V to 100,000 V, which is necessary to accelerate the movement across the tube.

The molybdenum focusing cup directs the electrons (cathode ray) from the cathode to the tungsten target of the anode.

The impact of the electrons striking the tungsten target converts the kinetic (motion) energy to x-radiation energy (1%) and heat (99%). The kilovolt (kV) controls the quality or penetrating power of the x-ray beam.

The x-rays travel through the porte (unleaded portion of the tube), the aluminum filter, and the collimating devices (diaphragm and position-indicating device [PID]) and are directed at the patient to produce the images needed for dental diagnosis.

Circuitry

The two major circuits in the x-ray machine are the *filament circuit* and the *high-voltage circuit*. Each circuit uses a transformer to convert the line voltage and current. The filament circuit uses 3 V to 5 V; thus, the 110 V (or 220 V) line current is reduced by means of a step-down transformer (see Fig. 2.4). The heating of the cathode filament by the electric current is controlled by a rheostat in this circuit and is a function of the milliamperage. The milliamperage determines the quantity of the x-rays produced. The high-voltage circuit in the dental x-ray machine requires voltage in the range of 65,000 V to 100,000 V. This increase in voltage is achieved by the use of a step-up transformer that energizes the cathode ray to travel from the cathode to the anode. An autotransformer also is used in the circuit as a line compensator to control fluctuations in the line voltage.

Control Panel

The control panel of the older dental x-ray machines (Fig. 2.5) contain an on-off switch and indicator light, an exposure button and indicator light, timer dial, and kV and mA selectors. The exposure button is on a 6-ft retractable cord or linked to a remote station that is behind an acceptable barrier. Newer dental x-ray machines have preset, fixed milliamperage choices, usually 7, 10, or 15 mA. The kV values may be fixed or have a range from 60 to 100. Some units, instead of having numerical choices for kV, have icons or diagrams of a small, medium, or large patient, because the

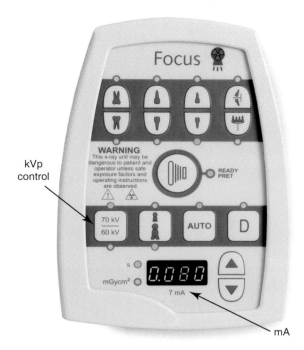

• **Figure 2.6** Icons on the control panel indicate kVp, mA, and patient size. (Courtesy KaVo Kerr, Charlotte, NC.)

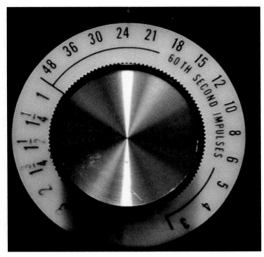

• **Figure 2.7** Timer dial. Note the increments in impulses (1/60 second). (From Langlais RP, Miller CS: *Exercises in Oral Radiology and Interpretation*, ed 5, St Louis, 2017, Elsevier.)

amount of kVs needed for penetration is linked to the size of the patient. Other units only have a choice of setting the patient size for an "adult" or "pediatric" patient (Fig. 2.6). In any event, when the size-of-the-patient icon is changed, the x-ray unit automatically adjusts itself to maintain the desired image density.

Timer

As previously discussed, the dental x-ray tube may emit a continuous stream of radiation or a series of impulses of radiation. The number of impulses depends on the number of cycles per second in the electric current being used. In a 60-cycle AC, there are 60 pulses of x-rays per second (Fig. 2.7). Each impulse lasts only 1/120 second because no x-rays are emitted in the negative half of the cycle when the polarity of the tube is reversed. The exposure time on newer-model dental x-ray machines are most likely represented in fractions of seconds rather than in impulses and have electronic timers. The old mechanical timers with increments of 3½ seconds, which were usually inaccurate by at least 2¾ seconds, are unacceptable for the shorter exposure times in use today for faster-speed film or digital sensors and in many instances are violations of the radiation code.

The x-ray machine should be turned off after use. Warm-up time is not a factor because it is almost instantaneous for the x-ray tube; thus, there is no need to keep the machine on during the entire work day. Most offices have definite settings for mA and kV that are used for all patients. As discussed in the next chapter, the kV is determined by the density of the object and the type of contrast desired, whereas the mA is determined by the speed

of the receptor, the exposure time, and the source-to-patient distance (or FFD).

X-Ray Beam

The x-ray photons produced at the target in the dental x-ray tube emanate from and leave the tube as a divergent beam. The x-ray at the center of the beam is called the **central ray**. The x-rays closest to the central ray are more parallel, and those farthest away are more divergent. The more parallel rays produce less magnification of the image; thus, they are the most useful (Fig. 2.8).

The x-ray beam is positioned or aimed at the receptor in the patient's mouth by an open-ended device, either a rectangle or a cylinder, called a **position-indicating device (PID)**. These PIDs should be lead-lined to prevent the escape of **scatter radiation** and are usually 8, 12, or 16 inches long (Fig. 2.9). In the past, dental x-ray machines had plastic, pointed cones as PIDs. To this day, people incorrectly refer to open-ended cylinders or rectangles as **cones**; the proper term to use in reference to this device is the *position-indicating device (PID)* or can sometimes also be referred to as a *collimator*.

The pointed cone was designed as a user-friendly aiming device, with the tip of the cone indicating the position of the central ray. This technique called for aiming the tip of the cone at the center of the film packet placed in the patient's mouth. One of the unfortunate outcomes of this type of instrumentation was that some practitioners came to believe that the x-ray beam was coming out only from the tip of the cone and that the size of the beam was that limited.

The problem with the pointed plastic cone is that secondary (scattered) radiation was produced by the interaction of the primary beam of x-ray photons with the plastic cone (Fig. 2.10). These secondary (scattered) x-rays increase the long-wavelength radiation exposure to the patient's face and

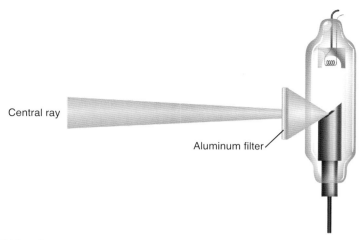

• **Figure 2.8** The divergent x-ray beam. The aluminum filter removes longer wavelength x-rays from the beam.

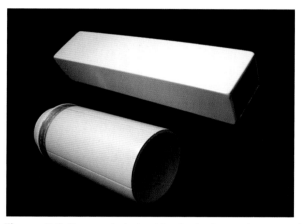

• **Figure 2.9** Open-ended, lead-lined circular and rectangular position-indicating devices (PIDs). (From Iannucci JM, Howerton LJ: *Dental Radiography: Principles and Techniques*, ed 5, St Louis, 2017, Elsevier.)

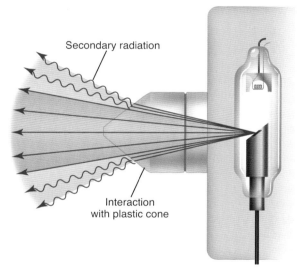

• **Figure 2.10** Production of secondary radiation resulting from interaction of the primary beam with the closed-end plastic cone.

degraded the diagnostic image on the film. X-rays interact with plastic, even though one might not consider plastic to be a very dense material.

X-rays interact and cause secondary radiation with any form of matter, from a piece of tissue paper to a bar of steel. The density of the material and the quality of the x-ray beam determine the type and extent of interaction. When the open-ended PID is used, there is no material at the end of the PID with which to interact. Novice students starting instruction in radiology have no more difficulty using open-ended PIDs than their predecessors had with the pointed models. Radiation protection codes have required the use of open-ended PIDs. The standard of care in radiation risk prevention calls for open-ended, lead-lined PIDs.

Quality and Quantity of X-Rays: The Difference Between Milliamperage and Kilovoltage

The three parameters of the dental x-ray beam are (1) the energy or penetrating power (quality) of the x-ray beam,

(2) the number of x-rays produced (quantity), and (3) the length of time for which these x-rays will be produced (exposure time).

Quality

The quality, wavelength, or penetrating power of the x-ray beam is controlled by the kilovoltage. In the past, the suitable range for dental radiography was 65 kV to 100 kV. You could adjust the kilovoltage in these units depending on the density of the area being exposed and the diagnostic needs of the patient. If the area was more dense, the kilovoltage would be increased; and if the area was less dense, the kilovoltage would be decreased. Contemporary units could have adjustable kilovoltage settings in the 60 kV to 100 kV range or have a preset kilovoltage (as seen in Fig. 2.6). Actually, with some x-ray units the name of the model can represent a detailed description of the machine. For example, a Gendex 765DC indicates that the machine is

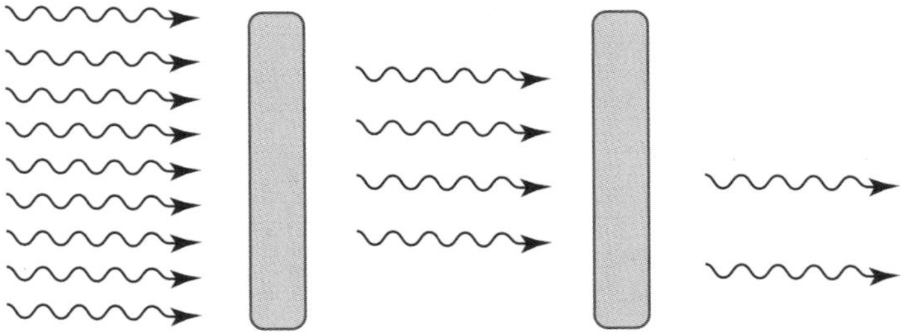

• **Figure 2.11** Half-value layer (HVL) of an x-ray beam. Note how the thickness of aluminum used reduces the intensity of x-ray photons by half.

preset at a mA setting of 7, a kilovoltage setting of 65, and operates on a DC.

Dental diagnostic radiology is generally within the 60 kV to 100 kV range. The density of the structures dealt with in dentistry (teeth, bone, etc.) determine the useful penetration range. Kilovoltage settings below 40 would not give adequate penetration of the object. Kilovoltage from 40 kV to below 60 kV would penetrate and produce a diagnostic radiograph but not without undue production of secondary x-radiation, and kilovoltage above 100 causes overpenetration. The overall objective of diagnostic radiology is to record differences in densities on the image receptors of the objects being radiographed. A kilovoltage range is chosen that will indicate the difference of penetration and absorption so that the differences in structural densities can be recorded. The choice of kilovoltage setting within the acceptable range is discussed in the section on density and contrast. Thus, a kilovoltage is selected that allows complete absorption of some x-rays, partial absorption of others, and passage of other x-rays through the object to reach the film or digital sensor.

Differential absorption of the x-ray beam by the object being radiographed produces the image. That is why less-dense structures, such as the dental pulp, appear radiolucent (dark or black) on the x-ray image, and highly calcified denser structures, such as the enamel, appear radiopaque (light or white). The less-dense areas in the object allow greater passage of x-rays than do denser areas, and more x-rays strike the film or sensor in these areas to darken them.

Half-Value Layer

The term half-value layer (HVL) is more appropriate than kilovoltage to describe beam quality and penetration. Kilovoltage is a description of the electric energy put into an x-ray tube. HVL represents the quality (penetration) of the x-rays emitted from the tube. Two similar x-ray machines operating at the same kilovoltage may not produce x-rays of the same penetration. The HVL is defined as the thickness of aluminum (measured in millimeters) that will reduce the intensity of the x-ray beam by 50%. For example, a dental x-ray beam could be described as having an HVL of 2 mm. This means that the energy of this particular beam is such that a thickness of 2 mm of aluminum would be necessary

to decrease its intensity by half (Fig. 2.11). A beam with an HVL of 1 mm would not be as energized, because only 1 mm of aluminum is necessary to decrease its energy by half. The normal HVL for a dental x-ray beam is about 2.75 mm of aluminum.

Quantity

The milliamperage determines the number of x-rays produced in a given exposure period by controlling the heating of the tungsten filament to produce electrons at the cathode of the tube. Just as the kilovoltage determines the quality (penetrating power) of the x-rays produced, the milliamperage determines the quantity (amount) of x-rays produced.

It is better to consider the concept of milliampere seconds (mAs) than milliamperage alone. An exposure, at a given kilovoltage, of 1 second using 10 mA is 10 mAs. A 2-second exposure, at the same kilovoltage, using 5 mA would produce an identical image, because the mAs are again 10 (10 × 1 = 10; 5 × 2 = 10).

The sensitivity of the receptor and the target-receptor distance (or focal-film distance [FFD]) is used to determine the mAs required at a given kilovoltage. The more sensitive the receptor is to radiation, the fewer mAs required. The advantage of higher milliamperage is that a shorter exposure time can be used. This does not represent a decrease in the patient's x-ray exposure but rather a decrease in the time necessary to expose the receptor. Ideally, the shortest exposure time with high milliamperage is the best way to achieve the desired mAs. The range of milliamperage on dental x-ray machines is usually from 5 to 15 mA. As mentioned, the limiting factor is the heat produced at the desired small target. Milliamperage higher than 15 produces too many electrons bombarding the target and thus too much heat. As mentioned, some x-ray machines in dentistry are made specifically for extraoral radiography and have rotating anodes. A rotating anode is a spinning disk composed of many tungsten targets instead of one stationary target, as found in the standard intraoral x-ray unit. Because the targets are rotating, they are struck by the electrons through only part of their 360-degree rotation. During the rest of the rotation, the targets can cool; thus, the heat is dissipated, preventing damage to the anode. (see Fig. 1.13).

Intensity

The beam *intensity* is affected by the kilovoltage, milliamperage, exposure time, and the target-receptor distance (or FFD). As shown, the kilovoltage determines the quality (penetration) of the x-ray beam, and the milliamperage determines the quantity of the x-rays produced. Quality and quantity are linked together with the target-receptor distance (or FFD) and exposure time in the expression of the intensity of the x-ray beam. The intensity of the beam is the product of the quality and quantity of the beam per unit of area per unit of exposure time. (The quality multiplied by the quantity divided by the product of beam area and exposure time equals the intensity of the beam.)

$$\text{Intensity} = \frac{(kV) \times (mA)}{(\text{area}) \times (\text{exposure})}$$

Higher kilovoltage and milliamperage settings increase the intensity of the beam, and an increase in exposure time will also increase the x-ray beam intensity. However, as the target-receptor distance (or FFD) increases, the intensity of the beam decreases because the divergence of the beam produces a larger field size or area. The larger the denominator (lower number in a fraction) with all other factors staying the same, the lower the intensity of the beam. This concept is applied clinically in Chapter 3 in the discussion of the inverse square law.

Filtration

As shown in Fig. 2.12, the x-ray beam that originates at the anode is not homogeneous because of the multiple bremsstrahlung reactions that occur at the target. The beam consists of a spectrum of long and short wavelengths. In fact, very few of the x-ray photons produced have energy or penetration power corresponding to the desired kilovoltage. In other words, only a few of the x-ray photons produced will correspond to the kilovoltage setting established in the dental x-ray unit. Almost all of the x-ray photons produced

will have wavelengths longer than those corresponding to the kilovoltage setting and thus will be less penetrating. This is partially the result of the electrons in the tube bombarding multiple atomic layers of the tungsten target with the resulting bremsstrahlung and characteristic x-ray production. As shown in the graph in Fig. 2.13, the x-ray beam is not homogeneous but rather heterogeneous, having a full range of wavelengths. The longer, lower-kilovoltage wavelengths do not penetrate tooth and bone and are absorbed by the skin or produce secondary radiation.

The function of the aluminum *filter* is to remove the long, nonpenetrating wavelength x-rays from the primary beam (see Fig. 2.8). After the primary beam has been filtered and collimated, it is referred to as the *useful beam*. There is some "inherent filtration" of the x-ray beam as it passes through the glass window and the insulating oil, which is equivalent to about 0.5 to 1 mm of aluminum. "Added filtration" is the thickness of aluminum disks that are added to achieve "total filtration."

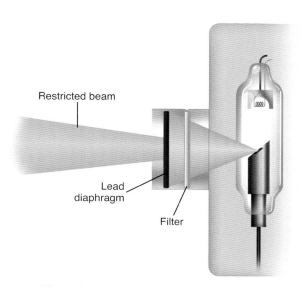

• **Figure 2.12** Collimation and filtration of x-ray beam.

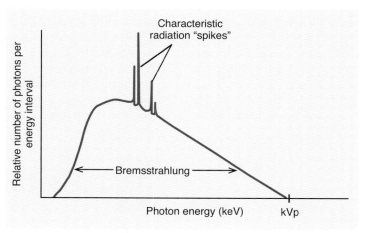

• **Figure 2.13** Spectrum of x-ray beam from dental x-ray machine operating at 65 kV. Note number of low-energy photons produced. Note where the characteristic x-rays occur. *keV,* kiloelectron volt.

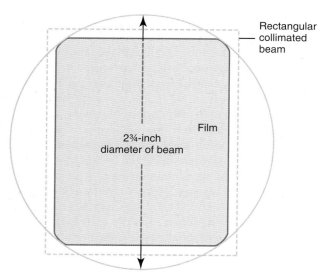

• **Figure 2.14** Relative size of adult receptor compared with x-ray beam 2¾ inches (7 cm) in diameter and rectangularly collimated beam.

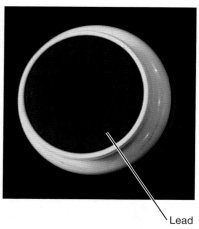

• **Figure 2.15** Lead diaphragm. (From Iannucci JM, Howerton LJ: Dental Radiography: *Principles and Techniques,* ed 5, St Louis, 2017, Elsevier.)

Federal regulations specify that for dental x-ray machines operating at kilovoltage up to 70 kV, 1.5 mm total filtration is required. For those machines operating at 70 kV and higher, 2.5 mm of total filtration is required.

Collimation

A collimating device (see Fig. 2.12) restricts the size and shape of the x-ray beam as it leaves the tube head. In intra-oral radiography, the beam should be just large enough to cover the film packet or digital sensor. Circular collimation allows a margin of error in receptor-beam alignment (Fig. 2.14). A beam size any larger than this would expose the patient's face to unnecessary primary radiation. Historically, in dentistry, the diameter of the x-ray beam measured at the patient's face has been decreasing. From no limitation at all in the early days of dental radiology, the beam diameter has gone to 3½ inches, to 3 inches, and presently to 2.75 inches (which is equivalent to 2¾ inches or 7 cm).

The collimating device often used is a lead diaphragm with a circular aperture for circular PIDs (Fig. 2.15) or a rectangular aperture for rectangular PIDs and the lead-lined PID. The size of the diaphragm's aperture at a selected target-receptor distance (or FFD) determines the beam size. The lead-lined PIDs, whether open-ended cylinders or rectangles, also serve as collimating devices. Federal regulations presently require that the x-ray beam not exceed 2.75 inches (2¾ inches or 7 cm) in diameter when measured at the patient's skin.

Rectangular Collimation

In the past, the shape of the dental x-ray beam most often was circular. The question can be asked, "Why is a circular beam used when the receptor is rectangular in shape?" The circular beam covers a greater facial area, and it exposes the patient to more primary radiation than a tightly collimated rectangular beam. The current movement in the dental profession is now toward rectangular collimation. It is taught as the primary technique at most dental schools and is recommended by the American Dental Association (ADA) and the American Academy of Oral and Maxillofacial Radiology. This change to rectangular collimation can be accomplished without an increase in collimator cutoff (formerly referred to as cone cutting) with the use of proper equipment. Collimator cutoff occurs when the beam is not centered on the film or sensor and thus part of the image is cut off. X-ray beams can be aligned to film or sensors easily using the XCP Beam Alignment System (Rinn Corp.), and the RAPD Positioning System can be used in conjunction with a rectangular PID collimator (Fig. 2.16). The use of these devices in rectangular collimation is illustrated and described in Chapter 9. Rectangular collimation is said to be the single most important factor in reducing radiation exposure to the patient, because it does not expose excess tissue to x-radiation. The utilization of rectangular collimation is thought to produce 60% less x-radiation exposure to the patient than the use of circular (cylindrical) collimation.

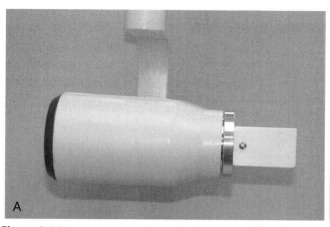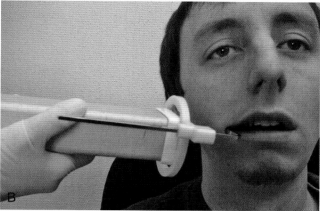

• **Figure 2.16** Rectangular position-indicating device (PID) collimator **(A)** with paralleling positioning device **(B).** (B, From Langlais RP, Miller CS: *Exercises in Oral Radiology and Interpretation*, ed 5, St Louis, 2017, Elsevier.)

Chapter Summary

- Electricity is the primary source of energy for the dental x-ray machine, used to create x-rays.
- Contemporary dental radiography utilizes machines that operate on a DC current rather than the older AC units.
- There are three transformers (step-up, step-down, and autotransformer) used in dental radiography to change the voltage in an electric circuit.
- The three important parameters of the dental x-ray beam that are set in the dental radiographic unit are the quality (or kV), quantity (or mA), and exposure time.

- The intensity of the x-ray beam is affected by the kilovoltage, milliamperage exposure time, and the target-receptor distance (formerly known as the FFD).
- Federal regulations specify that for dental x-ray units operating at 70 kV or higher, 2.5 mm of aluminum filtration is required.
- Federal regulations specify that the x-ray beam measured at the patient's face not exceed 2.75 inches (2¾ inches or 7 cm).

Chapter Review Questions

Multiple Choice

1. A dental x-ray machine operating on an AC blocks the reversal of the current and is therefore said to be (indicate all that apply):
   a. Electrically circuited
   b. Full cycled
   c. Self-rectified
   d. Half-wave rectified
   e. Independent
2. The transformer that is responsible for making minor changes in voltage in the dental x-ray machine is the:
   a. Step-over transformer
   b. Step-up transformer
   c. Step-down transformer
   d. Autotransformer
   e. Circuit transformer
3. For a dental x-ray unit that functions on an AC current, ¼ second exposure time would be equivalent to:
   a. 15 impulses
   b. 20 impulses
   c. 30 impulses

   d. 45 impulses
   e. 60 impulses
4. The x-ray in the middle of the divergent x-ray beam is known as the:
   a. Middle ray
   b. Utilized ray
   c. Central ray
   d. Attenuated ray
   e. Purposeful ray
5. The reason why the "pointed cone" is no longer used in dental radiography is because it produced secondary or scatter radiation that:
   a. Could increase radiation exposure to the patient
   b. Could cause fogging of the image
   c. Could degrade the diagnostic image
   d. Could increase long wavelength radiation exposure to the patient's face
   e. All of the above are correct

Critical Thinking Exercises

1. Explain how the flow of the electric current in the dental x-ray machine differs in a unit that operates on an AC as opposed to one that operates on a DC and the importance of both in x-ray production.
   a. Include *rectification* in your description.
   b. Include *voltage, amperage,* and *transformers* in your description.
2. The dental x-ray unit in the dental facility where you work has a unit that operates at 70 kV and has a PID that is cylindrical. What do the respective federal regulations require in terms of filtration and collimation of the x-ray beam in your dental facility?
   a. State the federal regulations for filtration of the dental x-ray beam of a unit that operates at a kilovoltage lower than 70 and a unit that operates at 70 kV or higher.
   b. State the federal regulations for collimation of the beam, including a discussion of the amount of skin exposure that cannot be exceeded and the advantage of rectangular collimation regarding patient exposure.

Bibliography

American Dental Association Council on Scientific Affairs: An update on radiographic practices: information and recommendations, *J Am Dent Assoc* 132:234–238, 2001.

FDA Department of Health and Human Services, 21 C.F.R., Subchapter J Radiological Health, General § 1000.1 (1994).

Iannucci JM, Howerton LJ: *Dental radiography: Principles and techniques,* ed 5, St Louis, MO, 2016, Elsevier Saunders.

Langland OE, Langlais RP: *Principles of dental imaging,* Baltimore, MD, 1997, Williams & Wilkins.

National Council on Radiation Protection and Measurements. NCRP Report No. 145, Radiation in Dentistry; 2004.

Thompson EM, Johnson ON: *Essentials of dental radiography for dental assistants and hygienists,* ed 9, Upper Saddle River, NJ, 2012, Pearson Education, Inc.

White SC, Pharoah MJ: *Oral radiology: Principles and interpretation,* ed 7, St Louis, MO, 2013, Mosby.

3

Image Formation

EDUCATIONAL OBJECTIVES

Upon completing this chapter, the student will be able to:

1. Define the key terms listed at the beginning of the chapter.
2. Discuss the following related to density and contrast:
   - Define *density* and *contrast*.
   - Know the differences between *short-scale contrast* and *long-scale contrast,* as well as the differences between *high contrast* and *low contrast,* and the kilovoltage (kV) settings for each of these types of contrast.
   - List the determining factors of object contrast.
   - List the causes of film fog and its effect on image contrast.
3. Discuss the factors that will produce diagnostic radiographs in terms of image sharpness, resolution, detail, and definition. In addition:
   - Define and discuss the differences between the umbra and penumbra.
   - Explain what is meant by a *recessed tube* or *recessed target*.
   - Explain the significance of the inverse square law in dental radiography and know how to calculate the mathematical equations associated with this law.
4. List and describe the factors that will minimize image distortion and enlargement, as well as explain the effect that movement during an exposure can have on the resultant image.

KEY TERMS

actual focal area
bisecting-angle technique
blurred image
contrast
detail
effective focal area
film fog
focal-film distance (FFD)
high contrast
illuminator (viewbox)
image

image density
intensity
inverse square law
long-scale contrast
low-contrast
magnification
object density
object-film distance (OFD)
object-receptor distance
paralleling technique
penumbra

radiolucent
radiopaque
recessed target
recessed tube
scale of contrast
sharpness
short-scale contrast
target-receptor distance
umbra

Introduction

This chapter emphasizes that, regardless of what imaging system is used to produce radiographs of dental and maxillofacial structures, the goal is to create an image with the proper degree of density and contrast, detail sharpness, and minimal enlargement and distortion. These factors enable the most diagnostic information for the amount of radiation expended.

Density and Contrast

The two types of related densities that are factors in image formation are the object density (teeth, bone, soft tissue), which is determined by the structure of the object being radiographed, and the image density, which is the degree of blackness on an image. Contrast is the difference in the degrees of blackness on the image between adjacent areas. When comparing a black area on an image with a white area, a great deal of difference, or high contrast, is seen. When comparing gray with white or gray with black areas or shades of gray, less or low contrast is seen. The density of an image is determined by the relative transmissions of the x-rays through parts of the object and the absorption of the x-rays in the receptor. These two factors, the object being radiographed (object contrast) and the properties of the receptor (receptor contrast), determine the overall density and contrast of the finished radiograph.

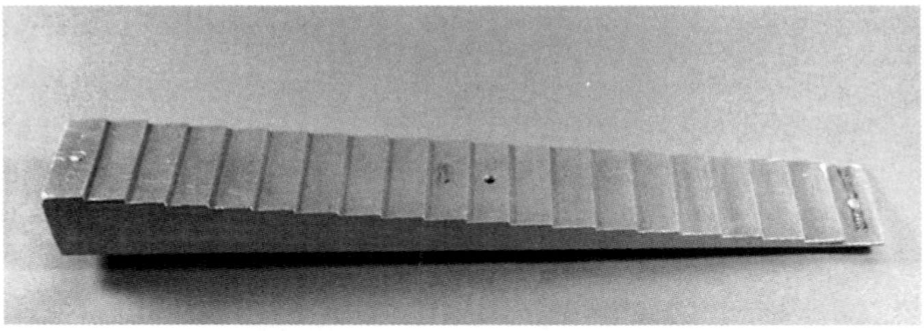

• **Figure 3.1** Aluminum step wedge.

Object Contrast

The object contrast is determined by: (1) the thickness of the object, (2) the density of the object, (3) the chemical composition of the object, (4) the quality of the x-ray beam, and (5) scatter radiation. The thickness, density, or atomic number of the structures being radiographed (teeth, bone, etc.) cannot be controlled. However, these parameters determine the range of kilovoltage that is used in dentistry. Therefore a kilovoltage range that produces a differential absorption pattern to portray differences in object density on the receptor is used. Using a kilovoltage setting greater than 100 kV in dentistry results in overpenetration, and using a kilovoltage below 40 kV results in underpenetration. In both cases, the selective penetration desired is not achieved.

This can be demonstrated with the use of an aluminum step wedge (Fig. 3.1). A step wedge consists of plates of increasing thickness. As the wedge gets thicker, there is a decrease in x-ray penetration due to the object density. The only variables of object contrast are the quality or penetration of the x-rays within the dental diagnostic penetration range of 60 kV to 100 kV and the scatter radiation produced. Clinically, the step wedge can be used to monitor film processing and the quality of the film and digital sensor. It can also be utilized in calibrating dental x-ray units.

The difference between x-ray images produced at the different kilovoltage settings in the dental range is the resulting contrast. By varying the kilovoltage and thus the quality of the radiation, and keeping scatter to a minimum, either high- or low-contrast images can be produced (Fig. 3.2). It should be noted again that kilovoltage in the 45 kV to below 60 kV range can produce a diagnostic image but should not be used because of the amount of secondary (scatter) radiation produced.

Short Scale

The scale of contrast refers to the range of densities seen in a dental radiographic image. High-contrast images appear mainly black and white with very few gray tones, and the densities (black and white) seen are easy to distinguish from each other. They also are referred to as short-scale contrast images and are produced by a lower kilovoltage range. These films are said to be "crisper" and more pleasing to the eye, but they may not reveal incipient pathologic changes. The short-scale image is a yes-or-no situation: either the x-ray

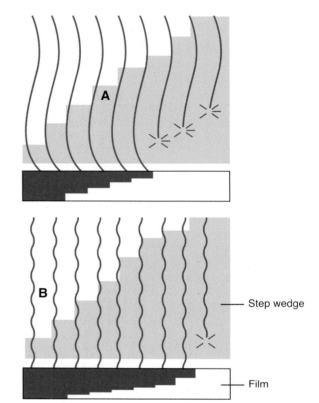

• **Figure 3.2** Relative penetrations of an aluminum step wedge by different energy x-ray beams and resulting density and contrast. *A,* 65 kV. *B,* 90 kV. Note the large gray areas with 90 kV and the large black and white areas with 65 kV.

beam penetrates the object or it does not. Areas appear black (radiolucent) or white (radiopaque), with few gray tones in the middle range (Figs. 3.3 and 3.4).

Furthermore, the lower kilovoltage ranges are undesirable because they result in increased facial absorption and scatter, potentially degrading the image, as a result of their less penetrating wavelengths.

Long Scale

The low-contrast images, also referred to as long-scale contrast, are produced by a higher kilovoltage range. In these images, there are many tones of gray in addition to the blacks and whites. The long-scale image is not as visually pleasing as the short-scale image. However, early changes

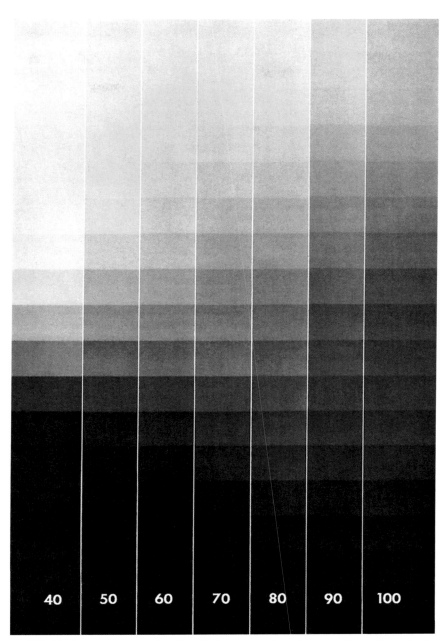

Figure 3.3 Aluminum step wedge densities. A step wedge of aluminum is radiographed using increasing kilovoltage peak (penetration). The thinner portion of the step wedge shows complete penetration of all kilovoltages. At the thicker portion of the wedge, the lower kilovoltage does not penetrate, whereas the higher kilovoltage penetrates, as shown by the gray tones. (Courtesy Eastman Kodak Co., Rochester, NY.)

in object density, such as early bone loss or incipient decay, may be seen in the gradation of the gray tones because of more selective penetration (see Fig. 3.4), which is not present in the high-contrast images.

HELPFUL HINT

Always remember that:
- Low kilovoltage range = High-contrast = Short-scale contrast = Black and white
- High kilovoltage range = Low-contrast = Long-scale contrast = Shades of gray

---

Contrast and Conventional Radiography
Scatter Radiation—Film Fog

In addition to its effect on other parts of the patient's body, scattered radiation produces a darkening over the image; in doing so, it reduces the contrast. Scatter radiation is one of the causes of **film fog** (an overall gray appearance due to diminished contrast); it degrades the diagnostic image when using film (as opposed to a digital sensor) as the receptor. Most scatter radiation originates in the object itself; thus, the larger the field, the more that object scatter becomes a factor. As noted in Chapter 13, grids are sometimes used to

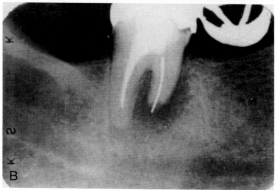

• **Figure 3.4 A,** High-contrast radiograph taken at 65 kV. Note the predominance of black and white tones. **B,** Low-contrast radiograph taken at 90 kV. Note the predominance of gray tones.

eliminate object scatter in extraoral radiography. In intraoral radiography, scatter radiation is reduced by using as small a beam as possible, open-ended position-indicating devices (PIDs), lead backing in the film packet (in conventional radiography), and higher kilovoltage settings.

Film Contrast (Conventional Radiography)

In the case of conventional radiography, film contrast is determined by (1) the amount of radiation transmitted (object contrast); (2) the properties of the film; (3) intensifying screens, if used; (4) film processing; and (5) viewing conditions. All of these factors are discussed in their respective chapters. It is important to remember that any secondary radiation or light that affects the film decreases the desired contrast, that is, it "fogs" the film and degrades the image.

Image Sharpness, Resolution, Detail, and Definition

Image sharpness is the visual quality or clarity of a radiograph (conventional or digital), which depends on the resolution, detail, or definition of a radiographic image. The sharpness of an image is determined by being able to distinguish the outlines of an object and the ability of the dental image to mimic the smallest details of an object or structure. The factors that influence sharpness (resolution, detail, and definition) are (1) size of the target or focal

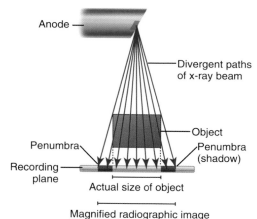

• **Figure 3.5** Image penumbra.

area; (2) target-receptor distance (or focal-film distance [FFD]); (3) object-receptor distance (or object-film distance [OFD]); (4) movement of patient, receptor, or x-ray machine; (5) type of intensifying screen, if used; and (6) image contrast.

The penumbra is the area of unsharpness or blurring that surrounds the edge of a radiographic image, whereas the umbra is the sharp area. It is desirable to keep the penumbra as small as possible. This is done by using a small focal spot, angulation of the target, an increased target-receptor distance, and a decreased object-receptor distance (Fig. 3.5). Definition can also be judged by the size of the penumbra that the image produces.

Size of Tube Focal (Target) Area

The smaller the focal area (spot) at the anode (see Fig. 1.12) of the x-ray, the better the image detail will be. As discussed in Chapter 1, the heat produced limits how small the focal area can be. The focal area in the tube is tilted, usually at an angle of 20 degrees to the cathode (Fig. 3.6). When viewed from below, the focal area appears to be smaller than it actually is and functions as the desired smaller focal area. This is called the effective focal area, in contrast to the actual focal area. The effective focal area is always smaller than the actual focal area. Most dental x-ray machines are equipped with the smallest fixed focal area possible given the heat production restrictions.

Target-Receptor Distance (Focal-Film Distance) and Object-Receptor Distance (Object-Film Distance)

> **NOTE**
>
> The terms *focal-film distance (FFD)* and *object-film distance (OFD)* were formerly used to represent the distance between the focal area and the film and between the object and the film. This text expresses these distances as the *target-receptor distance* and the *object-receptor distance* accompanied by the acronyms of the former terms in parentheses.

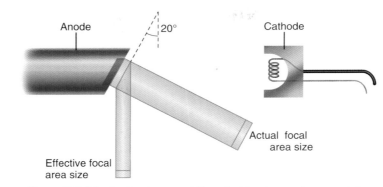

Figure 3.6 Effective focal area and the actual focal area of an x-ray tube.

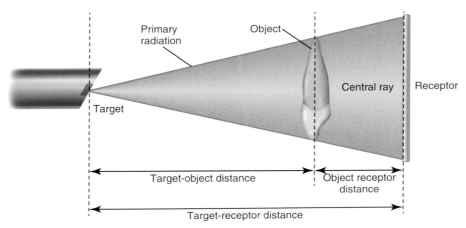

Figure 3.7 Relationships among target, object, and receptor.

The ideal radiograph of a tooth or other object—in terms of definition, image enlargement, and distortion—can be made by meeting the following criteria:

1. Establish a maximum target-receptor distance (or FFD). This is the distance between the target at the anode and the receptor in the patient's mouth or the focal area at the anode and the film (or receptor) in the patient's mouth. The maximal distance allows the more parallel rays from the center of the x-ray beam to strike the object and the receptor and not the more divergent x-rays from the periphery of the beam, which would cause enlargement of the image (Fig. 3.7).
2. Determine a minimal object-receptor distance (or OFD). The tooth and the receptor or the tooth and the film should be as close together as possible. The closer they are, the less enlarged the image is on the receptor (Fig. 3.8).
3. Position the object and the receptor (film or digital sensor) parallel to each other in their long axes and the central ray perpendicular to both. These are the optimal requirements. Because of anatomic constraints in intraoral radiography, it is sometimes difficult to meet all of these requirements at the same time.

Target-Receptor Distance (Focal-Film Distance)

The most common target-receptor distances (or FFDs) used in dentistry are 8, 12, and 16 inches. A target-receptor

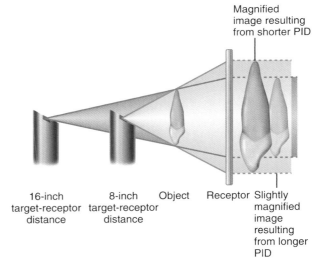

Figure 3.8 Comparison of 8-inch and 16-inch target-receptor distances (focal-film distances [FFDs]).

distance (or FFD) of less than 8 inches may cause **magnification** of the image that is larger than the receptor (see Fig. 3.8). As the target-receptor distance (or FFD) is increased to 12 or 16 inches, the magnification of the image decreases because the image is formed by the more parallel x-rays from the center of the beam. However, this decrease in magnification is not linear beyond 16 inches. Fig. 3.9

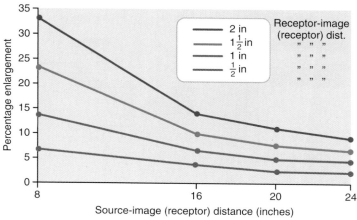

● **Figure 3.9** Relationship of image magnification to object-receptor distance (object-film distance [OFD]) and target-receptor (focal-film distance [FFD]).

shows that as the target-receptor distance (or FFD) increases beyond 16 inches, the percentage of magnification does not decrease significantly, and the difference cannot be seen by the naked eye. Therefore, using a 24-inch target-receptor distance (or FFD) does not give a significantly better image clinically than a 16-inch target-receptor distance (or FFD). The 16-inch target-receptor distance (or FFD) is the distance of choice. The extended or 16-inch target-receptor distance (or FFD) also results in exposure of less tissue volume (see Chapter 6, Fig. 6.10). The 16-inch target-receptor distance (FFD) produces a better image because of the decrease in magnification, with less radiation to the patient. For these reasons, its use is strongly recommended.

X-Ray *Tube Position*

The x-ray tube is positioned in the anterior part of the head of the machine, close to the PID (Fig. 3.10). The rest of the head of the x-ray machine contains electric circuitry and cooling devices. The open-ended, lead-lined, rectangle or cylinder PID placed on the head of the machine serves as the aiming device for the x-ray beam.

With the increasing popularity of the paralleling technique and the need for an extended target-receptor distance (or FFD; 16 inches), a new design for the tube head was introduced. Fig. 3.10 illustrates the operation of the new design. The x-ray tube is placed in the rear part of the machine's head, and the rest of the components are placed on both sides of the beam. This concept is known as a **recessed tube** or **recessed target**. The advantage of this design is in the extended focal distance and the elimination of the longer PID. Consequently, the machine with the short PID may actually have a long target-receptor distance (FFD), depending on the placement of the x-ray tube in the head of the machine.

Inverse Square Law

One factor that must be considered in choosing or changing a target-receptor distance (or FFD) is the **inverse square law** (Fig. 3.11), which states that "the **intensity** of radiation varies inversely with the square of the distance from the source of radiation." This is attributable to the fact that as

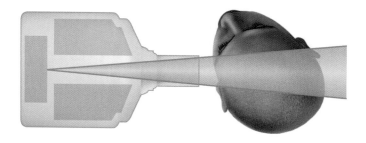

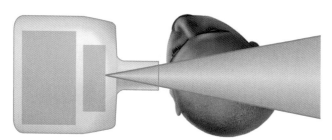

● **Figure 3.10** Long-beam tube head (*top*) and conventional tube head (*bottom*). Note different position of x-ray tube, which allows increased target-receptor (focal-film distance [FFD]).

the target-receptor distance (or FFD) increases, the intensity of the beam decreases because of the divergence of the x-ray beam, which produces a larger field size. More simply stated, if the target-receptor distance (or FFD) doubles, the intensity of the beam is decreased by one-fourth and the exposure time should be quadrupled to compensate for the decrease in intensity. Conversely, if the target-receptor distance (or FFD) decreases by half, the intensity quadruples and the exposure time is then decreased by one-fourth. This assumes that the milliamperage and kilovoltage remain the same. The inverse square law is discussed again in Chapter 7 regarding its relationship to radiation protection for the operator.

As seen in Fig. 3.11, the intensity of the radiation at 16 inches is much less than at 8 inches because it is spread out

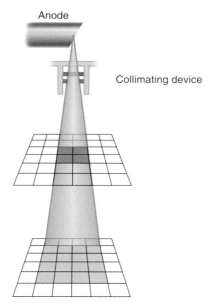

Anode

Collimating device

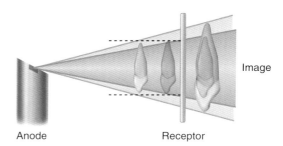

Image

Anode

Receptor

• **Figure 3.12** Comparison of object-receptor (object-film) distances and the effect on image magnification.

• **Figure 3.11** Inverse square law. The effect of distance on the intensity of the radiation.

over 16 boxes. To achieve the same intensity of radiation, the exposure time must be increased by a factor of 4.

Object-Receptor Distance (Object-Film Distance)

The closer the object (tooth, bone, etc.) is to the receptor, the better the detail and the less the enlargement (Fig. 3.12). The object-receptor distance (or OFD) is determined by the anatomy of the area of the mouth being radiographed and whether the paralleling or bisecting-angle technique is used. In the paralleling technique in some areas of the mouth (i.e., most of the maxillary periapical projections and the mandibular anterior periapical projections), the object-receptor distance (or OFD) has to be increased to position the receptor parallel to the long axis of the tooth, as discussed in a later chapter on the paralleling technique. Compare the object-receptor distance (or OFD) needed for parallelism in the mandibular molar area with that needed in the maxillary molar area. In the lower area, the receptor is very close to the tooth and still parallel, whereas in the upper area the receptor has to be positioned in the midline of the palate to achieve parallelism.

Image Distortion and Enlargement

In some cases, because of the mouth's anatomy, it is almost impossible to ideally satisfy criteria 2 and 3 (p. 29), which refer to object-receptor distance (or OFD) and parallelism between the object and the receptor. For example, if the receptor is held close to the teeth, then the parallelism is lost; if the teeth and receptor are to be parallel, then there must be an increased object-receptor distance (or OFD).

This is the basis for the two techniques used in receptor placement for intraoral radiography: the paralleling technique and the bisecting-angle technique. The clinical methods of performing these techniques, as well as their advantages and disadvantages, are described in Chapters 9 and 10. In

---

HELPFUL HINT

Inverse square law application equations:
A. Mathematical equation for calculating the effect that a change in the target-receptor distance (focal-film distance [FFD]) has on the beam intensity:

$$\text{Equation:} \quad \frac{\text{Original Intensity}}{\text{New Intensity}} = \frac{\text{New Distance}^2}{\text{Original Distance}^2}$$

Example: If the target-receptor distance (or FFD) is increased from 8 inches to 16 inches, what is the effect on the intensity of the beam? *Note:* Assume that the original intensity is 1 at 8 inches.

$$\frac{1}{x} = \frac{16^2}{8^2}$$

$$\frac{1}{x} = \frac{256}{64}$$

$$\frac{1}{x} = \frac{4}{1}$$

$$x = \frac{1}{4}$$

Therefore, the beam will be one-fourth as intense when the target-receptor distance is increased from 8 inches to 16 inches.
B. Mathematical equation for calculating the change in time when the target-receptor distance is changed:
   Example: If the target-receptor distance (or FFD) is 8 inches and the exposure time is set at 2 impulses, what would the new exposure time be at a target-receptor distance (or FFD) of 16 inches with the kilovoltage and milliamperage remaining the same.
   1. What is the difference in distance: 8 to 16 inches; = **2**
   2. Square the difference in distance: 2^2 = **4**
   3. Original time = 2 (impulses); 2 × 4 = **8** (impulses)
   Therefore, the new time at a target-receptor distance (or FFD) of 16 inches instead of 8 inches is 8 impulses.
   Remember: If the distance increases, the time increases and if the distance decreases, the time decreases in an inverse square law equation.

the paralleling technique, the first principle states that the receptor is held parallel to the long axis of the tooth. This results in an increased object-receptor distance (or OFD) in most areas of the mouth; that is, for the receptor to remain parallel to the tooth, it must be positioned away from the tooth (Fig. 3.13). The compensation for enlargement caused by the increased object-receptor distance (or OFD) is using an increased target-receptor distance (or FFD): 12 to 16 inches. The second principle of the paralleling technique states that the central ray is directed perpendicular to the tooth and the receptor (which are parallel to each other). In the bisecting-angle technique, the receptor is held as close to the tooth as possible. At this point, the long axis of the tooth and the plane of the receptor cannot be parallel. An imaginary line is drawn that bisects the angle formed by the long axis of the tooth and the plane of the dental receptor (Fig. 3.14). The central ray of the x-ray beam is then directed perpendicularly to this bisecting line. This projects the proper linear dimensions of the tooth onto the receptor without elongation or foreshortening.

Movement

Image detail is affected by patient movement, receptor movement, and x-ray source movement during exposure (Fig. 3.15). Patient and receptor movement are controlled by good chairside technique and are discussed later in the book. Source movement, or tube and arm movement, is caused by improper upkeep and quality control of x-ray equipment. If the arm or tube head moves or vibrates during an exposure, image quality is compromised, causing a blurred image. An effective quality control program should be able to detect this type of malfunction. In many jurisdictions, tube or arm movement is a violation of the Radiation Health Code.

Viewing Conditions

When viewing digital images, the practitioner can employ the image-enhancing options on the digital system in use. There are options for magnifying the image and for changing the contrast and density of the image to assist in optimal viewing of the digital images.

When viewing film-based, conventional radiographs, the practitioner should always view the processed radiograph on an illuminator or viewbox (Fig. 3.16). A magnifying glass can be used to examine fine changes. A darkened room

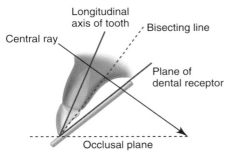

• **Figure 3.14** Relationships of central ray, tooth, and receptor in the bisecting-angle technique.

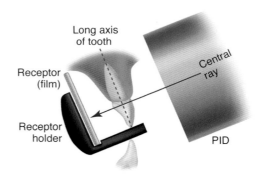

• **Figure 3.13** Relationships of central ray, tooth, and receptor in the paralleling technique. *PID,* Position-indicating device.

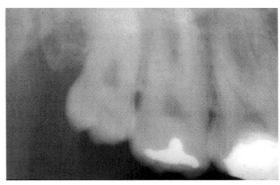

• **Figure 3.15** Radiograph showing movement (blurred image).

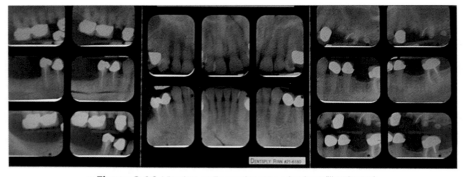

• **Figure 3.16** Viewing radiographs on a viewbox (illuminator).

for using an illuminator is the ideal setting for viewing radiographs. The darkened room may not be practical in all dental offices, but certainly viewing radiographs on an illuminator is always feasible. Holding radiographs up to the light on the unit or ceiling or in front of the window is not an acceptable substitute for an illuminator. Valuable information can be lost or never seen if the proper viewing conditions are not used and maintained.

Chapter Summary

- The density of an image is determined by the relative transmissions of the x-rays through the object and the absorption of the x-rays in the receptor.
- The scale of contrast refers to the range of densities seen in the dental radiographic image.
- Kilovoltage has a direct effect on the overall contrast of the radiographic image. Low kilovoltage produces an image with high contrast, also known as *short-scale contrast,* mostly consisting of an image composed of blacks and whites. High kilovoltage produces an image with low contrast, also known as *long-scale contrast,* consisting of an image showing shades of gray.
- A step wedge is made of aluminum and consists of plates of increasing thickness. It is used to exhibit short-scale and long-scale contrast arrangements.
- Contrast can be reduced by "film fog," which is described as an overall gray appearance due to diminished contrast and has various causes (scatter radiation, faulty safelight, light leaks, etc.).
- The factors that influence detail, definition, sharpness, and resolution are the size of the focal area, the target-receptor distance (or FFD), the object-receptor distance (or OFD), and movement during exposure.
- The ideal radiograph can be achieved using a small focal area, a long target-receptor distance (or FFD), a short object-receptor distance (or OFD), and by placing the receptor parallel to the tooth being exposed.
- The inverse square law states that the intensity of the radiation varies inversely with the square of the distance from the source of radiation. This is comparable to the intensity of a flashlight beam at a long distance projected on a wall and then decreasing the distance and observing an increase in the intensity of the beam. See the mathematical examples in the chapter for a better understanding of calculating the inverse square law.
- Image detail is affected by movement of the patient, receptor, PID, or x-ray source during an exposure.

Chapter Review Questions

Multiple Choice

1. A step wedge device can be used in a dental clinical setting to (indicate all that apply):
   a. Monitor film processing
   b. Monitor the quality of the film and digital sensor
   c. Calibrate dental x-ray units
   d. Test safelights in the darkroom
   e. Test the quantity of processing solutions in the automatic processing machine
2. Object contrast is determined by:
   a. The thickness of an object
   b. The density of the object
   c. The chemical composition of the object
   d. The quality of the x-ray beam
   e. All of the above answers are correct.
3. Film fog can be caused by scatter radiation exposure to the receptor that can be reduced by (indicate all that apply):
   a. Using an open-ended PID
   b. Using as small a beam as possible
   c. Using lead backing in a film packet in the case of conventional radiography
   d. Using high kilovoltage settings
   e. Using a long receptor object distance
4. The two basic principles of the paralleling technique are:
   a. The receptor should be placed as close to the tooth as possible
   b. The receptor should be placed parallel to the tooth
   c. The central ray should be directed perpendicular to the tooth and the receptor
   d. Both a and c are correct.
   e. Both b and c are correct.
5. Image detail is greatly affected by movement during a dental radiographic exposure. Movement of the patient, receptor, or x-ray source will result in a fogged image. (Indicate all that apply.)
   a. Both statements are true.
   b. Both statements are false.
   c. The first statement is true and the second statement is false.
   d. The first statement is false and the second statement is true.
   e. The statements are related.

Critical Thinking Exercises

1. If the target-receptor distance (or FFD) is decreased from 16 inches to 8 inches and the exposure time is set at 12 impulses, what would the new exposure time be with the kilovoltage and milliamperage remaining the same?
   a. What is the difference in distance?
   b. Square the difference in distance.
   c. What is the new time (in impulses) at the adjusted target-receptor distance (or FFD)?

2. Explain the relationship of kilovoltage to the contrast on the radiographic image.
   a. What effects does a low kilovoltage have on the image contrast?
   b. What effects does a high kilovoltage have on the image contrast?

Bibliography

American Dental Association Council on Scientific Affairs: An update on radiographic practices: information and recommendations, *J Am Dent Assoc* 132:234–238, 2001.

Iannucci JM, Howerton LJ: *Dental radiography: principles and techniques*, ed 5, St Louis, MO, 2016, Elsevier Saunders.

Langland OE, Langlais RP: *Principles of dental imaging*, Baltimore, MD, 1997, Williams & Wilkins.

National Council on Radiation Protection and Measurements: NCRP Report No. 145, Radiation in Dentistry, 2004.

New York City Health Code: Article 175, February 1998.

Thompson EM, Johnson ON: *Essentials of dental radiography for dental assistants and hygienists*, ed 9, Upper Saddle River, NJ, 2012, Pearson Education, Inc.

White SC, Pharoah MJ: *Oral radiology: principles and interpretation*, ed 7, St Louis, MO, 2013, Mosby.

4

Image Receptors

EDUCATIONAL OBJECTIVES

Upon completing this chapter, the student will be able to:

1. Define the key terms listed at the beginning of the chapter.
2. Discuss the evolution of the dental x-ray "packet" from 1896 until today.
3. Discuss the following related to film packets:
   - List the components of the film packet and the respective function of each component.
   - Discuss the composition of the film itself.
   - Define and describe the concepts of film speed and film sensitivity.

- Explain what is meant by the term *film fog*, and discuss the sources of fogging.
4. Summarize the duplicating process in dental radiography.
5. Summarize the imaging system used in conventional extraoral radiography known as a *film-screen system*.
6. Differentiate between the sensors and the process utilized in direct versus indirect digital radiography.

KEY TERMS

active pixel sensor (APS)
American National Standards Institute (ANSI)
calcium tungstate
charge-coupled device (CCD)
complementary metal oxide semiconductor (CMOS)
direct digital imaging
double-film packet

duplicating film
emulsion
film base
film fog
film packet
film-screen system
film speed (film sensitivity)
fluorescence
image receptor

indirect digital imaging
intensifying screen
orientation dot
phosphor
photostimulable phosphor (PSP)
rare earth elements
sensor
silver bromide
silver halide

Introduction

The image receptors used in dentistry today include film, film-screen combinations, duplicating film, electronic sensors used in direct digital imaging, and computed tomography (CT) scanning and phosphor plates used in indirect digital imaging. All of these receptors are used to produce images in dental radiography. This chapter discusses the receptor options available and the mechanisms by which radiographic images are created with each of the receptors mentioned.

History of Dental X-Ray Film

Although advances in technology and the rise of the utilization of digital imaging may eventually entirely replace conventional film-based radiography, it is still useful to acquire

information about this technique and its importance in dental radiography.

Dental x-ray film has evolved since the discovery of x-rays in 1895 and the taking of the first dental radiograph in 1896. To appreciate how far dental radiography has come in reducing radiation exposure and in improving the diagnostic image, a review of the evolution of dental x-ray film is essential. In the early days, from 1896 through 1913, the *x-ray packet* consisted of glass photographic plates or film cut into pieces and hand-wrapped by the dentist in black paper or a rubber dam. These packets were prepared by the dentist just before use. The corners of the packets were square, and the packets were thick and rigid, resulting in a great deal of patient discomfort.

In 1913, the Eastman Kodak Company introduced the first commercially available prepackaged dental x-ray film. The film packets were still made by hand and consisted of two pieces of film but with the emulsion coating only on one side of each film. In 1921, the first machine-made packet was placed on the market, and the packet began to resemble the one used today in that it was flatter, contained a thin sheet of lead to prevent backscatter, had rounded edges, and was easier to open. All of these factors led to greater patient comfort and easier usage for the operator.

By 1923, Kodak was producing dental film packets in two speeds: regular and extra-fast. In 1925, double-coated emulsion film was introduced, which greatly reduced the amount of exposure necessary because of the more efficient use of the radiation. Film speed has increased over the years, the x-ray emulsion has been made less sensitive to darkroom safelighting, and the packet itself has been made more flexible. Contemporary dental radiographic films are also faster, giving less radiation exposure to the patient and produce improved diagnostic images.

Film Packet

Intraoral **film packets** come in five basic sizes—the higher the designated number, the larger the film packet (Fig. 4.1): #0, child size; #1, narrow anterior film; #2, adult size (standard film size); #3, preformed bitewing film; and #4, occlusal film. All of the film packets must be light-tight and resistant to moisture. These packets must have some degree of flexibility and should be easy to open in the darkroom.

The dental x-ray film packet is composed of four separate components: (1) an outer vinyl package wrapper, (2) a black paper film wrapper, (3) an x-ray film, and (4) a lead-foil backing.

The outer vinyl package wrapper protects the film from exposure to light and salivary seepage. Inside the outer plastic

covering is the black paper film wrapper, which directly protects the film from exposure to light. The actual x-ray film that is inside the black paper wrapping records images of oral structures when exposed to x-radiation. In addition, the packet contains a lead-foil backing that is placed behind the film in the packet and is meant to absorb any unused radiation, thus protecting the patient and protecting the film from backscatter that can also cause film fog (Fig. 4.2). Some film packets can be encased in a clear plastic barrier envelope that protects the packet from contamination, and this barrier envelope is discussed further in Chapter 8. A film packet may contain one or two pieces of film. The so-called **double-film packet** requires more exposure time than the single-film packet. Some dental offices prefer using the double packet, because it provides an automatic second original film or series of original films even though the exposure time is increased, thereby increasing the overall x-radiation exposure to the patient. These double packets

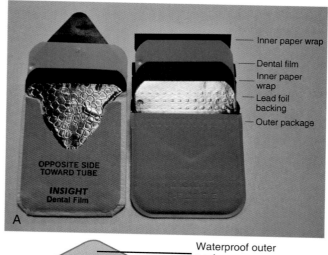

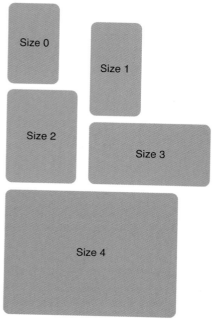

• **Figure 4.1** Intraoral film packet sizes: child (#0), narrow anterior (#1), adult size (#2), preformed bitewing (#3), and occlusal (#4).

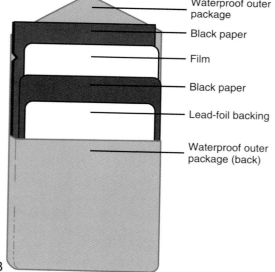

• **Figure 4.2** Photo **(A)** and illustration **(B)** of dental film packet. (A, Courtesy Carestream Health Inc, Rochester, NY.)

eliminate the need for duplicating films. Incidentally, many insurance companies require films for preauthorization of patient treatment. However, the dental facility should always have an original set of images in the patient's records.

Film Composition

X-ray film is composed of a flexible polyester film base that is coated with an emulsion of silver halide (usually silver bromide) grains suspended in a layer of gelatin (Fig. 4.3) that contains radiosensitive dyes as well. The emulsion with its protective coating is attached to the film base by an adhesive. The emulsion is sensitive to x-rays, visible light, and static electricity. The film base is coated on both sides; thus it is referred to as a *double-sided emulsion.* Less radiation is used with a doubled-sided emulsion than with the antiquated, single-sided emulsion film. Clinically, this means that a radiograph can be viewed correctly from either side. Previously, with single-emulsion film, the film had to be viewed from the side with the emulsion on it only. The film also has a "button", or orientation dot, on it (Fig. 4.4). This is a small, convex-concave area that indicates which side of the film was facing the tooth and the source of radiation and helps to orient the developed film in mounting (see

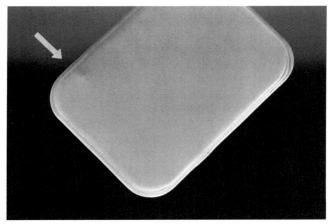

• **Figure 4.3** The orientation marker *(dot)* on the film packet.

Chapter 19). The raised portion of the orientation dot is on the white side or front of the film packet.

> **HELPFUL HINT**
>
> Remember to always try to have the white side of the film packet toward the tooth, toward the source of radiation, and toward you! Don't expose unless you see the white of the film!

Film Sensitivity (Speed)

The size of the silver halide crystals, the thickness of the emulsion, and the presence of special radiosensitive dyes determine the film speed, or film sensitivity. Film sensitivity determines how much radiation and for what period of time the radiation is needed to produce an image on the film.

More sensitive films require less exposure time and are said to have greater film speed; these are the fast films. Films that require more exposure time are less sensitive to radiation and are called *slow films.* The size of the silver bromide crystals is the main factor in determining the film speed: *The larger the crystals, the faster the film.* Film sensitivity is compared or expressed by means of a characteristic curve (Hurter and Driffield [H & D] curve, Fig. 4.5). The curve expresses the relationship between radiation exposure to the film and resulting film density. A fast film requires less exposure to produce a desired density than a slow film. The presence of radiosensitive dyes in the film emulsion influences the speed of the film as well.

Different film manufacturers give different brand names to their various film speed types. Film speed is formally designated by group by the American National Standards Institute (ANSI) using the letters A through F—*A* for the slowest film and *F* for the fastest. F-speed film is the fastest film available. To obtain comparable film sensitivities when changing from one manufacturer to another, one should consult the ANSI speed group ratings found on the package and not be misled by descriptive names.

The American Dental Association (ADA) and the American Academy of Oral and Maxillofacial Radiology

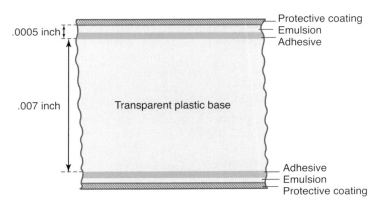

• **Figure 4.4** Cross-sectional diagram of film base and emulsion

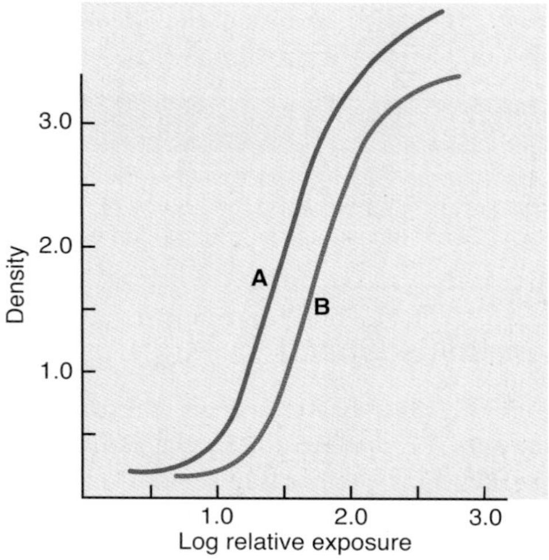

Figure 4.5 Characteristic curve. Note that film *(A)* requires less exposure to achieve a given film density than film *(B)*.

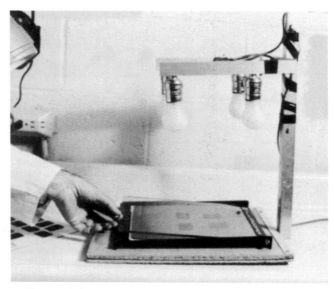

Figure 4.6 Outdated, "homemade" setup for radiographic duplication.

recommend that F-speed film be used. For example, group E film is twice as fast as group D; thus, the patient receives half the radiation exposure for a comparable diagnostic film. The new F-speed film reduces radiation exposure by 20% and 70% when compared with E-speed film and D-speed film, respectively.

Film Fog

X-ray **film fog** is an overall gray appearance to the film due to diminished contrast. It occurs when all or part of the radiograph is darkened by sources other than the primary beam of radiation to which the film was exposed. Fogging degrades the diagnostic image; use of a good-quality assurance program should minimize its deleterious effects. Sources of fogging may include the following:

- Chemical fog results from an imbalance or exhaustion of processing solutions (see Chapter 11).
- Light fog results from unintentional exposure from light leaks, cell phone light, and improper safelighting to which the film emulsion is sensitive, either before or during processing (see Chapter 11).
- Scatter radiation fog results from radiation striking the film from sources other than the intentional exposure of the primary beam. Examples are scatter from the patient or unprotected storage of films before or after exposure (see Chapter 11).

Duplicating Film

The use of radiographic **duplicating film** can satisfy requests for duplicate radiographs without adding to the radiation exposure of the patient. Duplication of radiographs is a relatively easy process that requires only a few additions to normal darkroom equipment. Figure 4.6 shows an outdated "homemade" photographic printing frame that is the antiquated version of the contemporary commercially available duplicating machines and duplicating process, as pictured in Figure 4.7.

Radiographic duplicating film is readily available from dental supply firms. It is generally supplied in 8 × 10-inch or 5 × 12-inch sheets. The photographic duplicating emulsion is present on only one side of the film; thus, one must be careful in identifying the emulsion side when positioning the film. Under safelight conditions, the emulsion side appears dull when compared with the shiny, non-emulsion side. The duplicating film has a direct positive emulsion; therefore, if more film density is needed (darker film), the exposure time is shortened. Conversely, if decreased film density is desired (lighter film), the exposure time is increased. This is the opposite of time requirements for exposing dental film to x-rays. The key to remembering this fact is to think the opposite of what would be done normally with x-rays.

Procedure

Under safelight conditions, the radiographs to be duplicated are placed in close contact with the emulsion side of the duplicating film positioned so that the raised part of the mounting dot faces the light source first. When a commercial duplicating device is used, the manufacturer's recommendations should be followed, especially concerning the time of light exposure.

After the light exposure is completed, the duplicating film is processed in the same manner as radiographs, by using either manual or automatic technique (see Chapter 11). Close positive contact between the original radiograph and duplicating film is essential or image definition will be compromised. The original films should always be removed from their mounts to achieve tight contact and acceptable image definition.

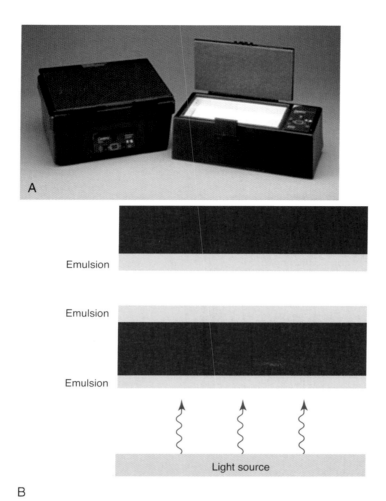

Emulsion

Emulsion

Emulsion

Light source

B

• **Figure 4.7** **A,** Radiographic duplicator. **B,** Duplication. Note that the originals are placed between the light source and the emulsion side of the duplicating film. (A, Courtesy Dentsply Rinn, York, PA.)

Film-Screen Combination

The imaging system used in conventional extraoral radiography is a film-screen system. The film is used in combination with intensifying screens. The film used is more sensitive to the light emitted by the intensifying screens than it is to radiation. However, the film used has to be sensitive to the type of light emitted by the particular screen (e.g., blue light or green light).

Extraoral film is available in 5 × 7 inches or 8 × 10 inches, as well as the panoramic sizes, 5 × 12 inches and 6 × 12 inches (Fig. 4.8).

Intensifying Screens

Cassettes used in extraoral and panoramic radiography contain intensifying screens (Fig. 4.9). The rigid, nonflexible cassettes have the intensifying screens mounted on the inside of the front and back of the cassette, and the flexible screens are removable (Fig. 4.10). As the name implies, these screens intensify or increase the radiation and thus decrease the exposure time needed. The screens are coated with a substance that has the property of fluorescence. Such

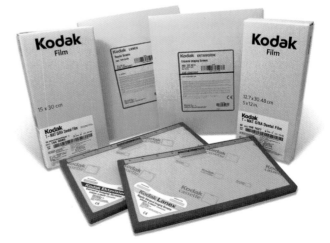

• **Figure 4.8** Extraoral film. (Courtesy Carestream Health Inc, Rochester, NY.)

a substance emits light when struck by x-radiation and is called a phosphor.

The intensifying screens produce light in the same pattern as the x-rays that have penetrated the object so that the film sandwiched inside the cassette between the intensifying screens is affected by both x-rays and light from the intensifying screen. However, a loss of image detail can result from this intensification of the x-ray beam, because the light may produce a halo at the periphery of the field (Fig. 4.11) that diffuses the borders of the image and thus decreases image sharpness to a certain extent.

Intensifying screens vary in their speed or exposure time requirements. The speed of the screen depends on the type of phosphor and the size of the crystal: The larger the crystal, the faster the screen. Originally, the most common type of phosphor was calcium tungstate, which produces blue light. New phosphors, the rare earth elements, which produce green light, are now used in intensifying screens instead of calcium tungstate. The rare earth elements are four times more efficient in converting x-ray energy into light than calcium tungstate crystals; thus, the screens are faster and require less exposure time. Rare earth screens must be used with a compatible film that is sensitive to the light in the green portion of the light spectrum. It is recommended that the rare earth screens with their corresponding film be used in preference to calcium tungstate screens.

When cassettes are loaded or unloaded in the darkroom, operators should take care not to scratch the intensifying screens with sharp objects. If an intensifying screen is badly scratched and the phosphor removed, a dark streak will appear on the film taken with this screen. Damaged screens and cassettes should be discarded. Screens should be cleaned with a solution of soapy water. Maintenance and monitoring of screens are part of a quality-control program.

Because neither the film nor the intensifying screens have orientation dots, as the intraoral film does, metallic "R"

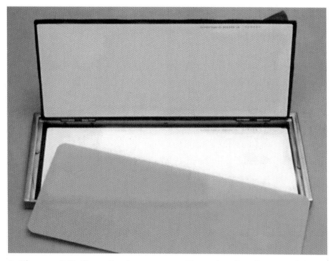

• **Figure 4.9** Cassette in open position showing front and back intensifying screens and piece of film. (From White SC, Pharoah MJ: *Oral Radiology: Principles and Techniques,* ed 7, St Louis, 2014, Mosby.)

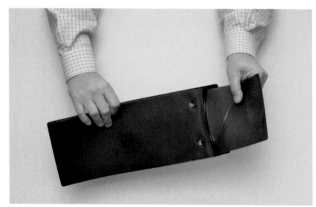

• **Figure 4.10** Flexible 5 x 12-inch panoramic cassette. (Courtesy KaVo Kerr, Charlotte, NC.)

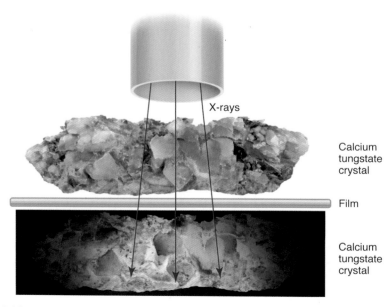

X-rays

Calcium tungstate crystal

Film

Calcium tungstate crystal

• **Figure 4.11** Effect of x-rays on intensifying screens. Note halo of light produced at the periphery that reduces radiographic definition.

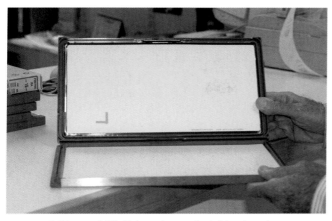

• **Figure 4.12** Extraoral cassette left lead marker.

and/or "L" markers are placed on the inside of the cassette (Fig. 4.12) to assist in identifying the right ("R") and left ("L") sides of the patient's oral cavity.

Digital Imaging

The field of dental imaging is continually changing, with more dental professionals using the most recent digital x-ray technology in their everyday practice. The driving force behind this transition has been the advantages of digital radiographic systems over film-based systems, including increased work flow, high-quality images for improved diagnoses, and reduced radiation exposure for patients. There are two types of digital imaging systems utilized in dentistry. They are direct digital imaging and indirect digital imaging.

Direct Digital Imaging Receptors

In direct digital imaging, the sensor is used as the image receptor, producing an instantaneous radiographic image.

The sensors that are utilized in intraoral digital imaging are comparable in size to the #0, #1, #2, and #4 size conventional films. These direct digital receptors send information directly to a computer by means of imaging software. Direct digital sensors may be "wired" or directly connected by a cable of varying lengths to a computer or may use a Wi-Fi system (technology for wireless local area networking) to send the image data to a computer. Wireless sensors are usually more expensive and thicker than wired sensors.

There are basically two types of direct digital sensors in dental digital imaging. They are the charge-coupled device (CCD) and the complementary metal oxide semiconductor (CMOS) also known as an active pixel sensor (APS). These two types of sensors will be discussed in detail in Chapter 15.

Indirect Digital Imaging Receptors

In indirect digital imaging, the photostimulable phosphor (PSP) plate is used as the image receptor. This receptor is not directly connected to the computer. They are used in both intraoral and extraoral digital imaging. This PSP plate is exposed to radiation and then converts the x-ray energy to light energy and records data used for diagnosis. The plates are then put into an electronic scanner that allows a laser to scan the plate and within minutes (depending on the unit used) produces an image on the computer monitor. This method takes more time than direct digital radiography, but the advantage of this method is that the PSP plates are more comfortable for the patient because they are thinner, flexible, and more similar to conventional films. They are also less expensive than direct digital imaging receptors. Direct, indirect, panoramic, and three-dimensional (3D) digital imaging is discussed in later chapters.

Chapter Summary

- The image receptors used in dentistry include film, film-screen systems, duplicating film, electronic sensors, and phosphor plates.
- Advances in digital dental radiographic technology will eventually entirely replace conventional film-based radiography.
- Dental x-ray film has evolved considerably since its inception in 1896. The film packet is available in five sizes: #0 (pediatric), #1 (narrow anterior), #2 (adult size), #3 (preformed bitewing film), and #4 (occlusal film).
- There are four separate components of the film packet: (1) an outer vinyl wrapper, (2) a black paper film wrapper, (3) an x-ray film, and (4) a lead-foil backing. There may be an additional clear plastic barrier envelope around the film packet to protect it from contamination and is used for infection control procedures.

- The film is composed of an emulsion that contains silver halide (silver bromide) crystals that affects the film's sensitivity to radiation.
- Film fog is an overall gray appearance to an image that is caused by the receptor being darkened by sources other than the primary x-ray beam.
- Film duplication is an option in producing a duplicate set of images when needed for insurance reasons, a patient's change in address, or another dental professional's opinion.
- A film-screen system is used in extraoral conventional radiography with the purpose of reducing the time needed for an exposure, which ultimately reduces the overall radiation exposure to the patient.
- The field of digital radiography is changing the scope of dental radiography with the use of digital sensors and phosphor plates as the x-ray receptors.

Chapter Review Questions

Multiple Choice

1. In 1913, the Eastman Kodak Company introduced the first commercially available:
   a. Film holder
   b. X-ray unit
   c. Duplicating machine
   d. Film packet
   e. Film-screen system

2. If you are exposing a periapical radiograph of the lower anterior teeth of a patient with a narrow arch, the size film packet you would most likely use would be:
   a. #0
   b. #1
   c. #2
   d. #3
   e. #4

3. The sensitivity of the x-ray film is dependent on the presence of (indicate all that apply):
   a. Radiosensitive dyes in the emulsion
   b. Protective coating in the emulsion
   c. Adhesive on the film base
   d. Size of the silver bromide crystals in the emulsion
   e. Flexible polyester film base

4. Indicate all of the statements below that are true concerning film duplication:
   a. Duplicating film is generally supplied in 5 ×12-inch or 8 ×10-inch sheets.
   b. Duplicating film has emulsion on only one side of the film.
   c. Duplicating film has a direct negative emulsion.
   d. The films that are being duplicated should be taken out of their mounts.
   e. There should be a close contact between the original films and the duplicating film.

5. Direct digital sensors send information directly to a computer by means of imaging software. Direct digital sensors may be connected directly to the computer by a cable or may use a Wi-Fi system to send the image data to the computer. (Indicate all that apply.)
   a. Both statements are true.
   b. Both statements are false.
   c. The first statement is true, and the second statement is false.
   d. The first statement is false, and the second statement is true.
   e. The statements are related.

Critical Thinking Exercises

1. The insurance company requests that a duplicate set of radiographs be sent to them to establish your patient's eligibility for the treatment recommended by your dental facility. You are given the responsibility of duplicating the radiographs taken.
   a. Would you be working in white light or safelight conditions?
   b. What is the correct placement of the original radiographs and duplicating film on the duplicating machine?
   c. What is the next step following the light exposure?
   d. What adjustment to the light exposure time in the duplicating machine would be made if more density (darker film) is needed on the duplicate?
   e. What adjustment to the light exposure time in the duplicating machine would be made if less density (lighter film) is needed on the duplicate?

2. The imaging system used in conventional extraoral radiography is a film-screen system. Explain this concept.
   a. What is the film in this system used in combination with?
   b. What substance is coated on the screen that allows it to produce light when it is struck by x-radiation? What is the property of emitting light when exposed to x-radiation called?
   c. Explain the concept of the compatibility of the screens with a certain film depending on the color of the light that is emitted from the screen when struck by x-radiation.
   d. Name the two types of screens available, what color light they each emit, and which is considered to be faster than the other.

Bibliography

American Academy of Oral and Maxillofacial Radiology: Recommendations for quality assurance in dental radiography, *Oral Surg Oral Med Oral Pathol* 55:421–426, 1983.

American Dental Association Council on Scientific Affairs: An update on radiographic practices: information and recommendations, *J Am Dent Assoc* 132:234–238, 2001.

Frommer HH, Jain RK: A comparative clinical study of group D and E dental film, *Oral Surg Oral Med Oral Pathol* 63:738–742, 1987.

Iannucci JM, Howerton LJ: *Dental radiography: principles and techniques*, ed 5, St Louis, MO, 2016, Elsevier Saunders.

Kantor ML, Reiskin AB, Lurie AG: A clinical comparison of x-ray films for detection of proximal surface caries. Erratum, *J Am Dent Assoc* 112:310, 1986.

Langland OE, Langlais RP: *Principles of dental imaging*, Baltimore, MD, 1997, Williams & Wilkins.

Ludlow JB, Platin E: Densitometric comparisons of Ultra-speed, Ektaspeed, and Ektaspeed Plus intraoral films for two processing conditions, *Oral Surg Oral Med Oral Pathol Oral Radiol Endod* 79:114–116, 1995.

New York City Health Code, Article 175, February 1998.

Platin E, Nesbit SP, Ludlow JB: The influence of storage conditions on film characteristics of Ektaspeed Plus and Ultra-speed films, *J Am Dent Assoc* 130:211–218, 1999.

Silha RE: Methods for reducing patient exposure combined with Kodak Ektaspeed dental x-ray film, *Dent Radiogr Photogr* 54:80–87, 1981.

Thompson EM, Johnson ON: *Essentials of dental radiography for dental assistants and hygienists*, ed 9, Upper Saddle River, NJ, 2012, Pearson Education, Inc.

Thunthy KH, Weinberg R: Sensitometric comparison of Kodak Ektaspeed Plus, Ektaspeed, and Ultra-speed dental films, *Oral Surg Oral Med Oral Pathol Oral Radiol Endod* 79:114–116, 1995.

White SC, Pharoah MJ: *Oral radiology: principles and interpretation*, ed 7, St Louis, MO, 2013, Mosby.

5

Biologic Effects of Radiation

EDUCATIONAL OBJECTIVES

Upon completing this chapter, the student will be able to:

1. Define the key terms listed at the beginning of the chapter.
2. Describe the historical concern about the effects of ionizing radiation.
3. Discuss the ways in which x-rays interact with matter and the difference between direct and indirect effects of radiation.
4. Explain the difference between the definitions of exposure and dose and the units of radiation measurement for both,

including their respective International System of Units (SI) conversions.
5. Define the basic terms and concepts related to the biologic effects of ionizing radiation on human tissue.
6. Discuss the factors that are related to a particular human tissue's sensitivity to radiation exposure.
7. Define and give examples of *background radiation*.

KEY TERMS

absorption
acute (short-term) effects
ALARA principle (concept)
attenuation
background radiation
cell recovery
chronic (long-term) effects
clusters
Compton effect
coulomb per kilogram (C/kg)
critical organ
cumulative effects
deterministic effects
direct effect
dose
dose equivalent
dose rate

dose–response curve
effective dose
exposure
free radical
genetic effects
gray (Gy)
indirect effect
interaction
ionizing radiation
ions
latent period
localized exposure
nonstochastic effects
osteoradionecrosis
period of injury
photoelectric effect
progeny

quality factor
radiation absorbed dose (rad)
radiation caries
radiobiology
radioresistant
radiosensitive
risk factors
roentgen (R)
roentgen equivalent man (rem)
sievert (Sv)
somatic effect
stochastic effects
threshold erythema dose (TED)
tissue sensitivity
total body exposure

Introduction

Ionizing radiation can have an effect on living tissue in various ways. In this chapter, we discuss the effects that ionizing radiation can have on living tissue, including the harmful effects x-radiation can cause. The information contained in this chapter covers the basic concepts of radiation biology, the units of radiation measurement, and the varying degrees of sensitivity of human tissues to x-radiation.

Historical Concern About the Effects of Ionizing Radiation

Much attention has been given, not only in scientific journals but also in the media, to the effects of ionizing radiation,

both artificial and naturally occurring, on human beings and the environment. This continual concern about the biologic effects of ionizing radiation is not limited to the scientific community but is evident in the public sector as well. Events such as the near-fatal nuclear accident at Three Mile Island, Pennsylvania (March 28, 1979), the catastrophe at Chernobyl (April 26, 1986) in the former Soviet Union, and the more recent Japanese tsunami and nuclear accident (March 11, 2011) have heightened public awareness of the dangers of ionizing radiation. The ongoing concern with the high incidence of cancers in certain geographic areas, referred to as clusters, and revelations about human exposure to nuclear testing during World War II and the Cold War have kept radiation exposure in the news. To add to the mix is the fear of terrorism, with its possible nuclear threat. A "dirty bomb" producing ionizing radiation is now considered a weapon of mass destruction. The uncertainty aroused by these events may cause some patients concern, and they may be hesitant to accept the necessary diagnostic radiographic examinations. Health professionals must be informed about the risks and benefits of dental radiation exposure and the extent of its relationship to these events so that they may anticipate and allay unfounded fears.

Information about ionizing radiation that reaches the public from the media can be misleading and confusing. The 2006 National Council on Radiation Protection and Measurements (NCRP) data indicate that radiation from medicine and dentistry accounts for about 48% of the average annual dose equivalent to the US population. This is the largest source of artificial radiation to which the population is exposed. At the same time, in learning about the risk of exposure, one should consider the diagnostic benefits and health-preserving or lifesaving consequences of diagnostic radiation exposure.

Patient reaction can vary from questioning the need for dental radiographs to outright refusal. The dental professional must face this patient reaction calmly and be able to explain to the patient the biologic effects of dental x-ray exposure and the diagnostic benefits that are derived. Proper dentistry cannot and should not be done without adequate diagnostic radiographs. This is an accepted standard of care for dental practice. A patient may refuse to have radiographs, but the dentist also can refuse to treat that patient without up-to-date diagnostic radiographs available.

> **NOTE**
>
> Treating a patient without the appropriately prescribed diagnostic radiographs available is like putting a blindfold over the dental professionals' eyes while they're working! Just as a building cannot be built without detailed blueprints drawn up by a licensed architect, a dental patient cannot be treated by a licensed dental professional without adequate diagnostic dental radiographs! Ionizing radiation does produce biologic changes in living tissue; thus patients should not be misled into believing that dental x-rays have no effect on human cells. The reply used in the past to patient queries regarding radiation safety stating that "dental x-rays are safe because the dosage is so small it doesn't matter" no longer satisfies current, well-informed health care consumers.

The question is no longer whether dental x-rays pose a risk but rather how much of a risk exists. In determining whether radiographs should be used, the dentist must weigh the potential harm of dental x-rays against the benefit that the diagnostic information will yield. In dental radiography performed under optimal conditions and when indicated, diagnostic benefits far outweigh potential risks.

The dental professional's objective for the patient is to use the least possible amount of radiation to obtain the greatest diagnostic yield (known as "radiation hygiene"). For dental professionals, the objective is to achieve occupational radiation exposure as close to zero as possible as well. To achieve these objectives, they must fully understand the subjects of radiation biology and protection. Explanations to patients then will be meaningful, and the dental professional will feel at ease working in an environment in which diagnostic radiation is used.

Interaction of X-Rays with Matter

X-rays interact with all forms of matter. This interaction can result in absorption of energy and thus attenuation of the x-ray beam (a reduction in the intensity of the x-ray beam) and the production of secondary radiation. The x-ray energy absorbed by the tissue causes chemical changes that result in tissue damage. The two mechanisms for this change are ionization and free radical formation.

Primary radiation is radiation that emanates from the focal (target) area resulting from the high-speed electrons hitting the target of the anode in the x-ray tube. Secondary radiation is the result of the interaction of primary radiation with any form of matter (see Fig. 6.1). Scatter radiation is a type of secondary radiation. When x-rays are absorbed by matter, positive and negative ions and secondary radiation are formed from previously neutral atoms. The amount and type of absorption that takes place depend on the energy of the x-ray beam (the wavelength) and the composition of the absorbing matter. The thicker the material that an x-ray beam must penetrate, the more x-rays will be absorbed. However, more than thickness determines x-ray absorption. The atomic configuration—the number of orbiting electrons and the numbers of protons and neutrons in the nucleus of the atom—also determine x-ray absorption. Heavy elements (those with greater mass) are more likely to absorb the radiation than lighter elements. The more electrons available in an absorbing material, the more x-ray photons are absorbed. Heavy metals with high atomic numbers (the atomic number indicates the number of protons in the nucleus of the atom), such as lead, readily absorb x-ray photons.

An important detail is that when x-rays are absorbed by any material, that material does not become radioactive, because x-rays have no effect on the nucleus of the absorbing atom, affecting only the atom's orbiting electrons. This means that the equipment or walls in a dental operatory do not become radioactive after continuous exposure to radiation.

At the atomic level, four possibilities can occur when an x-ray photon interacts with tissue; two of these will result in ionization, which is one of the basic mechanisms for the effect of radiation on tissue.

These four possibilities are as follows:

1. ***No interaction (pass through).*** The x-ray photon can pass through the atom unchanged and leave the atom unchanged (Fig. 5.1A). This happens about 9% of the time in dental radiography.

2. ***Thompson scatter (unmodified or coherent scatter).*** In this instance, the x-ray photon has its path altered by the atom. There is no change to the absorbing atom, but a photon of scattered radiation is produced (see Fig. 5.1A). This accounts for about 8% of the interactions that take place in dental radiography.

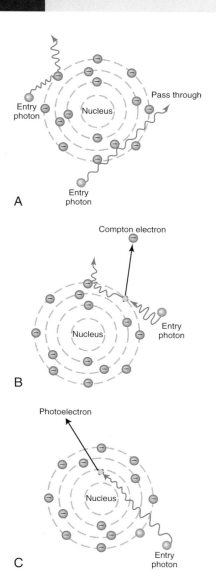

A

B

C

• **Figure 5.1** Interaction of x-rays with matter. **A,** Pass through and Thompson scatter. **B,** Compton effect. **C,** Photoelectric effect.

3. **Photoelectric effect.** The x-ray photon can collide with an orbiting electron, giving up all its energy to dislodge the electron from its orbit. The photoelectron that is produced has a negative charge, and the remaining atom has a positive charge. This, as mentioned, is an example of classic ionization (see Fig. 5.1C). This interaction takes place about 30% of the time in dental radiography.
4. **Compton effect.** The x-ray photon can collide with a loosely bound electron in an outer shell of the atom and only give up part of its energy in ejecting the electron from its orbit. This results in a negatively charged, ejected Compton electron, a photon of scattered radiation, and a remaining atom that is now positively charged. This occurrence is also considered to be a form of ionization (see Fig. 5.1B). However, this interaction takes place about 62% of the time in dental radiography.

In both the Compton and photoelectric interactions, the ejected high-speed electron interacts with other absorbing tissue and causes further ionization, excitation, or breaking of molecular bonds, all of which produce adverse tissue effects.

Effects of Ionizing Radiation

Radiobiology is the study of the effects of ionizing radiation on biologic tissue. When a dental radiograph is taken, not all of the x-rays reach the receptor, and some even penetrate beyond it. Some of the x-ray energy of the primary beam is absorbed by the skin, bones, teeth, and other body tissues that lie in its path. Tissues that do not lie in the path of the primary beam absorb the energy of the secondary (scatter) radiation that comes from the patient as a result of the interaction of the primary beam. The differential absorption (density) of the x-ray photons by the hard tissues, teeth, and bones enables the practitioner to distinguish various structures on a diagnostic radiograph.

What, then, is the effect of this x-ray energy absorption on the various tissues, and how is it manifested? Human tissue is composed primarily of water (H_2O). X-ray photons separate the water into ions (HOH and an electron). These ions may recombine into water or go on to other reactions that result in free radical formation (OH, H, O). A free radical is an uncharged molecule with a single unpaired electron in its outer shell. These free radicals are very unstable and exist for only a short time before they stabilize themselves by (1) recombining to form a stable molecule that will not cause tissue damage (H_2O) or (2) combining with other free radicals, which causes changes or the production of a tissue toxin, such as hydrogen peroxide (H_2O_2).

Direct and Indirect Effects

Damage to biologic molecules by radiation can occur by either a direct or indirect effect, with indirect being by far the most prevalent mechanism. In the direct mechanism, the x-ray photons directly hit critical areas within the cell and cause damage to those particular cells (e.g., deoxyribonucleic acid [DNA]). In the indirect mechanism, the free radicals that are formed as the result of the ionization of water go on to form toxins that injure or alter cells.

Units of Radiation Measurement

Before logically discussing the potential effects of dental radiation, we will first consider a quantitative means of measuring radiation. The dental x-ray machine settings are not units of measurement for the x-ray energy (ionizing radiation) produced. The kilovoltage and milliamperage are indications of the quality and quantity of the electric energy put into the x-ray machine, and the time is set to provide a reading of how long the ionizing radiation is produced. The half-value layer (HVL), although a characteristic of the x-ray beam, describes the penetration and quality of the beam, not its effect on tissue.

TABLE 5.1	Radiation Units				
Conventional Unit	Definition	SI Unit	Definition	Conversion
Roentgen (R)	1 ESU/cc³ of air	Coulomb/kg (C/kg)	1 C/kg = 3876 R	
Rad	100 erg/g	Gray (Gy)	1 J/kg	1 Gy = 100 rad
Rem	rad × Q	Sievert (Sv)	Gy × Q	1 Sv = 100 rem

ESU, electrostatic unit; Rad, radiation absorbed dose; Rem, roentgen equivalent man.

The units of measurement that commonly have been employed and are referred to as the conventional or traditional units are the roentgen (R), the radiation absorbed dose (rad), and the roentgen equivalent man (rem; Table 5.1). To standardize units to the metric system, these conventional units have been replaced by those of the International System of Units (SI). However, the conventional units are still used widely both in presentations and in the literature. The metric system conversions employed are the coulomb per kilogram (C/kg), the gray (Gy), and the sievert (Sv) respectively. This text uses both the conventional units and the SI units to express the measurements of radiation exposure and dose.

Exposure

Exposure is defined as the measure of the ionization in air produced by x-ray or gamma radiation. The conventional unit used to measure the amount of energy, or ionizing radiation, produced by the x-ray machine is the roentgen (R). The milliroentgen (mR) is 1/1000 of a roentgen; because exposures in dental radiology are small, they are often expressed in milliroentgens (1000 mR = 1 R). The SI unit for exposure is the coulomb per kilogram (1 C/kg = 3.88×10^{-3} R).

The roentgen or coulomb per kilogram are units that measure ionization in air. In clinical application, an ionization chamber is placed in front of the position-indicating device (PID) of a dental x-ray machine to measure the x-ray exposure emanating from the machine (Fig. 5.2). This is called the *exposure rate* or *output* of the machine. Because it is an expression of ionization in air, it is measured in roentgens or coulombs per kilogram per second. A well-calibrated dental x-ray machine has an output in the range of 0.7 to 1 R/sec. If a patient had a radiograph taken with such a machine and the exposure time was 1 second, the facial exposure of the patient would be 0.7 R (0.7 R/sec × 1 = 0.7 R).

Dose

The critical factor in discussing the effects of radiation is not the amount of radiation at a point in air but rather the amount of energy absorbed by tissue at a specific point. The term dose is defined as the amount of radiation energy

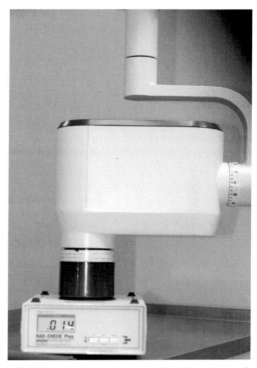

• **Figure 5.2** Ionization chamber measuring the output of a dental x-ray machine.

absorbed per unit mass of tissue at a particular site. To express the amount of energy absorbed by a tissue, the rad or gray (SI unit) is used. The rad is a unit of absorbed dose and is defined as 100 ergs of energy per gram of absorber (tissue). The millirad is 1/1000 of a rad. The unit for the absorbed dose in SI units is the gray (1 rad = 0.01 Gy or 1 Gy = 100 rad).

Dose Equivalent

Different types of radiation on a rad-for-rad basis have different effects on living tissue. Neutrons, for example, have a greater effect on tissue than x-rays or gamma radiation. A rad of x-radiation does not have the same effect on human tissue as a neutron rad. The term dose equivalent is meant to illustrate this difference; it is defined as the dose multiplied by the quality factor and is expressed in rems. The millirem is 1/1000 of a rem. The unit for the dose equivalent in SI units is the sievert (1 rem = 0.01 Sv or 1 Sv = 100 rem). The quality factor by definition for x-radiation and gamma radiation is 1, so the dose equivalent in rems (Svs) is equal to the dose in rads (Gys).

Basic Concepts

Exposure and Dose

Although the terms are often interchanged, there is a very definite distinction between radiation exposure and dosage. As previously mentioned, exposure is the amount of ionization in the air produced by x-rays or gamma radiation; it is the quantity of radiation in an area to which the patient is exposed. The radiation dose is the amount of energy absorbed per unit mass of tissue at a particular site. In dentistry, the patient is exposed to a certain amount of radiation, some of which is absorbed by tissue in different parts of the body; this is the *dose* to the area. Thus, there is a skin dose, a thyroid dose, a gonadal dose, and so on. Exposure should be expressed in roentgens (C/kg), and dose should be expressed in rads (Gys) or rems (Svs).

Localized Radiation and Total Body Exposure

It is important to differentiate between localized radiation and total body radiation exposure (Fig. 5.3). When a dental radiograph is taken, the patient's face is exposed to an x-ray beam that is 2¾ inches (2.75 inches or 7 cm) in diameter (with circular collimation). This is a localized exposure and represents less than 1% of the total area of the body. A rad (Gy) of radiation to the localized area means that each gram of body tissue in that area absorbs 1 rad (Gy). A rad (Gy) of total body exposure means that each gram of tissue in the entire body absorbs 1 rad (Gy). In dentistry, the x-ray machine delivers a localized exposure that results in a total body exposure much less than the facial exposure. In fact the total body exposure from a dental radiograph is approximately 1/10,000 of the facial exposure.

Dose–Response Curve

The dose–response curve is an important concept because it illustrates the possible biologic responses to a harmful agent such as ionizing radiation. The responses can be *linear* or *nonlinear*, and they can be *threshold* or *non-threshold*. In a linear dose–response relationship, the response is directly proportional to the dose. In a nonlinear relationship, the response is not proportional to the dose. Fig. 5.4A is a threshold curve with both linear and nonlinear responses, indicating that below a certain level (the threshold), there is no response to the agent. Applying this concept to dental radiation would yield a level below which radiographs would be "perfectly safe," because there would be no biologic response below that level. This is not thought to be the case for ionizing radiation (see Fig. 5.4B). This curve

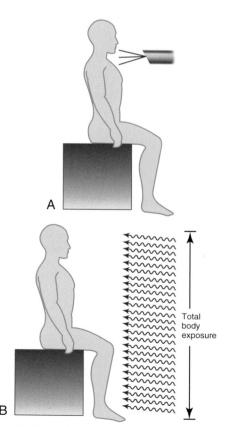

• **Figure 5.3** (A) Localized exposure. (B) Total body exposure.

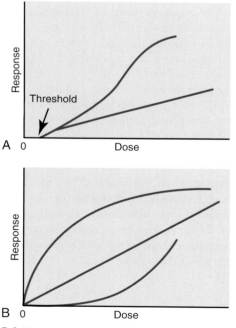

• **Figure 5.4** Linear and nonlinear dose–response curves. **A,** Threshold curve. **B,** Non-threshold type. (From National Council on Radiation Protection and Measurements [NCRP]. Ionizing radiation exposure of the population of the United States, Report No. 100. Washington, DC; 1989.)

indicates that any dose of radiation, regardless of how small and whether the response is linear or nonlinear, will produce some degree of biologic response. Therefore, dental x-rays do produce biologic changes in the tissues of patients who receive them, even though no signs or symptoms may be detected and no permanent damage is done to the tissue.

Most of the data that produces such a dose–response curve for humans comes from studying the effects of large doses of radiation on populations, such as atomic bomb survivors. In the low-dose range for humans, in which dental x-rays fall, little has been documented. The line is therefore an extrapolation based on the limited human data and animal and cellular experiments. The prevailing consensus is that low-dose, ionizing radiation is a linear, non-threshold relationship.

Somatic and Genetic Effects

All cells in the body, with the exception of the reproductive cells (sperm and ova), are included in the grouping of somatic tissue. Changes in these cells are not passed on to succeeding generations of the species. For example, a cancerous skin condition will not be passed on to an offspring. Somatic tissue can be affected by radiation, and some cells may die, be altered, or even recover, but none of these effects will be seen in the somatic tissue of the progeny (offspring). This is known as the somatic effect.

Changes in genetic cells cannot be detected in the exposed patient but are passed on to succeeding generations. These are referred to as genetic effects or mutations. There are many agents other than ionizing radiation that have been found to be mutagenic, including a variety of chemicals, certain drugs, and even elevated body temperatures. Background radiation (radiation in the environment) also accounts for a portion of naturally occurring mutations. Some of the mutations that have been manifested have been positive and have added to the so-called evolution of the species. A mutation may be recessive and carried in the progeny for many generations before becoming clinically evident.

Stochastic and Deterministic (Nonstochastic) Radiation Effects

Stochastic effects are the effects of radiation exposure that occur by chance and by changes in the DNA of body cells. These effects may occur without a threshold level (non-threshold) of dose, whose probability is proportional to the dose and whose severity is independent of the dose. Stochastic effects transpire due to the effect of radiation that causes ionization on chromosomes that result in damage to genetic cells (i.e., genetic mutations). In the context of radiation protection, the main stochastic effect is radiation-induced cancer.

Deterministic or nonstochastic effects increase in severity with increased absorbed dose and do have a threshold, unlike stochastic effects. Once the threshold has been exceeded, the severity of an effect increases with dose. However, because there is a specific threshold level, operators are encouraged to employ radiation safety guidelines in protecting themselves and their patients from harmful x-radiation exposure. Some examples of deterministic or nonstochastic effects and their respective threshold levels include hair loss (threshold: 2–5 Gy), cataracts (threshold: 5 Gy), and fetal abnormality (threshold: 0.1–0.5 Gy).

Acute and Chronic Effects

The acute (short-term) effects of radiation result from high doses of whole body radiation. The clinical effects of the exposure, which may vary from mild and transient illness to death, may occur minutes, hours, or weeks after the acute exposure. Obviously, dental radiographers are not concerned with acute radiation doses.

Chronic (long-term) effects of radiation may be seen years after the original exposures. Acute and/or chronic exposures may produce cumulative effects on the somatic cells over the patient's lifetime, as well as genetic effects on future generations.

Latent Period, Period of Injury, and Cell Recovery

The latent period is the time that elapses between the exposure to ionizing radiation and the appearance of clinical symptoms. This time may vary from hours to years, depending on the magnitude of the exposure and the tissues involved. It is also difficult, if not impossible, to single out radiation as the cause of a specific pathologic change that takes years to develop. As noted, there is no specific long-term radiation disease, and the conditions associated with radiation (e.g., cancer) have multiple etiologic agents. The period of injury occurs after the latent period, which can include changes in the cell's or tissue's function. However, not all radiation-induced changes in tissue cells are permanent. Depending on the time interval, dose, and sensitivity of the affected cells to radiation, the cells' repair processes may be sufficient to effect cell recovery (the process by which cells heal themselves) from the effects of radiation exposure. In addition, radiation exposure can produce cumulative effects or additive effects, as repetitive exposure can damage cells that are not repaired and can lead to health problems.

Dose Rate

The dose rate, the rate at which exposure to ionizing radiation occurs and absorption takes place, is a critical factor in determining the effects. Because cells do recover from radiation exposure, a specific dose produces less damage if it is extended in intervals over time. In dentistry, the time interval between exposures—excluding retakes and working films or images—is usually months or years, further minimizing the effects.

Long-Term Effects

The long-term effects of radiation manifest themselves years after the exposure. The latent period is very long. These delayed effects may be from an acute exposure or a series of low-level exposures.

Again, no specific disease has been associated solely with the long-term effects of radiation to date. Cancer can be caused by radiation, but it is also caused by other etiologic agents, such as smoking, chronic irritation, and exposure to certain chemicals.

Because there is no specific disease solely associated with radiation exposure, the long-term effects of radiation express themselves in human populations as a statistical increase in the incidence of certain diseases. One can study the incidence of diseases in irradiated populations and compare it with that in nonirradiated groups. A study of atomic bomb survivors and the incidence of leukemias among them is a good example of this type of evaluation of long-term effects. Evaluating the long-term effects of dental x-rays, for which the dose is low, would require large populations over a long period of time, because the latent period for radiation-induced cancer—even from large doses—ranges from years to decades.

Risk Estimates

There is no effective way of analyzing the cause of a radiation-induced cancer on a case-by-case basis; thus, dosages in irradiated populations are compared with the number of cancers in these populations. This number is then compared with that of nonirradiated populations, and the difference is expressed as the risk factor. Risk factors are expressed as the number of cases or deaths from a specific disease per million persons. The American Dental Association (ADA) recommends the use of rectangular collimation along with digital radiography as the most effective way of reducing radiation exposure to the dental patient. The ADA also endorses the use of selection criteria (radiation history and personal risk of dental disease) in prescribing dental radiographs.

Tissue Sensitivity

Tissue sensitivity is an important factor in determining the effects of ionizing radiation on the patient's tissue. Effective dose is a calculation that considers the difference in tissue sensitivity. It is the preferred method for comparing effective tissue sensitivity. Tissues vary widely in their sensitivity to ionizing radiation and thus the amount of radiation required to produce damage. The effect of radiation on certain tissues and organs has predictable disease manifestations, such as hematopoietic tissue giving rise to leukemia or exposure to the sun giving rise to skin cancer. The same dose of radiation has different degrees of effect on different types of cells in the same organism. Young, rapidly dividing, non-differentiated cells, such as those found in the abdomens of pregnant dental patients, are more radiosensitive than older

---

> **• BOX 5.1   Effect of Radiation on Tissues and Organs**
>
> **High Sensitivity**
> - Lymphoid organs
> - Bone marrow
> - Testes
> - Intestines
> - Skin
> - Cornea
>
> **Intermediate Sensitivity**
> - Fine vasculature
> - Growing cartilage
> - Growing bone
>
> **Low Sensitivity**
> - Salivary glands
> - Lungs
> - Kidneys
> - Liver
> - Optic lens
> - Muscle cells
> - Neurons

cells. Also, children are more prone to damage resulting from radiation exposure than adults are. In addition to the age of the cell and its rate of differentiation, tissues vary in their sensitivity to radiation.

A cell that is sensitive to radiation exposure is considered to be radiosensitive; a cell that is not sensitive to radiation exposure is said to be radioresistant. The determining factors associated with the sensitivity of a cell to radiation are the rate of cell metabolism, mitotic activity, and differentiation. Therefore, the cells, tissues, and organs that have a higher rate of metabolism, division, and differentiation are more sensitive to radiation exposure. The grouping of cells, tissues, and organs in descending order of sensitivity to radiation is shown in Box 5.1.

Critical Organs

Certain organs and tissues have been designated as critical, because they are exposed to more radiation than others in dental radiography. These critical organs and tissues, with their potential risks, are the skin (carcinoma), thyroid (carcinoma), lens of the eye (cataract), hematopoietic tissue (leukemia), and genetic tissue (congenital defects or mutations).

Background Radiation

Background radiation is a form of ionizing radiation, both naturally occurring and artificial, that is ever-present in the environment. Naturally occurring radiation always has been present on earth, but the artificial component has been increasing as a result of nuclear accidents, fallout from nuclear testing, and radioactive wastes from industry. It

TABLE 5.2	Annual Exposure of US Population	
Source		**Dose (mrem)**
Natural Sources		
Radon		200
Cosmic radiation		27
Soil and building materials		28
Internal radioactivity		39
Other Sources		
Occupational		0.9
Nuclear fuel cycle		0.5
Consumer products		9.0
Miscellaneous		0.06
Medical and dental		53.0

mrem, millirem.

would be helpful to know the level of background radiation and its sources so that dental radiation exposure can be put in its proper perspective. An estimate of the average personal exposure, weighted from different sources to approximate a "total body exposure," has been prepared and is shown in Table 5.2. This report shows an estimated average annual dose of 300 mrem (3 mSv) resulting from natural background sources. With the addition of the average contributions of medical and dental procedures, the total annual population exposure is about 360 mrem (3.6 mSv). This amount is increased at higher elevations, and the difference between these elevations and sea level is often used to make comparisons for the dose from dental exposures. Of the total background exposure, 55% is from exposure to radon, and because not all geographic areas have large amounts of radon gases, background radiation is sometimes considered to be about 100 mrem (1 mSv) per year. This data is helpful in comparing dental exposure with background exposure.

Patient Dosage

Ample evidence in the literature substantiates the adverse effects of radiation in high doses. The problem is that although no direct evidence exists of such effects from dental diagnostic doses, there is also no evidence for the absence of adverse effects. To treat a patient without current and diagnostic radiographs is a disservice to the patient and leaves the dentist unprotected against possible legal action for not adhering to the standard of care. Radiographs are an integral part of modern dental practice. The goal in dental radiography is to use the least amount of radiation to satisfy the patient's diagnostic needs, that is, minimize the exposure while maximizing the diagnostic yield. Efforts

to minimize the amount of radiation must be guided by the ALARA principle (concept), which means "as low as reasonably achievable." The radiation exposure to patients should be reduced as much as possible within the dental office without excessive cost or inconvenience to the patient.

Dental professionals and dentists, because of their involvement with low-level ionizing radiation, should be aware of the consequences of chronic exposure for their patients. In this manner, they are better equipped to make the essential risk–benefit decision before exposing their patients to x-radiation. Additionally, careful consideration must be dedicated to patient and operator protection during dental radiographic procedures.

The following examples of specific tissue effects from dental x-ray exposure and the critical levels for these tissues support the conclusion that the benefits derived from dental x-ray exposure, when used judiciously under proper conditions, far outweigh any possible risk.

Skin

Erythema (reddening of the skin) is the usual effect of radiation and is not a major risk in dental radiography. Its importance lies in the fact that the skin dose is the most commonly reported value for dental x-ray examinations. The skin dose has limitations in that (1) skin is easily penetrated and does not reflect a dose to deeper tissues, (2) the skin dose varies greatly with the kilovoltage used, and (3) the skin is less sensitive than many other tissues exposed during dental radiography. The threshold erythema dose (TED), the amount of radiation needed to produce an erythema or reddening of the most sensitive individual, is very high in comparison to the exposure received from dental radiographic procedures.

Eyes

Exposure of the lens of the eye to ionizing radiation in high doses can induce cataract formation. The lens of the eye is exposed to radiation during intraoral radiography, but the risk of cataract formation is extremely low.

Thyroid

The thyroid gland, which is particularly radiosensitive, may lie in the beam of primary radiation in some dental views. The dose to this radiosensitive tissue should be kept to an absolute minimum, especially in children. This can be accomplished, as shall be seen in the next chapter, by the use of a thyroid collar and the paralleling technique.

Bone Marrow

It is now thought that the greatest somatic hazard to patients from dental x-ray exposure is leukemia induction. The red bone marrow is one of the blood-forming organs of the body. The significant hematopoietic bone marrow exposed to dental x-rays is located in the mandible, the calvarium of the skull, and the cervical spine. The calvarium and cervical spine are exposed to primary radiation in extraoral and panoramic radiography. The bone marrow of the mandible and maxilla is also of concern in extraoral dental radiography. However, with judicious use of radiation and proper technique, the diagnostic benefit derived outweighs the slight risk.

Gonads

The reproductive cells (sperm and ova) are very radiosensitive. The dose to the gonads during dental radiographic procedures is in the form of secondary (scatter) radiation. Consequently, this area is shielded from x-ray exposure with use of a protective apron during dental radiographic procedures.

Pregnancy

As mentioned, the nondifferentiated rapidly dividing fetal cells are extremely radiosensitive; therefore, there is a concern about pregnant patients. A panel of dental radiologists in the early 1980s considered the appropriateness of dental radiography for pregnant patients. They concluded that the guidelines for taking radiographs (discussed in Chapter 6) need not be altered for the pregnant patient. They pointed out that the concept of avoiding radiography during pregnancy generally applies to procedures in which the fetus or embryo would be in or near the primary x-ray beam. In dentistry, the primary beam is limited to the head and neck region, and the only radiation the fetus would be exposed to would be secondary (scatter) radiation. Uterine doses for a full-mouth series without use of a lead apron have been shown to be less than 1 mrem. Radiographs, in some cases, may have to be deferred during pregnancy for purely psychological reasons or ill-founded recommendations of physicians. If this is the case, then no dental treatment should be rendered that would violate the standard of care, as stated previously.

A study was published that indicated a possible link between dental x-rays taken of women during their pregnancy and low-birthweight deliveries. This raises the possibility that x-ray exposure of the thyroid area could be linked to low birthweight. The dental profession through its many organizations was quick to point out that the use of a thyroid collar on any patient is routine procedure. It has restated its position that only radiographs that are essential to proper treatment should be taken for pregnant patients and that patients should be encouraged to return for complete treatment after they deliver. Again, it is a risk–benefit concept, because the overall health of the patient and the fetus can severely be affected by dental disease.

As shown in Chapter 7, no occupational hazard for the pregnant dental professional exists. When appropriate precautionary procedures are followed, the occupational dose is zero.

Radiation Caries

One of the accepted modalities for treatment of head and neck cancer is radiation. The high doses of radiation used (6000 rad) affect not only the malignant cells but also the soft tissue of the oral cavity, the mandible and maxilla, and the salivary glands, if they are in the field of radiation. The saliva production of the irradiated salivary glands is diminished and is more viscous; thus, it loses its lubricative function, leading to xerostomia (dry mouth). The altered quality and quantity of saliva make the patient more susceptible to a rampant type of radiation caries that is characterized by its circumferential pattern, because it affects all surfaces of the teeth at the cervical area. A well-taken health history and therapeutic measures—such as fluoride treatments, artificial saliva, and frequent recall visits—are all part of accepted means to manage this condition.

Another sequela of radiation therapy that dental professionals could contend with is osteoradionecrosis. Osteoradionecrosis is a possible complication following radiotherapy in which an area of bone does not heal from the high levels of radiation used in radiation therapy. This irradiation of bones causes damage to osteocytes and impairs the blood supply. Therefore, it is not the dental exposure that is the major cause of this infectious condition but rather the lowered resistance of the therapeutically irradiated tissue. One should understand that it is not the small dental dose of radiation that causes dental caries and osteoradionecrosis of bone, because the actual dental exposure is a minor factor.

Chapter Summary

- There has been a lot of attention given to the effects of both artificial and naturally occurring ionizing radiation on the environment and on humans.
- It is an accepted practice of care in dentistry that proper treatment cannot be accomplished without adequate diagnostic radiographic images.
- X-rays interact with matter in various ways.
- The Compton effect occurs most often (62% of the time) in dental radiography when an x-ray photon interacts with tissue and is one of the basic mechanisms for the effect of radiation on living tissue.
- Radiobiology is the study of the effects of ionizing radiation on biologic tissue.

- Radiation exposure is the measurement of the ionization in air produced by x-rays and is measured in roentgens or coulomb per kilograms (SI conversion). The dose of x-radiation is the measurement of the amount of radiation absorbed by tissue at a specific point and is measured in rads or grays (SI conversion). The rem or sievert (SI conversion) is used to measure the dose equivalent.
- There are various types of effects that radiation can have on the human body, including direct, indirect, somatic, genetic, stochastic, nonstochastic (or deterministic), acute, chronic, and long-term effects.
- Injury resulting from radiation exposure occurs in a series of events, including the latent period followed by

the period of injury and culminating in a period of cell recovery.

- The determining factors associated with the sensitivity of cells to radiation exposure are the rate of cell metabolism, mitotic activity, and cell differentiation.

- Background radiation is ionizing radiation that is ever present in the environment and can be naturally or artificially occurring.

- It can be concluded that the benefits derived from diagnostically sound dental x-ray exposure, when used judiciously and under safe and proper conditions, far outweigh any possible risks.

Chapter Review Questions

Multiple Choice

1. According to the 2006 data report of the National Council on Radiation Protection and Measurements (NCRP), what percentage of the annual dose equivalent radiation exposure is as a result of medical and dental exposure?
   a. 20%
   b. 15%
   c. 50%
   d. 48%
   e. 60%

2. Primary radiation is the radiation that is produced at the target of the anode in the dental x-ray tube. Secondary radiation is produced as a result of the interaction of primary radiation with any form of matter. (Indicate all that apply.)
   a. Both statements are true.
   b. Both statements are false.
   c. The first statement is true, and the second statement is false.
   d. The first statement is false, and the second statement is true.
   e. The statements are related.

3. The units of measurement that commonly have been employed and are referred to as the *conventional* (or traditional) units (as opposed to the SI conversions) of radiation exposure and dose are (indicate all that apply):
   a. Roentgen (R)
   b. Gray (Gy)
   c. Roentgen equivalent man (rem)
   d. Radiation absorbed dose (rad)
   e. Sievert (Sv)

4. It is the general consensus that low-dose, ionizing radiation, as in the case of dental x-rays, is a:
   a. Linear, threshold relationship
   b. Nonlinear, non-threshold relationship
   c. Linear, non-threshold relationship
   d. Nonlinear, threshold relationship
   e. Nonlinear, unknown threshold relationship

5. Which of the following tissues or organs have a high sensitivity to the effects of radiation? (Indicate all that apply.)
   a. Salivary glands
   b. Bone marrow
   c. Cornea
   d. Skin
   e. Neurons

Critical Thinking Exercises

1. There are four possibilities that could occur at the atomic level when an x-ray photon interacts with tissue.
   a. Name each of these four interactions.
   b. Explain what occurs at the atomic level in each one of these possible interactions.
   c. State whether each interaction is an example of ionization or not.
   d. State the percentage of time that each interaction occurs in dental radiography.

2. There are certain tissues and organs that are considered to be "critical organs" in dental radiography because they are specifically exposed to x-radiation more often than others during dental radiographic procedures. Provide information on the following:
   a. List the "critical organs."
   b. List the respective potential risks from exposing them to dental x-rays.
   c. Give a brief description of why you think that these organs are considered "critical" to consider in dental radiography based on your knowledge of anatomy, physiology, and dental radiology.

Bibliography

Budowsky J, Piro JD, Zegarelli EV, et al: Lack of effect of exposure to radiation during intraoral roentgenographic examination as evidenced by post examination blood studies, *J Am Dent Assoc* 55:199–204, 1957.

Gibbs SJ: Radiation dose to sensitive organs from intraoral dental radiography, *Dentomax Radiol* 17:15–23, 1987.

Hujoel PP, Bollen AM, Noonan CJ, et al: Antepartum dental radiography and infant low birth weight, *JAMA* 291(16):1987–1993, 2004.

Iannucci JM, Howerton LJ: *Dental radiography: principles and techniques*, ed 5, St Louis, MO, 2016, Elsevier Saunders.

Langland OE, Langlais RP: *Principles of dental imaging*, Baltimore, MD, 1997, Williams & Wilkins.

National Academy of Sciences, National Research Council: *The effects on population of exposure to low levels of ionizing radiation (Beir V)*, Washington, DC, 1990, National Academy Press.

National Council on Radiation Protection and Measurements. NCRP Report No. 145, Radiation in Dentistry, 2004.

Nolan WE: Radiation hazards to the patient from oral roentgenography, *J Am Dent Assoc* 47:681, 1953.

Thompson EM, Johnson ON: *Essentials of dental radiography for dental assistants and hygienists*, ed 9, Upper Saddle River, NJ, 2012, Pearson Education, Inc.

U.S. Department of Health and Human Services, Public Health Service, FDA: The selection of patients for dental radiographic examinations, 1987. HHS/PHS/FDA, 88-827310-21.

White SC: 1992 assessment of radiation risk from dental radiography, *Dentomaxillofac Radiol* 21:118–126, 1992.

White SC, Pharoah MJ: *Oral radiology: principles and interpretation*, ed 7, St Louis, MO, 2013, Mosby.

6

Patient Protection

EDUCATIONAL OBJECTIVES

Upon completing this chapter, the student will be able to:

1. Define the key terms listed at the beginning of the chapter.
2. Discuss patient protection and the ALARA principle (concept).
3. Discuss the role of the dental x-ray equipment in reducing radiation exposure to the patient before, during, and after the dental images are taken.
4. Describe the role of careful chairside techniques, processing techniques (when applicable), and image retrieval in reducing radiation exposure to the patient.
5. Define and recite the significance of radiation history, selection criteria, and the avoidance of administrative radiographs in patient protection.

KEY TERMS

administrative radiographs
ALARA principle (concept)
electronic timers
exposure time
film-holding device
film viewing
filtration
lead apron

operator concern
patient concern
primary radiation
radiation history
rectangular collimation
retake
scatter radiation
secondary radiation

selection criteria
shielding
thyroid collar
tube head drift
tube head leakage
useful beam

Introduction

Now that the mechanism of ionizing radiation and its effects on human tissue have been discussed, these principles can be applied to the clinical dental environment. The issue of radiation exposure and protection can be discussed from the perspectives of the two major concerns: patient concern and operator concern. This chapter discusses the techniques that are employed in the protection of the patient.

Patient Protection

In patient protection, the objective is to use the least amount of radiation to achieve the maximum diagnostic results, which is sometimes referred to as *radiation hygiene*. The patient must be protected from excessive or unnecessary primary radiation and the resulting secondary (scatter) radiation. This goal can be met by adhering to the ALARA principle (concept), which means "as low as reasonably achievable," through the use of safe, well-calibrated x-ray machines, rectangular collimation, receptor-holding devices, fast-speed film or digital imaging, lead aprons and thyroid collars, rare earth intensifying screens, proper shielding, effective chairside and darkroom techniques, and sound professional judgment in selection criteria.

Primary radiation is the x-rays that come directly from the target of the x-ray tube. The primary radiation is collimated by the lead diaphragm, and its softer, less penetrating wavelengths are removed by aluminum filters; it then can be referred to as the useful beam. All other radiation can be considered secondary radiation. Secondary radiation is defined as radiation that comes from any matter struck by primary radiation. The scatter radiation that results from the interaction of the useful beam and the patient's face is a form of secondary radiation (Fig. 6.1). Secondary radiation, besides being harmful to both patient and operator, can degrade the diagnostic image, because the scattered rays produce "film fog" on the radiographic image.

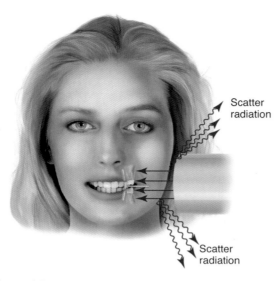

• **Figure 6.1** Production of scatter radiation of primary beam by interaction with a patient's face.

> **NOTE**
>
> The term *primary* means first, and primary radiation is the first radiation to leave the tube head. Secondary radiation comes after primary radiation, because it is produced when primary radiation interacts with matter. Scatter radiation is a form of secondary radiation that results from the interaction of the useful beam (primary radiation) with another form of matter (i.e., the patient's face) and scatters in different directions.

Equipment

All dental x-ray machines must meet federal diagnostic equipment performance standards. It is important to remember that the federal standards do not regulate diagnostic equipment users (such as, dentists, dental hygienists, and dental assistants) but rather only the equipment itself. However, most state or local governments also regulate equipment and have radiation health codes that pertain to the use of radiation. The federal government regulates the manufacture and installation of x-ray machines, whereas state and local governments may regulate the equipment and how the x-ray units are used. Depending on the local radiation code, dental offices, clinics, and dental schools may be inspected according to the regulatory guidelines to monitor equipment performance, processing equipment, and the barriers and procedures used when radiographs are taken.

Tube Head and Arm

Head Leakage

The term **tube head leakage** refers to radiation that escapes through the protective **shielding** of the x-ray tube head. The only radiation that should leave the tube head is the primary beam. Radiation leakage exposes the patient unnecessarily and should not occur in a properly functioning x-ray unit. Leakage is a violation of the federal performance standards

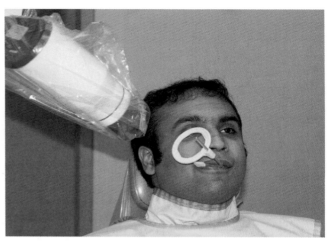

• **Figure 6.2** Tube head drift places the x-ray beam far from the receptor.

and local radiation codes. It is not a common problem, because most x-ray units are well built. If the unit is not abused in use or in positioning, head leakage is unlikely to occur.

Drift

Tube head drift (Fig. 6.2) is a common problem that is easily corrected. The tube head of the dental x-ray machine should not move, or drift, in any direction after positioning for an exposure (see Fig. 1.3). The movement can cause a blurred image if it occurs during exposure or can contribute to positioning the central ray off the receptor, resulting in a collimator cutoff ("cone cut"). If the tube head drifts, the arm can be stabilized by positioning the elbow of the unit's arm against a wall in the operatory. If this adjustment and all other attempts are unsuccessful, the cause of the drifting should be professionally repaired immediately. This can be addressed by just tightening the bolts that attach the tube head to the yolk or by adjusting another faulty component on the affected dental x-ray unit. The patient, the patient's companion, or the dental professional should never hold the tube head in place during an exposure to correct for tube head drift.

Checking for tube head drift in all directions is an important step in an office quality assurance program.

Kilovoltage and Milliampere Seconds

The equipment-related factors of kilovoltage and milliamperage control proper penetration and film density and contrast. As explained in Chapter 3, film speed and target-receptor distance (FFD) determine the contribution of milliamperes to the patient's radiation exposure. However, the choice of kilovoltage affects the contrast of the image and radiation dose. The patient's skin exposure decreases as the kilovoltage increases, but the dose to deeper tissues and the amount of scatter radiation increase. A kilovoltage that is best suited to the diagnostic requirements should be utilized. There is no question that kilovoltage below 60 should not be used, although it is possible to produce a

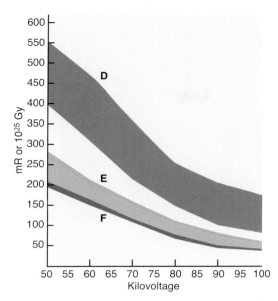

• **Figure 6.3** Acceptable x-ray exposure ranges for group D, E, and F films. Note the increased exposure in the low-kilovolt range and that the exposure with group E is about half that of group D. Gy, gray; *mR,* milliroentgen. (Courtesy Department of Health and Human Services. Modified by S. White.)

diagnostic image at that level. The exposure to the patient per exposure is increased when a kilovoltage setting below the acceptable range is used (Fig. 6.3).

Filtration

Because of the enactment and compliance of federal performance standards and the enforcement of local health codes, filtration is no longer a major concern in patient protection, because these regulations are generally easily met in dental facilities. The purpose of filtration is to remove the long (soft), nonpenetrating x-ray photons from the x-ray beam (see Chapter 2). These long wavelength photons either would be absorbed by the overlying tissues or give rise to secondary (scatter) radiation to the patient and degrade the diagnostic image. In order to meet the state and federal regulations for aluminum filtration, the inherent filtration is equivalent to 0.5 to 1.0 mm of aluminum and does not meet the standards alone. Therefore, for x-ray units operating at a kilovoltage below 70, aluminum discs (equivalent to 0.5 mm aluminum each) are added to produce a total filtration (inherent plus added filtration) up to 1.5 mm. For units operating at 70 kV or higher, the total aluminum filtration must be at a minimum of 2.5 mm with added aluminum discs.

NOTE

The kilovoltage (kV) setting has a direct effect on the amount of aluminum filtration needed to filter out the long wavelength, less energetic, and less penetrating x-rays.
- kV lower than 70 = 1.5 mm of total aluminum filtration
- kV at 70 or higher = 2.5 mm of total aluminum filtration

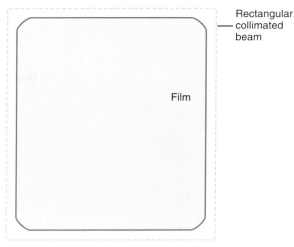

• **Figure 6.4** Rectangular collimation.

Collimation

The collimation of the x-ray beam limits the size and shape of the area exposed by the primary beam and the amount of scatter produced. The beam size is discussed in Chapter 2, and at present a 2¾-inch (2.75-inch or 7-cm) circular beam measured at the skin is required. If the size and shape of the x-ray beam is changed to a rectangle that is slightly larger than the receptor, the volume of tissue exposed could be reduced considerably. In fact, the skin exposure will decrease by 1 inch (¼ in on all four sides of the adult-size receptor) for each image exposed when compared with circular collimation. Actually, the utilization of rectangular collimation is said to produce 60 percent less x-radiation exposure to the patient's skin than the use of circular (cylindrical) collimation. The American Dental Association (ADA) and the American Academy of Oral and Maxillofacial Radiology (AAOMR) strongly recommend the use of rectangular collimation (Fig. 6.4). Rectangular collimation is said to be the single most effective factor in reducing radiation exposure to the patient.

Timing Device

The use of more sensitive x-ray film and digital sensors with extremely short exposure times makes the use of electronic timers imperative (see Fig. 2.5). All new x-ray machines come equipped with these recommended devices.

The mechanical timers existing on older machines are inaccurate at short exposures. These timers are usually calibrated down to ¼ second and can have a ¼-second margin of error. Only an electronic timer should be used as the standard of care in contemporary dental imaging.

Position-Indicating Devices

Open-ended, lead-lined (shielded) rectangles (Fig. 6.5A) or cylinders (see Fig. 6.5B) are the only types of position-indicating devices (PIDs) that should be used. The use of closed-ended, pointed cones is contraindicated (see Chapter 2). These cones increase scatter radiation to the patient

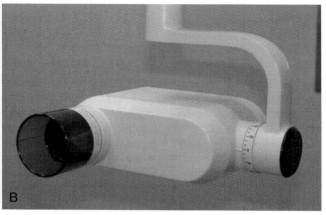

• **Figure 6.5 A,** Open-ended lead-lined rectangular collimator. **B,** Open-ended, lead-lined cylindrical collimator.

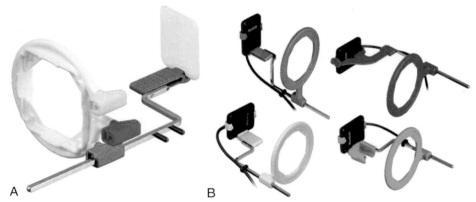

• **Figure 6.6** XCP-ORA **(A)** and conventional XCP **(B)** receptor holding devices that can be used with film or with digital sensors, as well as with circular and rectangular collimation. (Courtesy Dentsply Rinn, York, PA.)

because of the interaction of the primary beam with the closed end of the cone (see Fig. 2.10). Conversely, the use of open-ended, lead-lined rectangular or cylindrical (round) PIDs reduces the production of scatter radiation to the patient. Therefore, state or local health codes prohibit the use of closed-ended, pointed PIDs.

Receptor (Film) Holders

Film holders that align the x-ray beam with the receptor in the patient's mouth should be used. These film-holding devices (receptor-holding devices) also act to reduce the possibility of collimator cutoff. These devices can be used with circular and rectangular collimation and with conventional or digital imaging (Fig. 6.6). A receptor holder should never be held in place for the patient by the operator or by patients themselves. Some of the more commonly used film-holding devices are shown in Fig. 10.12.

Digital Sensors, Film, and Intensifying Screens

Decreasing exposure time by the use of a more sensitive receptor (digital sensors, fast-speed film, and film-screen combinations) is one of the most effective factors in reducing

radiation exposure to the patient. As will be discussed in Chapter 15, the use of digital imaging can reduce the patient's radiation exposure by up to 90% (when compared to the use of D speed film). These digital receptors are more sensitive to radiation and require less exposure time; therefore, they are an effective means of reducing radiation exposure to the patient.

If digital radiography is not used, fast-speed film is recommended. There has been a consistent improvement in decreasing patient exposure with the use of faster-speed film over time. Group E film, when compared with group D film, reduces the radiation exposure by 50% (see Fig. 6.3). The ADA recommends the use of F speed film (Insight), because it provides a major advance in patient protection when conventional radiography is used.

Extraoral projections (e.g., panoramic radiographs, lateral skull projections, etc.) should always be done using the fastest intensifying screen available with its respective compatible film. The use of intensifying screens reduces radiation exposure to the patient by providing exposure of the film to both x-radiation and the light emitted by the phosphor on the intensifying screen. Subsequently, the exposure time is decreased, thereby decreasing radiation exposure to the patient.

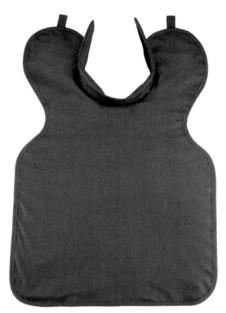

• **Figure 6.7** Lead apron with thyroid collar. (Courtesy Dentsply RINN, York, PA.)

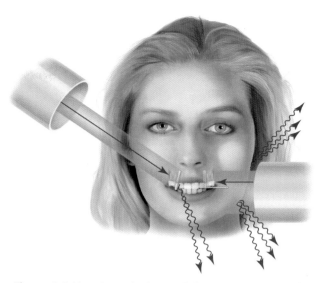

• **Figure 6.8** X-ray beam in the paralleling and bisecting methods and scatter radiation to the thyroid gland.

Lead Aprons and Thyroid Collars

All patients should be draped with a lead apron and wear a thyroid collar for every intraoral exposure (Fig. 6.7). This rule holds regardless of the patient's age or the number of projections exposed. The use of lead aprons and thyroid collars can reduce radiation to the thyroid and gonads by up to 94%. The apron should cover the patient from the thyroid to the gonadal area. Lead aprons with attached cervical (thyroid) shields are available. Separate thyroid collars can be purchased to use with existing lead aprons as well. The aprons available are usually the equivalent of 0.25-mm lead or lead equivalent, relatively flexible, and not too uncomfortable for the patient. The dose to the gonads is very small during dental exposures but can be reduced even further with the lead apron. The thyroid gland—except with rectangular collimation and, more specifically, with the bisecting-angle technique—may lie in the path of the primary beam. The dose may be small but can be decreased significantly with the use of the thyroid collar. There are also lead-free aprons available for intraoral and extraoral radiographic procedures. These aprons provide ample protection for the patient, weigh less than leaded aprons, and are comfortable and easy to handle. There is no valid reason not to use a barrier apron and collar for every intraoral and extraoral exposure. Many states have enacted legislation that makes this procedure mandatory. Patients react favorably to the apron, because they feel protected and are reassured that the dental office is up-to-date and concerned about radiation safety.

Lead aprons should not be folded but rather hung up or draped over a rounded surface when not in use. Folding eventually cracks the lead and allows leakage. For taking panoramic projections, the positioning of the front and back lead aprons must be modified and thyroid collars are not recommended for use, as discussed in Chapter 12.

Technique

Retakes

One of the major sources of unnecessary exposure to radiation in the dental office is retaking films as a result of poor technique. Every retake represents an unnecessary doubling of radiation exposure to the patient for that projection. Dental professionals are obligated to perfect their intraoral technique so that retakes can be avoided. This professional improvement can be accomplished by ensuring that office personnel are well trained and respectful of the patient in working with x-radiation. Every error should be analyzed regarding its cause and rate of occurrence and what must be done to correct the error. Colleagues should critique each other's work and help to correct errors in technique.

Paralleling Technique

In addition to producing a more accurate diagnostic image with dimensional accuracy, the paralleling technique results in lower dose levels to the thyroid gland and the lens of the eye (Fig. 6.8). In the paralleling method, the x-ray beam for all projections is very close to being parallel to the floor, whereas the bisecting method results in an x-ray beam that has steep vertical angulations that may put the thyroid gland and lens of the eye in the path of the primary x-ray beam as well as the secondary (scatter) radiation.

Target-Receptor Distance (Focal-Film Distance)

Increased target-receptor distances (or FFDs), up to 16 inches, are recommended with the paralleling technique

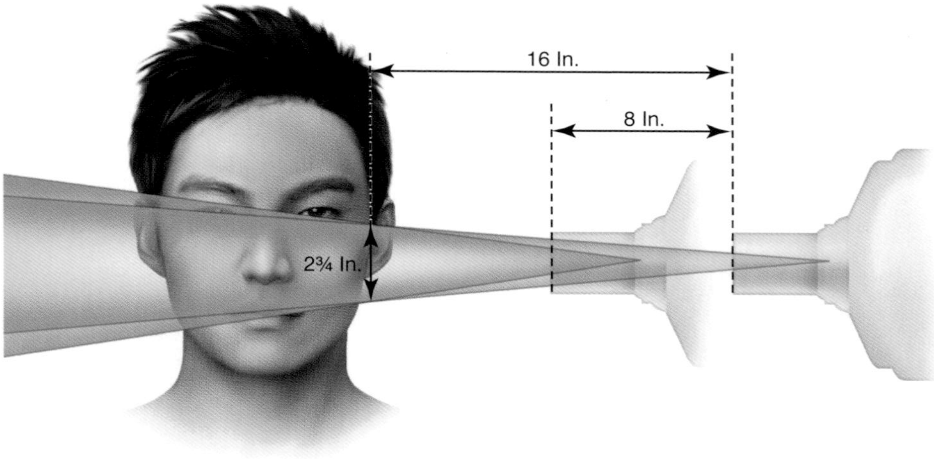

• **Figure 6.9** Focal-film distance (FFD) and tissue volume exposed. Shaded areas represent tissue exposed at 8-inch FFD but not in the beam at 16-inch FFD because of the more parallel and less divergent x-rays..

to compensate for the magnification of the image caused by the increased object-receptor distance (see Chapter 3). Another important advantage of an increased target-receptor distance (or FFD) is that less total tissue volume is in the path of the primary beam at 16 inches than at 8 inches. As the distance increases from 8 inches to 16 inches (Fig. 6.9), the x-ray beam becomes less divergent and less total body area is irradiated by the primary beam after it penetrates the skin. The shorter target-receptor distance (or FFD), with a more divergent beam, irradiates a far greater volume of tissue. The maximum diameter of the primary beam should still not exceed $2\frac{3}{4}$ inches (2.75 inches or 7 cm) at the skin level in both cases. The difference is in beam divergence after skin entry and film exposure.

Processing and Viewing With the Use of Conventional Film

Darkroom

Every effort should be made to establish darkroom procedures that produce films with the maximum diagnostic yield when employing conventional radiography. For example, when a film is overexposed, it is not acceptable to then underdevelop the film to compensate for the overexposure to the patient. In addition, there is no excuse for darkroom errors that can cause film retakes. This subject is discussed thoroughly in Chapter 11.

Viewing Finished Radiographs

To obtain maximum diagnostic yield for the radiation expended, the manner of film viewing for interpretation is extremely important. The only proper way to view a conventional radiograph is in front of an illuminator (view box), preferably with a variable light source (see Fig. 3.16). Using sunlight in front of a window or the lamp on the

dental unit is unsatisfactory. The film mount used for the full-mouth survey should cover the entire illuminator, and empty windows in the mount should be covered with an opaque material (such as, the black paper in the film packet). This prevents light that escapes around the periphery or through the mount from distracting the viewer. Ideally, radiographs should be viewed in a darkened room to avoid excessive reflection when this can be achieved in the average dental facility.

Clinical Judgment

Radiation History

Specific questions regarding the patient's previous radiation exposures should be part of every history. This radiation history should include medical, dental diagnostic, and therapeutic radiation. Patients should be asked when their last radiographs were taken, how many were taken, and what type of radiographs were taken at that time. Questions of this type may help determine whether dental radiographs have been taken recently that might be available and still diagnostically valid. These radiographs also provide historical data, show previous dental disease, and indicate the result of treatment. Such historical data will influence the selection criteria evaluation, in which certain positive historical findings will indicate a need for radiographs. A history of radiation therapy is important because of risk of the added dental dose and because of interest in the areas irradiated. As mentioned in Chapter 5, radiation to the head and neck region may leave the patient susceptible to xerostomia, radiation caries, and osteoradionecrosis, and a preventive protocol should be instituted. The radiation history contains valuable and pertinent information in treatment planning.

Selection Criteria

Selection criteria are descriptions of clinical conditions (signs and symptoms) and historical data that identify patients who are most likely to benefit from a particular radiographic examination. The dental professional should look in the patient's oral cavity with a mouth mirror, as well as interviewing the patient in order to develop a sense of the patient's risk for dental disease. The selection criteria aid the dentist, as this is the dentist's decision, to select which patients need radiographs and determine which radiographs are needed. The final decision rests with the individual dentist and is determined by professional judgment.

An expert panel of dentists sponsored by the Public Health Service had developed guidelines for the prescription of dental radiographs. The guidelines have been revised recently by another select panel of the ADA and US Food and Drug Administration (Fig. 6.10). Using these guidelines, the dentist can decide when, what type, and how many radiographs should be taken. The practice of taking dental radiographs based on a time interval rather than on patient needs, as determined by clinical examination and dental history, is not considered an appropriate way to practice dental radiography. The dentist should decide whether to take radiographs after examining the patient. There are no routine dental radiographs. Radiographic needs are not determined by the calendar alone but rather by evaluating the overall health needs of a patient after a clinical examination and history is taken. Positive findings in these categories would change the radiation needs of a patient and reclassify the patient from the asymptomatic to the symptomatic category, for which radiographs would be indicated and the guidelines would not be operative. This is true for new patients, emergencies, and recall visits.

These guidelines for patients who are asymptomatic are shown in chart form in Fig. 6.10 and are from a report that covers three general categories of patients: (1) patients with positive historical findings, (2) those who are symptomatic, and (3) those who are asymptomatic. Asymptomatic patients are divided into three main categories: (1) children with primary or transitional dentition; (2) adolescents with permanent dentition; and (3) adults, including dentulous and edentulous patients. Each patient category is further divided into new-patient and recall-patient categories. In addition, the recall-patient category is subdivided into clinical caries or high-risk factors for caries, no clinical caries or high-risk factors, periodontal disease, growth and development assessment, and patients with other circumstances.

Using these guidelines, it is clear that all new patients should have a recent radiographic survey of some type on file before treatment is instituted. The radiographs may be taken by the current dentist or may be duplicates of those taken by a previous dentist. The resulting survey is essential for case planning, baseline data for future reference, and medicolegal reasons.

Recall radiographs should not be taken for all patients as a matter of routine. As seen in Fig. 6.10, very few patients

The recommendations in this chart are subject to clinical judgment and may not apply to every patient. They are to be used by dentists only after reviewing the patient's health history and completing a clinical examination. Because every precaution should be taken to minimize radiation exposure, protective thyroid collars and aprons should be used whenever possible. This practice is strongly recommended for children, women of childbearing age, and pregnant women.

TYPE OF ENCOUNTER	PATIENT AGE AND DENTAL DEVELOPMENTAL STAGE				
	Child with Primary Dentition (prior to eruption of first permanent tooth)	Child with Transitional Dentition (after eruption of first permanent tooth)	Adolescent with Permanent Dentition (prior to eruption of third molars)	Adult, Dentate or Partially Edentulous	Adult, Edentulous
New patient* being evaluated for dental diseases and dental development	Individualized radiographic exam consisting of selected periapical/occlusal views and/or posterior bitewings if proximal surfaces cannot be visualized or probed. Patients without evidence of disease and with open proximal contacts may not require a radiographic exam at this time.	Individualized radiographic exam consisting of posterior bitewings with panoramic exam or posterior bitewings and selected periapical images	Individualized radiographic exam consisting of posterior bitewings with panoramic exam or posterior bitewings and selected periapical images. A full-mouth intraoral radiographic exam is preferred when the patient has clinical evidence of generalized dental disease or a history of extensive dental treatment.		Individualized radiographic exam, based on clinical signs and symptoms
Recall patient* with clinical caries or at increased risk for caries†	Posterior bitewing exam at 6- to 12-month intervals if proximal surfaces cannot be examined visually or with a probe			Posterior bitewing exam at 6- to 18-month intervals	Not applicable
Recall patient* with no clinical caries and not at increased risk for caries†	Posterior bitewing exam at 12- to 24-month intervals if proximal surfaces cannot be examined visually or with a probe		Posterior bitewing exam at 18- to 36-month intervals	Posterior bitewing exam at 24- to 36-month intervals	Not applicable

• **Figure 6.10** Guidelines for prescribing dental radiographs. (From American Dental Association, US Food & Drug Administration. The Selection of Patients for Dental Radiograph Examinations. November, 2004 http://www.ada.org/en/~/media/ADA/Science%20and%20Research/Files/Professional_Topic_Radiography_X-Rays.)

Continued

TYPE OF ENCOUNTER	PATIENT AGE AND DENTAL DEVELOPMENTAL STAGE				
	Child with Primary Dentition (prior to eruption of first permanent tooth)	Child with Transitional Dentition (after eruption of first permanent tooth)	Adolescent with Permanent Dentition (prior to eruption of third molars)	Adult, Dentate or Partially Edentulous	Adult, Edentulous
Recall patient* with periodontal disease	Clinical judgment as to the need for and type of radiographic images for the evaluation of periodontal disease. Imaging may consist of, but is not limited to, selected bitewing and/or periapical images of areas where periodontal disease (other than nonspecific gingivitis) can be identified clinically.				Not applicable
Patient for monitoring of growth and development	Clinical judgment as to the need for and type of radiographic images for evaluation and/or monitoring of dentofacial growth and development		Clinical judgment as to the need for and type of radiographic images for evaluation and/or monitoring of dentofacial growth and development. Panoramic or periapical exam to assess developing third molars	Usually not indicated	
Patient with other circumstances including, but not limited to, proposed or existing implants, pathologic conditions, restorative/endodontic needs, treated periodontal disease, and caries remineralization	Clinical judgment as to the need for and type of radiographic images for evaluation and/or monitoring in these circumstances				

*Clinical situations for which radiographs may be indicated include but are not limited to the following:

A. Positive historical findings
1. Previous periodontal or endodontic treatment
2. History of pain or trauma
3. Familial history of dental anomalies
4. Postoperative evaluation of healing
5. Remineralization monitoring
6. Presence of implants or evaluation for implant placement

B. Positive clinical signs/symptoms
1. Clinical evidence of periodontal disease
2. Large or deep restorations
3. Deep carious lesions
4. Malposed or clinically impacted teeth
5. Swelling
6. Evidence of dental/facial trauma
7. Mobility of teeth
8. Sinus tract ("fistula")
9. Clinically suspected sinus pathologic condition
10. Growth abnormalities
11. Oral involvement in known or suspected systemic disease
12. Positive neurologic findings in the head and neck
13. Evidence of foreign objects
14. Pain and/or dysfunction of the temporomandibular joint
15. Facial asymmetry
16. Abutment teeth for fixed or removable partial prosthesis
17. Unexplained bleeding
18. Unexplained sensitivity of teeth
19. Unusual eruption, spacing, or migration of teeth
20. Unusual tooth morphology, calcification, or color
21. Unexplained absence of teeth
22. Clinical erosion

†Factors increasing risk for caries may include but are not limited to:
1. High level of caries experience or demineralization
2. History of recurrent caries
3. High titers of cariogenic bacteria
4. Existing restoration(s) of poor quality
5. Poor oral hygiene
6. Inadequate fluoride exposure
7. Prolonged nursing (bottle or breast)
8. Frequent high sucrose content in diet
9. Poor family dental health
10. Developmental or acquired enamel defects
11. Developmental or acquired disability
12. Xerostomia
13. Genetic abnormality of teeth
14. Many multisurface restorations
15. Chemo/radiation therapy
16. Eating disorders
17. Drug/alcohol abuse
18. Irregular dental care

• Figure 6.10, cont'd

need radiographs at 6-month intervals. Caries susceptibility, for example, is a major factor in determining the time frame for recall radiographs. The diagnostic radiographic needs of a decay-prone teenager are quite different from those of a middle-aged periodontal recall patient whose last filling was placed 20 years earlier.

Administrative Radiographs

Administrative radiographs are those taken for reasons not related to the patient's immediate health needs. Included in this category are teaching films, those required by state examination and licensing authorities, and radiographs taken to verify treatment for compensation by insurance companies or other third-party carriers. Radiographs should never be taken for administrative reasons. If it produces no diagnostic benefit to the patient, the radiograph should not be taken. This is not to say that radiographs should not be submitted to insurance carriers; images taken for diagnostic purposes, or their duplicates, can be submitted because no unnecessary radiation is used. Many states have laws that prohibit the use of administrative radiographs, and the US Food and Drug Administration recommends that insurance carriers and others refrain from requiring administrative radiographs.

Postoperative radiographs are indicated only when they have diagnostic value, such as for confirming the retrieval of a root tip in surgery or the placement of filling materials in endodontic procedures. The use of radiographs to check the fit, contact, contour, and seating of restorations or seating of implant fixtures is strongly discouraged. These evaluations can be done with a mirror, explorer, and floss, thus saving the patient the radiation exposure.

Working or operative images in endodontics, surgical implant placement, and restorative post and pin preparations may be necessary for proper treatment, but every effort should be made to keep the number of exposures to a minimum.

Chapter Summary

- The goal in radiation patient protection is to use the least amount of radiation to achieve the maximum diagnostic yield.
- The patient is exposed to both primary and secondary (scatter) radiation. Efforts to protect the patient from unnecessary x-ray exposure addresses both primary and secondary sources.
- All dental x-ray equipment must meet federal diagnostic equipment performance standards, which includes avoiding head leakage and tube head drift. In addition, the kilovoltage, milliamperage, and exposure time must be set properly in order to avoid unnecessary x-ray exposure and still produce diagnostically acceptable images.
- The proper filtration and collimation must follow federal performance standards as well. If the kilovoltage is set at a level of 70 or higher, 2.5 mm of total aluminum filtration is required. The measurement of the circular beam aimed at the patient's face should not exceed 2.75 inches (2¾ inches or 7 cm). Rectangular collimation is highly recommended to reduce radiation exposure to the patient. All PIDs should be open ended and lead lined.
- The patient should not hold the receptor with the finger. Instead, receptor holders should be used to hold the respective receptor.

- Digital receptors, high-speed film, and intensifying screens reduce the time needed to expose them and, therefore, ultimately decrease radiation exposure to the patient.
- Protective aprons and thyroid collars should be placed on patients to ensure their safety against unnecessary x-ray exposure.
- The paralleling technique is recommended to reduce exposure to the patient's thyroid gland and lens of the eye when compared to the bisecting angle technique. Dental professionals are strongly encouraged to avoid retakes due to poor exposure techniques and, in the case of conventional radiography, poor darkroom techniques as well.
- Dental radiographs are prescribed according to the patient's immediate dental health needs based on the patient's radiation history and relative risk for dental diseases. Dental professionals are encouraged to follow the selection criteria guidelines and are warned to avoid taking administrative and routine radiographs.

Chapter Review Questions

Multiple Choice

1. Primary radiation is the x-radiation that is produced at the target of the anode in the dental x-ray tube. Tertiary radiation is the radiation that comes from any matter struck by primary radiation. (Indicate all that apply.)

   a. Both statements are true.
   b. Both statements are false.
   c. The first statement is true, and the second statement is false.
   d. The first statement is false, and the second statement is true.
   e. The statements are related.

2. The removal of soft, long, nonpenetrating x-ray photons from the heterogeneous x-ray beam is known as:
   a. Collimation
   b. Thermionic emission
   c. Exposure time
   d. Filtration
   e. Intensification

3. Paralleling receptor-holding devices that help align the x-ray beam with the receptor in the patient's mouth also help reduce the possibility of:
   a. A reversed film
   b. Elongation
   c. Foreshortening
   d. Double exposure
   e. Collimator cutoff

4. Which of the following should be **avoided** when taking radiographs of patients? (Indicate all that apply.)
   a. Radiographic retakes
   b. Selection criteria
   c. Administrative radiographs
   d. Routine radiographs
   e. Paralleling receptor holders with localizing rings

5. A patient's **radiation history** should include (indicate all that apply):
   a. Medical diagnostic radiation exposure
   b. Dental clinical examination
   c. Dental diagnostic radiation exposure
   d. Therapeutic radiation
   e. Medical yearly clinical examination

Critical Thinking Exercises

1. A patient presents at your dental facility for a series of radiographs and is concerned about the x-radiation exposure to be received. What could you say that will help to allay the patient's fears? Include in your discussion:
   a. The protective barriers you place on the patient
   b. The federal regulations that protect the patient
   c. The receptor-holding devices that are used
   d. The use of fast-speed film or digital sensors
   e. The prescription of the necessary radiographs
   f. Any other information that you can provide to help the patient feel safe and protected

2. What would be the radiographic prescription for the following three patients? Utilize the Selection Criteria Guideline chart accordingly.
   a. *Patient #1:* A 59-year-old edentulous patient presents to a dental office seeking new dentures. The patient's dentures were made in that office 5 years ago after radiographs revealed the necessity of multiple extractions. Following the extractions, the tissue healed uneventfully, and the dentures were fabricated. At the present time the clinical examination yields negative results and the patient's only concern is the lack of retention of the dentures. What would be the radiographic prescription for this patient?
   b. *Patient #2:* A 14-year-old patient presents for a 6-month recall examination. At the last visit, three teeth needed restorations. What would be the radiographic prescription?
   c. *Patient #3:* A new edentulous patient presents seeking new dentures and dental care. Intraoral examination suggests the presence of retained root tips. What would be the radiographic prescription?

Bibliography

American Dental Association Council on Scientific Affairs: An update on radiographic practices: information and recommendations, *J Am Dent Assoc* 32:234–238, 2001.

FDA Department of Health and Human Services, 21 C.F.R., Subchapter J Radiological Health, General § 1000.1 (1994).

Iannucci JM, Howerton LJ: *Dental radiography: principles and techniques*, ed 5, St Louis, MO, 2016, Elsevier Saunders.

Langland OE, Langlais RP: *Principles of dental imaging*, Baltimore, MD, 1997, Williams & Wilkins.

National Council on Radiation Protection and Measurements: NCRP Report No. 145, Radiation in Dentistry, 2004.

Recommendations on administratively required dental examination, *Fed Reg* 45:40976–40979, 1980.

Thompson EM, Johnson ON: *Essentials of dental radiography for dental assistants and hygienists*, ed 9, Upper Saddle River, NJ, 2012, Pearson Education, Inc.

US Department of Health and Human Services: Public Health Service, FDA: The selection of patients for dental radiographic examinations, HHS/PHS/FDA, 88-827310-21, 1987.

White SC, Pharoah MJ: *Oral radiology: principles and interpretation*, ed 7, St Louis, MO, 2013, Mosby.

7

Operator Protection

EDUCATIONAL OBJECTIVES

Upon completing this chapter, the student will be able to:

1. Define the key terms listed at the beginning of the chapter.
2. Discuss concepts related to operator dosage and protection, including maximum permissible dose (MPD), exposure technique, radiation monitoring, protective barriers, and the ALARA principle (concept).
3. Discuss how to deal with patients' concerns about and possible fear of dental radiographs.

KEY TERMS

ALARA principle (concept)
barrier
cumulative effective dose (CUMEfd)
exposure technique

film badge
maximum permissible dose (MPD)
monitoring devices
pocket dosimeters

primary radiation
secondary radiation

Introduction

This chapter addresses the steps that should be taken to protect the dental professional from unnecessary radiation exposure in the dental occupational facility. It is of utmost importance for operators to follow radiation safety regulations while working with x-radiation in their workplace. There are radiation safety regulations at both the federal and state levels in the United States. However, the state-governed radiation safety regulations vary from state to state. Consequently, dental professionals should be familiar with their state's regulations.

Operator Dosage and Protection

The sources of potential exposure to the dental professional are the primary beam, head leakage from the tube, and secondary (scatter) radiation originating from the patient, x-ray machine, or objects in the operatory. Through the use of careful technique in a well-designed, well-equipped, and well-monitored office, the occupational exposure of dental professionals to ionizing radiation can be kept to a minimum. In effect, the occupational dose should be zero.

Maximum Permissible Dose

The National Council on Radiation Protection and Measurements (NCRP) defines the maximum permissible dose (MPD) as the maximum amount of whole-body radiation that an occupationally or nonoccupationally involved person can receive within a specific period of time without experiencing injury. At present, the NCRP's recommendation regarding the MPD of whole-body radiation for persons occupationally concerned with ionizing radiation, such as dental professionals (including dentists), is 50 mSv (5000 mrem) per year. This is in contrast to the current recommended MPD of 5 mSv/year (500 mrem/year) for the general public (nonoccupationally involved persons) if the exposure is infrequent. Additionally, the NCRP states that for pregnant dental professionals, the recommended MPD should not exceed 0.5 mSv (50 mrem) per month during the pregnancy.

It is also recommended by the NCRP that dental personnel should not exceed a maximum accumulated lifetime dose known as the cumulative effective dose (CUMEfd). The NCRP states that for an occupationally involved individual, it should not be in excess of N (the person's age) × 10 mSv. For example, if the dental radiographer is 28 years old, the radiographer's CUMEfd would be 28 × 10 mSv (1000 mrems), which is 280 mSv (28,000 mrems). However, another option in calculating a maximum accumulated lifetime dose is to use the following equation:

$$(N = age) - 18 \times 50 \text{ mSv} (5000 \text{ mrems})$$

In this equation, the first 18 years of one's life is removed from the lifetime dose, because it is not recommended that a person work with x-radiation before the age of 18 years old.

Another regulating organization, the International Commission on Radiation Protection (ICRP) has recommended that the yearly MPD for occupationally involved personnel be 20 mSv (2000 mrem). They also recommend an MPD of 1 mSv (100 mrem) per year for the general public. Both recommendations are set lower than the MPD for occupationally involved individuals and the general public set by the NCRP. However, the NCRP, in its most recent report, has chosen to maintain its suggested MPD for dental personnel as stated previously (5000 mrem/year; 50 mSv/year). Ultimately, dental professionals (including dentists) should strive for an occupational dose of zero. If one's occupational dose is zero, any downward change in the MPD would produce no cause for concern because zero is zero. Zero exposure is not difficult to achieve in a dental facility that is well designed, well equipped, and well monitored and whose members have an awareness of radiation hygiene. A dental professional should not fear working with x-rays but should be knowledgeable regarding their safe use and potential abuse.

> **HELPFUL HINT**
>
> When working with x-radiation, it's better to be safe than sorry! Protect yourselves and your colleagues from unnecessary exposure in the workplace.

Exposure Technique

Dental professionals (including dentists) should never be in the path of the primary beam. They should not hold any receptor (film packet, digital sensor, or phosphor plate) in the patient's mouth nor should a drifting tube head be held by the dental radiographer, patient, or any other person (e.g., patient's companion). There should not be any exceptions to this rule. Ideally, for proper exposure technique, the operator should be a minimum of 6 feet (2 meters) away from the tube head (the source of radiation) and behind a suitable (acceptable) barrier when the exposure is made.

Federal and state regulations require that every x-ray machine be equipped with an activated exposure switch that allows operators to properly position themselves 6 feet (2 meters) away from the source of radiation (i.e., the tube head). Although not as crucial as distance and shielding, knowing the areas of minimum scatter is important to the operator. These areas are at right angles (perpendicular) to the x-ray beam and toward the back of the patient (Fig. 7.1). The areas of highest scatter are in back of the tube head and behind the patient. Correct positioning of the operator still necessitates the minimum 6-foot distance and adequate barrier protection (Figs. 7.2 and 7.3). Also, operators must make sure that coworkers are not in the way of the primary beam or scatter radiation. Operators should check that the work area in all directions is clear before pressing the exposure button.

Radiation Monitoring

How can dental professionals and dentists know the amount of occupational exposure of radiation that they receive? Concerned personnel can use two methods to measure the levels of radiation and potential exposure. First, a Certified Radiation Equipment Safety Officer (CRESO) can perform a radiation survey using ionization chambers to determine radiation levels during exposures at all locations in the

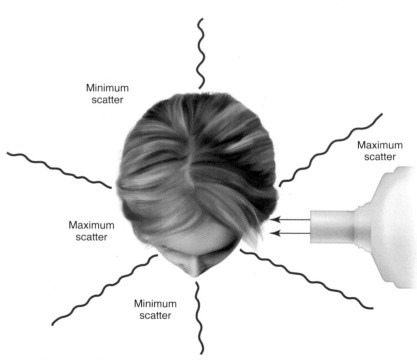

• **Figure 7.1** Areas of minimum and maximum scatter during dental x-ray exposure.

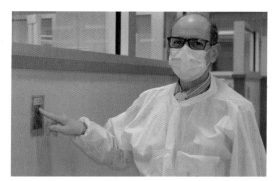

• **Figure 7.2** The dental professional must stand outside the path of the primary beam. Here, the operator is outside the operatory for safety.

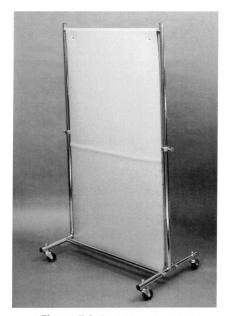

• **Figure 7.3** Portable x-ray shield.

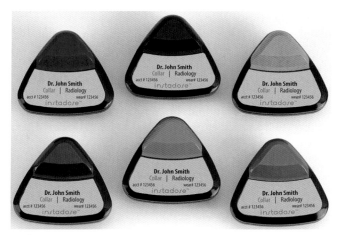

• **Figure 7.4** A direct ion storage (DIS) dosimeter measures the ionizing radiation exposure dose incident by calculating the amount of proportional change in the voltage across the memory cells. (Courtesy Mirion Technologies, Dosimetry Service Division, Irvine, CA [www.mirion.com].)

provide an accurate reading of occupational exposure. Each operator should have one's own badge, which should not be shared with other members of the dental facility. If clipped to a pocket, it should not be covered with a pen or piece of jewelry that might shield the badge. Dental professionals should not wear the badge outside the office, especially in sunlight, and they should remove it if they are having medical or dental x-rays because it is intended to measure only occupational exposure.

Protective Barriers

The walls, floor, and ceiling of the x-ray operatory must be of such construction that the surrounding areas are shielded from both primary and secondary radiation. This does not mean that they must be lead lined. Many materials used in construction today in the proper thickness provide adequate protective shielding. Because of the relatively low workload and the low x-ray energies used (60–90 kV), dental offices with concrete or cinder block walls have enough inherent shielding in wall construction materials. Drywall construction, if of proper thickness, is also sufficient for dental shielding.

The shielding or barrier requirements are based on such factors as workload, use and occupancy factors, maximum kilovoltage, and distance from the tube head. The formula $W \times U \times T$ is used to calculate the guide number. In this formula, W is the workload (in milliampere minutes per week), and U is the use factor. The walls in dental radiography have a higher use factor ($\frac{1}{4}$) than the floors or ceiling ($\frac{1}{16}$), because the central ray is never directed straight up or down. T is the occupancy factor, which accounts for whether a person is behind the barrier all the time, as is one seated at a desk (T = 1); sometimes, as in a waiting room (T = $\frac{1}{4}$); or occasionally, as in a passageway (T = $\frac{1}{8}$). The guide number is correlated with the proper kilovoltage and distance in reference tables found in Report 35 by

office. This type of survey, which is very much like a survey done by local or state agencies, checks the reliability of the x-ray machine and protective barriers. It does not monitor the day-to-day activity of the concerned personnel.

The second method is to have personnel wear monitoring devices, such as pocket dosimeters or film badges. Of the two methods, film badges are less expensive and more widely used. Film badge service is readily available from many radiation survey companies at a nominal monthly cost. The badge (Fig. 7.4) is usually worn for a specified period of time. It contains a sensor that is labeled with the wearer's name and, in some cases, the wearer's identification number as well. At the end of the prescribed reporting period, the film badge is returned to the survey company, where it is processed. The density on the receptor is compared with standards, and the exposure is determined. The report that is returned to the dental office contains not only the exposure for the reporting period but also the accumulated quarterly, yearly, and (if available) lifetime exposure of the individual. The film badge should be worn in the office at all times to the NCRP. These tables give the specifications of materials necessary for adequate shielding for the given conditions.

Pregnancy

The pregnant dental professional, in relation to occupational exposure, should not be compared with the pregnant patient, as discussed in Chapter 5. In a well-designed and well-monitored dental office, the occupational exposure should be zero. If a pregnant dental professional or dentist follows proper procedure in such an office, there is no risk to the fetus. A pregnant worker should wear a film badge to document occupational exposure and allay any fears. The courts have held that there is no reason to change chairside or other duties during pregnancy because of concern about radiation exposure. As previously mentioned, the NCRP states that for pregnant dental professionals, the recommended MPD should not exceed 0.5 mSv (50 mrem) per month during the pregnancy. However, there are specially designed lead aprons available for pregnant operator usage if they are requested by the operator or deemed necessary.

ALARA Principle (Concept)

As discussed in Chapter 6, the ALARA principle (concept) is an acronym for "as low as reasonably achievable. This principle applies to both patient and operator protection in the field of dental radiography. The clinical application of this concept to the dental practice encourages dental professionals to minimize radiation exposure to their patients and to themselves while maximizing the diagnostic capabilities of x-ray exposure.

Patient Concerns and Education

Dental professionals and dentists should understand and be sensitive to patients' concerns about and possible fear of dental radiographs. Recent years have been marked by a rise in members of the public who are more aware of the risks associated with x-radiation exposure. The media have been replete with stories warning of the danger of medical and dental radiographs.

Dental professionals, through knowledge and understanding, must be able to allay patients' fears and explain the necessity of radiographs for proper dental treatment. A patient is likely to question the dental supportive staff, as well as the dentist, about the potential danger of radiography. It may be helpful to explain to the patient how essential radiographs are in the detection and management of diseases and treatment planning. It is important to stress that the benefit of a dental radiographic examination in a safe and protected environment outweighs the risks of exposure. Patients also can be informed of federal and local laws enacted for their protection. The patient should be informed that the radiographs that are exposed are "prescribed" according to their immediate dental health needs, risk factors for dental diseases, and radiation history. They can be reminded of the various ways that they are protected against unnecessary radiation exposure, such as wearing a protective (lead or lead equivalent) apron and thyroid collar, the use of digital sensors or fast-speed film, and the avoidance of retakes by employing proper radiographic techniques. It may also be helpful to emphasize that the film or sensor is being held by a receptor-holding device rather than by the patient's finger. In addition, there are also printed educational materials that can be distributed to the patients either in support of or in place of an informal chairside discussion.

Chapter Summary

- The potential sources of radiation exposure to the dental professional are head leakage from the x-ray tube head; the primary beam of radiation; and secondary (scatter) radiation originating from the patient, the x-ray machine, or objects in the x-ray operatory.
- Technically, the x-ray exposure to the dental professional in a well-monitored, well-designed, well-equipped office should be zero if all of the radiation safety precautions are adhered to accordingly.
- The maximum permissible dose (MPD), as developed by the National Council on Radiation Protection and Measurements (NCRP) and the International Commission on Radiation Protection (ICRP), is defined as the maximum amount of whole-body radiation that an occupationally or nonoccupationally involved individual can receive within an established period of time without experiencing injury.
- The operator should be 6 feet away from the x-ray source and/or behind an acceptable barrier while exposing a patient to x-radiation.
- Dental radiographers can wear a personal monitoring device, such as a pocket dosimeter or film badge, to detect any radiation exposure that they may have received in the working environment.
- There are specific recommendations for pregnant dental professionals who are in a working environment where dental radiographs are being exposed.
- Dental professionals should be prepared to obtain the knowledge and understanding necessary to allay a patient's concerns and fears pertaining to dental radiography.

Chapter Review Questions

Multiple Choice

1. The MPD for whole-body ionizing radiation exposure for occupationally involved persons is currently:
   a. 500 mSv per year
   b. 5 mSv per year
   c. 5000 mSv per year
   d. 50 mSv per year
2. It is recommended that dental personnel not exceed a maximum accumulated lifetime radiation dose known as the:
   a. Cumulative maximum allowance
   b. Cumulative dose allowance
   c. Cumulative effective dose
   d. Cumulative regulated dose
   e. Cumulative exposure dose equivalent
3. The areas of minimum scatter while exposing radiographs are (indicate all that apply):
   a. Areas that are at right angles to the primary beam
   b. Toward the front of the patient
   c. In the back of the tube head
   d. Behind the patient
   e. Toward the back of the patient

4. The acronym CRESO pertaining to radiation monitoring stands for:
   a. Certificate for Radiation Effects Systems Organizer
   b. Contracted Radiation Efficiency Systems Officer
   c. Certified Radiation Equipment Safety Officer
   d. Contracts for Radiation Equipment State-based Organization
   e. Certified Radiation Efficiency Systems Organizer
5. The ALARA principle (concept) refers to minimizing radiation exposure to the patient only. Operator protection is not a concern when abiding by the ALARA principle (concept). (Indicate all that apply.)
   a. Both statements are true.
   b. Both statements are false.
   c. The first statement is true, and the second statement is false.
   d. The first statement is false, and the second statement is true.
   e. The statements are related.

Critical Thinking Exercises

1. The barrier or shielding requirements for those surfaces involved in workplace radiation protection are based on several factors.
   a. Name these factors.
   b. Explain what the equation $W \times U \times T$ is used to calculate.
   c. Explain what each of the components in the equation $W \times U \times T$ stand for and how they are related to establishing safe barriers and shielding in a dental facility.
2. One of your coworkers just found out that she is pregnant and is concerned about exposing dental radiographs on patients in the dental facility where you both work.

What information could you provide to her regarding her current status? Include all of the following in your explanation:
   a. What is the risk to the fetus in a well-designed and well-monitored dental office?
   b. What is the risk to the fetus if the dental professional follows proper radiographic procedures?
   c. What personal radiation devices can be worn to document occupational exposure and protect the pregnant dental professional?
   d. What do the courts recommend?
   e. What is the NCRP-recommended MPD for pregnant dental radiographers?

Bibliography

American Academy of Dental Radiology, Quality Assurance Committee: Recommendations for quality assurance in dental radiography, *Oral Surg* 55:421–426, 1983.

American Dental Association: *The benefits of x-rays.* Chicago, IL, 1993, American Dental Association.

Goren AD, Lundeen RC, Deahl ST 2nd, et al: Updated quality assurance self assessment exercise in intraoral and panoramic radiology, American Academy of Oral and Maxillofacial Radiology,

Radiology Practice Committee, *Oral Surg Oral Med Oral Pathol Oral Radiol Endod* 89:369–374, 2000.

Macdonald JCF, Reid JA, Berthory D: Dry wall construction as a dental radiation barrier, *Oral Surg* 55:319–326, 1983.

National Council on Radiation Protection and Measurements. NCRP Report No. 145, Radiation Protection in Dentistry, 2004.

National Council on Radiation Protection and Measurements. NCRP Report No. 116, Limits of Exposure to Ionizing Radiation, 1993.

Plunket L: When an employee becomes pregnant, *N Y State Dent J* 62:9–11, 1996.

8

Infection Control in Dental Radiography

EDUCATIONAL OBJECTIVES

Upon completing this chapter, the student will be able to:

1. Define the key terms listed at the beginning of the chapter.
2. State the primary purpose of infection control procedures, discuss the significance of cross-contamination in the office setting, and summarize the significance of taking an accurate medical history of your patient.
3. Define the meaning of a *pathogen*, and explain its relevance to an infection control protocol in the dental office.
4. Describe what the term *personal protective equipment (PPE)* means in reference to dental office infection control programs, as well as what the advised PPE requirements are for dental radiography.

5. Discuss the barriers used for sterilization, disinfection, digital radiography, film packets, processing solutions, and panoramic radiography in the dental office. In addition, perform the following procedures and discuss infection control protocol for each:
   - Chairside Exposure Procedures
   - Processing Procedures (Conventional Radiography)
   - Procedure for Daylight Loaders
6. Decide when antibiotic prophylaxis is required for dental radiographic procedures and what vaccinations are required for dental personnel.

KEY TERMS

acquired immunodeficiency syndrome (AIDS)
antibiotic prophylaxis
antiseptics
autoclaving
barrier envelope
Centers for Disease Control and Prevention (CDC)

cross-contamination
disinfection
hepatitis
human immunodeficiency virus (HIV)
immunizations
infection
microorganism

Occupational Safety and Health Administration (OSHA)
pathogen
personal protective equipment (PPE)
semi-critical devices
sterilization
universal precautions
vaccination

Introduction

Infection control has become a major concern of patients, regulatory agencies, and health care workers in the practice of dentistry. The primary purpose of infection control procedures is to prevent infectious disease transmission. Disease transmission in the dental practice can occur from a dental professional to a patient, from a patient to the dental professional, or even between patients. The dental professional should practice infection control at all times, because dental personnel and patients are at risk from pathogens. A pathogen is a microorganism capable of causing disease. Pathogens can be transmitted by infection from cuts, breaks in the skin, and contact with body secretions and inhalants. The emergence and identification of acquired immunodeficiency syndrome (AIDS) in 1981, the highly infectious hepatitis B and C viruses (HBV and HCV), and the resurgence of tuberculosis brought this public health issue to the forefront. Diseases such as tuberculosis, hepatitis,

and herpes always have been a risk for dental professionals, but it took the fatal consequences of AIDS in the 1980s to heighten the interest and awareness of the public, the government, and the profession to the importance of infection control in the dental office. Federal and state agencies at all levels are currently imposing requirements for office procedures and required courses in infection control. As a result, dental personnel are encouraged to employ universal infection control procedures when dealing with all of their dental patients.

Infection Control in Dental Practice

Any comprehensive infection control policy in dentistry must include protocols for radiology, including both chairside technique and, when applicable, darkroom procedures as well. Radiology is not exempt from infection control, even though radiographic procedures are not considered to be "invasive" procedures and do not involve the aerosol spray produced by the dental handpiece, needles, or the cutting of tissue and splatter of blood. Infectious disease can be transmitted by the cross-contamination of equipment, supplies, and receptors used to expose or process radiographs. In addition, dental radiographic procedures are in almost all cases performed in the same dental chairs and units that are used for more invasive procedures, with the potential for cross-contamination. Also, lead aprons and thyroid collars should be disinfected after each use to avoid contamination from one patient to the next. The American Dental Association (ADA), the Centers for Disease Control and Prevention (CDC), and the Occupational Safety and Health Administration (OSHA) all state that gloves must be worn when contact with blood, saliva, or other potentially infectious material, items, or surfaces is anticipated. Masks and eyewear are technically required only when splatter is anticipated. However, masks, eyewear, and protective clothing should potentially be used at all times, because these precautions will prevent potential cross-contamination where applicable.

> **NOTE**
>
> Personal protective equipment (PPE), such as gloves and protective clothing, are required when contact with blood or other bodily fluids is anticipated. However, protective eyewear and masks are considered optional for dental imaging procedures when aerosol and spatter of saliva and blood do not usually occur. There is a possibility of facial contact with blood and saliva during radiographic procedures, however. Therefore, it is recommended to wear a mask and protective eyewear, because it is better to be safe than sorry.

If infection control is understood and practiced, then patients, coworkers, and dental care providers themselves can be protected from harm. The objective is to be educated with the most up-to-date procedures so that work can be conducted in the safest possible manner. Proper infection control procedures should be followed before, during, and after dental radiographic exposures are made. Infection control steps for chairside dentistry should be followed in addition to the specific steps advised for dental radiographic procedures.

The following is a list of terms and definitions that are used in this discussion of infection control in the dental setting:

antiseptic: A substance that inhibits the growth of bacteria

autoclaving: The process of sterilization using steam

barrier: A substance used to protect the patient or worker from infective or contaminated substances

blood-borne pathogen: A pathogen present in blood that can cause infection in humans

critical instrument: An instrument used to penetrate soft tissue or bone

disinfection: The process of destroying disease-causing microorganisms by physical or chemical means (e.g., hand washing)

noncritical instrument: An instrument that does not come in contact with mucous membranes (e.g., position-indicating device [PID], exposure button, control panel)

occupational exposure: Contact of the skin or mucous membranes by blood or other infectious material that results from performing dental and other health care procedures

parenteral exposure: Exposure to blood or other infectious material that results in skin puncture

semi-critical instrument: An instrument that comes in contact with the mucous membrane but does not penetrate (e.g., x-ray receptor holding device)

sterilization: The process used to destroy all pathogens, including highly resistant bacteria and spores

universal precautions: An infection control protocol that is followed for all patients regardless of their history and clinical condition

Patient Medical History

The dentist or dental professional should document every patient's current medical history. This history should be obtained at the initial or recall visit using a questionnaire and/or direct questioning of the patient. Information gained by the history alerts the dental team to the presence or history of infectious disease or to potentially high-risk situations. Unfortunately, many potentially infectious patients cannot be identified by history or examination. Thus, a rational infection control policy should not distinguish between patients who are known to be infected and those who are not. Every patient should be treated in the same manner, with universal precautions carried out at all times. There should be no exceptions and therefore no surprises.

Sources of Infection

Through contact with saliva, blood, and nasal and respiratory secretions, many instruments and pieces of equipment can become the means of pathogen transmission. A pathogen is a microorganism that can cause disease. After the dental professional's gloves are contaminated by oral cavity fluids during radiographic procedures, everything that person touches is a possible transmitter of pathogens. Our concern, then, is with receptor-holding devices, instruments, receptors (including films and digital sensors), the x-ray machine, PID, tube head, control panel, exposure switch, clothing, countertops, dental chair, lead apron, light handle, walls, doorknobs, processors, patient records, and the computer keyboard. In short, any object that the operator touches after placing the packet in the patient's mouth can be considered contaminated and a source of transmission to the operator or other patients. On the other hand, any object that the operator touches before working in the mouth is a potential source of transmission to the patient. Thus, barriers to the transmission of infective microorganisms must be used. Personal barriers or personal protective equipment (PPE)

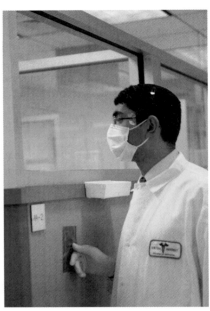

• **Figure 8.1** Operator exposing radiographs while wearing gloves, eyeglasses, mask, and protective clothing.

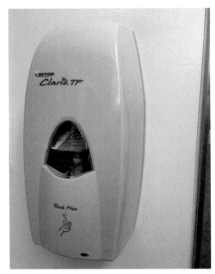

• **Figure 8.2** Instant hand sanitizer.

includes gloves, masks, protective eyewear, protective clothing, and surface coverings. If contamination does occur, as it does in the dental office, steps must be taken to remove or destroy the pathogen and the contaminated item to prevent further transmission.

Personnel

Dental personnel always should wear gloves, masks, protective eyewear and protective clothing (PPE) when working on patients (Fig. 8.1). Just as there is no excuse for not protecting yourself from radiation exposure (i.e., by standing 6 feet away from the x-ray machine), there is no excuse for not protecting oneself from infection. Blood is the most common and easily recognized transmission route of infectious microorganisms (i.e., microorganisms associated with **human immunodeficiency virus [HIV]**, HBV, and HCV). Although HIV has been isolated in the saliva of some patients, saliva alone is not considered to be a risk for HIV transmission, but because saliva is often contaminated with blood, there is a potential for transmission. It is true that no cases of HIV transmission have been documented via the salivary route by casual contact, but this should not be an excuse for not wearing gloves, masks, and protective clothing and eyewear. Saliva can be contaminated by blood and therefore poses the potential for transmission.

Protective Clothing

Any dental professional involved in direct patient care should wear a clean, long-sleeved, three-quarter-length uniform, jacket, or disposable gown with a closed collar. Protective clothing should not be worn outside of the dental care area or facility and should ideally be laundered immediately after professional use if it is not disposable.

Masks/Eye Protection/Plastic Face Shields

Face masks and protective eyewear (preferably with solid side shields) or plastic face shields that extend to the chin should be worn by dental professionals whenever they perform any intraoral radiographic procedures. Masks and eyewear or face shields should be in place before a practitioner washes hands and dons gloves, and should not be removed until the unit is cleaned after the completion of patient care.

Gloves/Hand Washing

Dental professionals must wear gloves when they perform intraoral procedures; there is no exception to this rule. Before putting on gloves, hands should be washed with an antimicrobial soap or a hand sanitizer (Fig. 8.2). This process should be repeated after gloves are removed at the completion of the patient's treatment. While gloved, one should not touch items, such as pens, pencils, x-ray mounts, charts, computer keyboards/mouse pads, or telephones. Paper towels may be used as barriers between these items and the gloved hands.

Barriers

Any object that the operator touches after placing the receptor in the patient's mouth must be covered with a removable barrier or disinfected after the patient leaves. A good maxim to remember is, "The less you touch, the less you have to worry about." There is a complete line of dental wrap with adhesive backing made specifically for barriers. Barrier material should be placed over the chair, headrest, countertop, arm and PID ("collimator") of the x-ray machine, control panel, computer keyboard, and exposure button before the

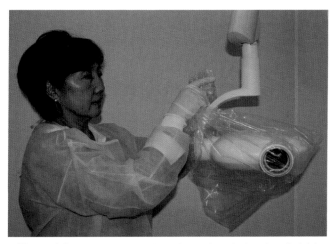

• **Figure 8.3** A plastic bag is slipped over the tubehead, pulled tight, and secured. (From Bird DL, Robinson DS: *Modern Dental Assisting,* ed 12, St Louis, 2018, Elsevier.)

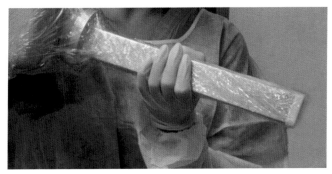

• **Figure 8.4** Plastic wrap covering the position-indicating device (PID). (From Langlais RP, Miller CM: *Exercises in Oral Radiology and Interpretation,* ed 5, St Louis, 2017, Elsevier.)

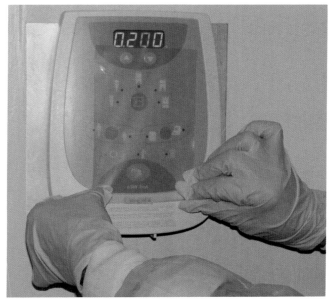

• **Figure 8.5** Plastic wrap covering the control panel and exposure switch. (From Bird DL, Robinson DS: *Modern Dental Assisting,* ed 12, St Louis, 2018, Elsevier.)

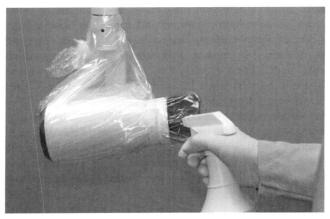

• **Figure 8.6** Barriers are preferred over disinfecting sprays that may not reach all surfaces or may affect electrical connections.

patient is seated (Figs. 8.3 to 8.5). The barriers are easily removed after the radiographic procedure is completed. If barriers are not used, these objects must be disinfected after the radiographic procedure is completed. Disinfecting solutions, such as iodophor or any other Environmental Protection Agency–registered chemical germicide, have the drawback that they may not reach irregular surfaces of the dental x-ray machine and have the potential to affect electrical connections in the head of the machine (Fig. 8.6). These irregular surfaces should be covered as opposed to sprayed with a disinfectant to prevent cross-contamination.

Sterilization and Disinfection

Sterilization produces the absence of all microorganisms, including spores. The most common method of sterilization used in the dental office is steam autoclaving. The radiographic instruments are sterilized in bags or appropriate cassettes in the same manner as other dental instruments.

Disinfection is the process that results in the absence of pathogenic organisms but not spores. Disinfecting agents are usually employed on surfaces but not on human tissue. Iodophors, chlorines, and synthetic phenolic compounds

are examples of disinfectants commonly used in the dental office.

"Cold sterilization" of instruments with quaternary ammonium compounds or glutaraldehyde is still used in the dental office but requires up to 6 hours of immersion to achieve sterilization. This method does not seem practical in a busy office and might lead to shortcutting time requirements. Furthermore, some instruments, such as plastic receptor holders, bite blocks, or localizing rings, may be damaged if not handled correctly during heat sterilization. The majority of radiographic devices manufactured today are autoclavable and are clearly marked as such.

Antiseptics are agents used on human tissue that are either bacteriostatic or bacteriocidal. In dentistry, they are used mainly for hand washing. In dental radiography, the use of sterilization, disinfection, and antiseptic agents results in a rational, workable infection control policy.

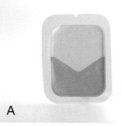

• **Figure 8.7** Digital sensor with barrier sheath in place.

Digital Radiography

Digital radiography receptor (directly wired or wireless sensors and phosphor plates) are considered to be semi-critical devices, because they are used intraorally and come into contact with mucous membranes. The direct digital sensors (charge-coupled device and complementary metal oxide semiconductor sensors) and phosphor plate sensors (indirect digital sensors) cannot be placed into an autoclave or immersed in contact disinfectants. It is recommended that U.S. Food and Drug Administration–approved hygienic barriers must be used to meet infection control standards and prevent cross-contamination (Fig. 8.7). It is important to cover the digital sensor and any cords that may come into contact with intraoral surfaces of contaminated hands (gloves). Finger cots can be used in addition to the barrier sheaths for added protection. It is also important to adequately clean and disinfect the sensor before and after use.

> ### NOTE
> To disinfect the sensor, only disinfecting wipes or a solution containing intermediate-level disinfectant should be used. It is also important to follow the manufacturer's directions for cleaning and disinfecting. Some manufacturers warn against using chlorine-based products (i.e., bleach), because they may be too corrosive for the sensors. Furthermore, digital sensors should never be soaked overnight, and barrier sheaths or envelopes must also never be reused. Care should be taken to clean, disinfect, and cover the computer keyboard/mouse being used according to infection control protocols as well.

Film Packets

Other than the operator's hands, the film packet or digital sensor is the main vector of cross-contamination. The receptor remains in the patient's mouth; when removed, it is coated with saliva or possibly with blood.

In the case in which the receptor is a film packet (as opposed to a digital sensor), it is handled carefully in the

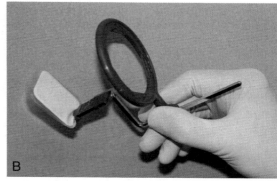

• **Figure 8.8** Barrier envelope. **A,** With film packet. **B,** In film holder. (A, Courtesy Carestream Dental, Rochester, NY.)

operatory and then transported to the darkroom. The following three methods can theoretically prevent transmission of microorganisms by the film packet to other parts of the operatory or the darkroom: (1) sterilization or disinfection of the exposed packet, (2) use of barrier protection for the packet, and (3) proper handling technique.

1. Sterilization and disinfection of the film packet are not advised, because they are impractical and time-consuming and may degrade or ruin the radiographic image. Autoclaving the film packet can also destroy the image. Immersing the packet in a disinfecting solution for the required time results in penetration of the solution to the film emulsion. Thus, neither sterilization nor disinfection is recommended.

2. Barrier envelopes for film packets are available in the dental market for x-ray films and may be purchased with the film packet already inserted into the barrier envelopes, or the barrier envelopes may be purchased separately and individual film packets may be inserted in them before exposure (Fig. 8.8).

The film packet is exposed in the barrier envelope, dried of saliva, and then brought to the darkroom in some type of a receptacle without the barrier envelope. The operator wears gloves to open the barrier envelope, taking care not to touch the film packet, and the packet is allowed to drop into a clean receptacle (i.e., cup) or surface. The gloves and the barrier envelope are then discarded, and the operator opens the film packet and processes the film with either bare hands or new, unused gloves.

3. If the barrier film packet technique is not used, after the exposure is made, the film packet that is contaminated by saliva or blood should be wiped dry and placed in a receptacle that is outside the operatory and carried to the darkroom when all the exposures have been made.

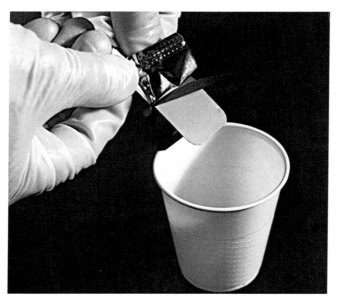

• **Figure 8.9** Opening contaminated film packet in the darkroom.

This film transport to the darkroom can be performed after the contaminated gloves are disposed of and a clean receptacle (i.e., cup) carrying the contaminated films are brought to the darkroom. Once operators are in the darkroom and have put on new gloves, they can open the film packets under safelight conditions. They should take care not to touch the films as they are dropped onto a clean surface (Fig. 8.9). The gloves that they handled the contaminated packets with are then discarded, and the films are processed either manually or automatically. If there are two people in the darkroom (admittedly, this is not common in most offices), one gloved person can open the contaminated packet and the other can remove the film from within the packet without touching the outside (Fig. 8.10). This process will also prevent contamination of the film.

Processing Solutions

The developing and fixing solutions used in the darkroom have not been shown to act as sterilizing agents. It is a

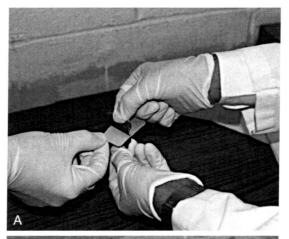

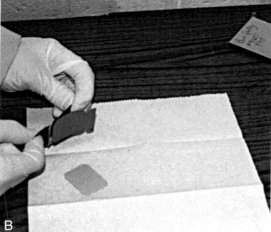

• **Figure 8.10** **A** and **B**, Two-operator technique for removing film from a contaminated packet.

common misconception that they do. Any contaminated film that is processed emerges from the processing procedure still contaminated. It has been shown that microorganisms can remain viable on radiographic equipment for at least 48 hours. In automatic processors, the rollers and tracks can be contaminated by the film, as can the film hangers in manual processing.

PROCEDURE 8.1

Chairside Exposure Procedures

1. Cover all appropriate surfaces with a plastic barrier. This should include but not be limited to the PID and arm of the x-ray machine, the control panel, the exposure button, the computer keyboard/mouse, and the working surfaces where unexposed receptors are placed (Fig. 8.11). Plan in advance, setting out all anticipated supplies (receptors, receptor holders, cotton rolls, and so on).

2. Seat the patient and drape with the lead apron and thyroid collar in the appropriate manner. Make sure that the protective apron and thyroid collar have been cleaned and disinfected before placing them on the patient.
3. Wash hands thoroughly with soap or an approved instant hand sanitizer (e.g., Purell) and put on gloves.
4. Make the required exposures, taking care to touch only the covered surfaces. If the procedure is interrupted and

Continued

PROCEDURE 8.1—cont'd

Chairside Exposure Procedures

you have to leave the room and touch anything, remove the gloves, dispose of them, and put on a new pair before resuming work. Each exposed receptor should be wiped dry of saliva and placed in a clean receptacle (i.e., cup) outside of the cubicle.

5. If no other dental procedures are to be done, dismiss the patient. Dispose of all contaminated barriers and supplies in the operatory; then, disinfect the lead apron/collar and other appropriate surfaces.
6. Remove the contaminated gloves.

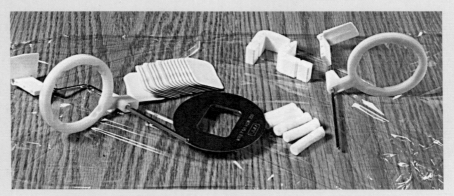

• **Figure 8.11** Plastic wrap covering necessary items on a work surface.

PROCEDURE 8.2

Processing Procedures (Conventional Radiography)

1. Put on new gloves.
2. Under safelight conditions with gloved hands, remove the films from the film packet or the film packets from the barrier envelopes by allowing them to drop onto a clean surface. Do not touch the film with gloved hands. The gloves are considered to be contaminated because they touched the film packet.
3. Dispose of the film packet wrappers and carrying cup and remove and dispose of the gloves.
4. Process the uncontaminated film on the clean surface either manually or automatically.
5. The film is not contaminated; thus, gloves are not needed for processing or mounting.

Automatic Processing (Conventional Radiography)

Operators should load film into an automatic processor with the same concern and method for avoiding cross-contamination as with manual processing film hangers. The problem is with the automatic processors used with daylight loaders. Use of daylight loaders creates a situation in which it is very difficult to avoid contamination as a result of the tight-fitting hand baffles, which serve as a source of cross-contamination (Fig. 8.12). This is not the case if one is using the barrier packs. It is also very difficult to remove the film from the film packet and to put on one's gloves within the confined space of the daylight loader, then take

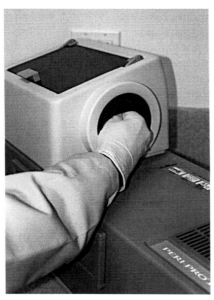

• **Figure 8.12** The sleeves of an automatic processor have been contaminated by the operator's contaminated gloves.

off the contaminated gloves and feed the film into the uptake slots. An operator who must use a daylight loader when the barrier packets are not available should follow the protocol found in Procedure 8.3.

Panoramic Radiography

Because panoramic radiography is an extraoral procedure, fewer areas are contaminated by the patient's saliva. In both conventional and digital panoramic radiography, the patient

PROCEDURE 8.3

Procedure for Daylight Loaders

1. Prepare the interior of the daylight loader by placing a barrier on the bottom surface. Place the cup with the exposed film packets, a pair of gloves, and a second cup inside the daylight loader and then close the top of the daylight loader.
2. Place clean hands through the sleeve baffles and put on the gloves.
3. Open packets, allowing the films to drop into the second cup.
4. Remove gloves and place the uncontaminated films in the processing slots; then, remove ungloved hands through the sleeves.
5. Open the top of the loader and wrap all trash in the barrier and remove.
6. Wash hands.

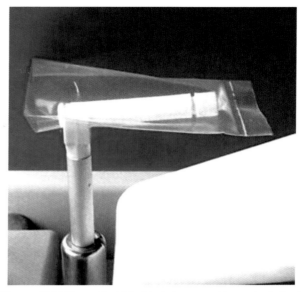

• **Figure 8.13** The patient bite block is covered by a plastic barrier cover.

bite block should be covered by a plastic barrier cover (Fig. 8.13) and the lead apron should be disinfected. Plastic barrier wrap should also be used on the chin rest, ear rods, patient handgrips, the control panel, and the computer keyboard/mouse. In conventional panoramic radiography, processing does not present a problem, because the cassette does not contact the patient; thus, the procedure for preventing film contamination is not necessary. The only possible contaminant in the darkroom would be the operator's gloves. These gloves should be removed before the cassette is taken from the panoramic unit.

Antibiotic Prophylaxis

It is an accepted and required procedure to provide prophylaxis with antibiotics for certain patients before dental procedures. Any procedure, including probing, that might produce bleeding should be considered invasive. The question then arises regarding whether intraoral radiography is an invasive procedure, because in rare instances it may produce bleeding. The American Medical Association suggests that prophylaxis is not necessary before taking radiographs; however, because of the immense risk to the patient, it is prudent to provide prophylaxis if any bleeding is expected. In clinical practice, however, most patients needing antibiotic prophylaxis will have been provided with prophylaxis, because it is rare that the only procedure done at a specific appointment is the taking of radiographs.

Immunization

All dental personnel should have the appropriate immunizations (e.g., tetanus, influenza, varicella), including that for the hepatitis B virus. OSHA's standard covering blood-borne pathogens requires health care employers to offer a three-injection HBV vaccination series free to all employees exposed to blood or other potentially infectious fluids or materials. The OSHA standard also states that if routine booster doses of the hepatitis vaccine are recommended at some future date, then the employer also should make these boosters available to employees at no cost.

Chapter Summary

- The primary purpose of infection control procedures in a dental practice is to prevent infectious disease transmission.
- Federal and state agencies at all levels are currently imposing requirements for dental office procedures and required courses in infection control.
- Infectious disease can be transmitted by the cross-contamination of equipment, supplies, and receptors used to expose or process radiographs.
- Every dental patient should be treated in the same manner, with universal precautions carried out at all times.

- Any object that the operator touches after placing the receptor in the patient's mouth must be covered with a removable barrier or disinfected after the patient leaves.
- Digital sensors and computer keyboards should be wiped and covered before use and wiped after use as well.
- Barrier envelopes are used to prevent cross-contamination by the film packet, and there are various ways of handling films during processing, depending on whether they have barrier envelopes on them or not.
- All dental personnel should practice the appropriate infection control procedures for all dental procedures, including dental radiography.

Chapter Review Questions

Multiple Choice

1. A pathogen is:
   a. An organism that attaches itself to another organism
   b. An autoimmune mechanism for disease
   c. A microorganism capable of causing disease
   d. A pathologic psychosis
   e. A person with a serious pathology

2. The personal protective equipment (PPE) strongly suggested for dental professionals to wear while exposing digital radiographs is:
   a. A mask
   b. Protective eyewear
   c. Protective clothing
   d. Gloves
   e. All of the above

3. Which of the following statements regarding "barrier envelopes" is false?
   a. Some films come with barrier envelopes.
   b. You can manually place a film packet in a barrier envelope.
   c. You can remove the barrier envelope and process with the same gloves.
   d. Digital sensors are covered with barrier sheaths, which are comparable in design and use to the barrier envelopes used with conventional film.
   e. Barrier envelopes help protect the film packet from contamination.

4. The American Medical Association suggests that antibiotic prophylaxis is:
   a. Necessary for all patients
   b. Necessary when bleeding is expected
   c. Not necessary for radiographic procedures
   d. a and b only
   e. b and c only

5. The primary purpose of infection control procedures in a dental practice is to prevent infectious disease transmission. The main vector for cross-contamination in dental radiography other than the operator's glove is the image receptor.
   a. Both statements are true.
   b. Both statements are false.
   c. The first statement is true, and the second statement is false.
   d. The first statement is false, and the second statement is true.
   e. Not enough information is given to answer this question correctly.

Critical Thinking Exercises

1. A new patient who requires antibiotic prophylaxis comes to your office for the first time. The only procedure that your patient is currently scheduled for is digital radiographs. The patient refuses to take the premedication "just for radiographs to be taken." Discuss how you would handle this situation, including the following:
   a. The American Medical Association's suggestion on this matter
   b. The procedure(s) that this patient is scheduled for
   c. The need for a clinical oral examination of the patient's periodontium
   d. The risks the patient will be taking if not premedicated
   e. The rationale behind your decision-making process in this particular situation

2. You are scheduled to expose a full series of radiographs on your patient utilizing film-based dental radiography. The patient has no known infectious diseases. You will be processing the radiographs in an automatic processor with a daylight loader. Describe the infection control steps you will take to protect your patient and yourself. Include in your discussion:
   a. Universal precautions
   b. The handling of the exposed film packets with barrier envelopes while exposing the radiographs
   c. The handling of the exposed film packets during the processing procedure
   d. The PPE that you will be wearing
   e. The preparation of the operatory
   f. What you will do with the XCP receptor-holding devices when you have completed the radiographic procedure

Bibliography

American Academy of Oral and Maxillofacial Radiology infection control guidelines for dental radiographic procedures, *Oral Surg Oral Med Oral Pathol* 73:248–249, 1992.

Bartoloni JA, Chariton DG, Flint DJ: Infection control practices in dental radiology, *Gen Dent* 51:264–271, 2003.

Eastman Kodak Co: *Infection in modern practice*, Rochester, NY, 1999, Health Science Division.

Glass BJ: Infection control in dental radiology. Current and future, *N Y State Dent J* 60:42–45, 1994.

Hastreiter RJ, Jiang P: Do regular dental visits affect the oral health care provided to people with HIV, *J Am Dent Assoc* 133:1343–1350, 2002.

Iannucci JM, Howerton LJ: *Dental radiography: Principles and techniques*, ed 5, St Louis, MO, 2016, Elsevier Saunders.

Infection control recommendations for the dental office and the dental laboratory. ADA Council on Scientific Affairs and ADA Council on Dental Practice, *J Am Dent Assoc* 127:672–680, 1996.

Jones GA, Woods MA, Burton EL, et al: Radiographic protocol for patients needing antibiotic prophylaxis: dental schools report no consensus, *J Am Dent Assoc* 125:602–604, 606, 1994.

Kohn WG, Harte JA, Malvitz DM, et al: Guidelines for infection control in dental health care settings—2003, *J Am Dent Assoc* 135:33–47, 2004.

Kohn WG, Collins AS, Cleveland JL, et al: Guidelines for infection control in dental health-care settings—2003, *MMWR Recomm Rep* 52(RR–17):1–61, 2003.

Langland OE, Langlais RP: *Principles of dental imaging*, Baltimore, MD, 1997, Williams & Wilkins.

Thompson EM, Johnson ON: *Essentials of dental radiography for dental assistants and hygienists*, ed 9, Upper Saddle River, NJ, 2012, Pearson Education, Inc.

White SC, Pharoah MJ: *Oral radiology: Principles and interpretation*, ed 7, St Louis, MO, 2013, Mosby.

9

Intraoral Radiographic Technique: The Paralleling Method

EDUCATIONAL OBJECTIVES

Upon completing this chapter, the student will be able to:

1. Define the key terms listed at the beginning of the chapter.
2. Discuss the following related to the radiographic survey:
   - Know the importance of radiographs in treatment planning and diagnosis.
   - Explain what factors are involved in "prescribing" dental radiographs.
   - State the components of a general full-mouth survey (FMS), a pediatric FMS, and an edentulous FMS.
   - Describe what should be seen on periapical and bitewing projections and what the indications for use are for both projections.
   - Know the 8 criteria for acceptable intraoral radiographs.
3. List the principles, advantages, and disadvantages of the paralleling technique.
4. Recite the routine in preparing for and exposing dental radiographs, and explain the purpose of having a systematic sequence when exposing radiographic images.

5. Discuss the advantage of using a paralleling receptor-holding device (i.e., extension cone paralleling [XCP] instrument) when exposing intraoral radiographs.
6. Discuss the following related to the paralleling method:
   - List the six factors that must be considered in any periapical projection.
   - Know what factors are considered in determining the exposure time setting for dental radiographic exposures.
   - Be able to apply the principles of the paralleling intraoral radiographic technique to exposing all periapical and bitewing radiographs indicated for their dental patients.
7. Know the causes, appearances, and remedies for the discussed exposure errors, as well as list the three most common bitewing errors, including their causes, appearance, and remedies.

KEY TERMS

bitewing projection
chair position
collimator cutoff (cone cutting)
dimensional accuracy
dimensional distortion
double exposure
elongation
exposure routine
extension cone paralleling (XCP)
   technique

film reversal
foreshortening
full-mouth survey (FMS)
hemostat
horizontal angulation
localizing ring
long axis
long cone technique
occlusal plane
overexposure

overlapping
patient movement
periapical projection
point of entry
receptor position
right-angle technique
sagittal plane
underexposure
vertical angulation
vertical bitewings

Introduction

The radiographic examination is an integral component of formulating a diagnosis and treatment plan for the dental patient. It is of the utmost importance that the radiographic images of the patient's oral structures be diagnostically acceptable. It is the dental professional's responsibility to produce the most diagnostically acceptable radiographs possible while keeping the patient's exposure to x-radiation at a minimum. Furthermore, only those radiographs that address the patient's immediate dental health needs should be taken. Radiographers should refine their technique in an effort to reduce the number of retakes and ultimately the amount of radiation exposure to their patients. This chapter discusses the types of intraoral radiographs available; the paralleling exposure technique; receptor-holding devices; and the appearance, cause, and remedy for various common exposure errors in dental radiography. Film-based and digital radiographic techniques are discussed here; the digital radiographic techniques are further discussed in Chapter 15.

The Radiographic Survey

Intraoral radiography is a dental imaging technique utilized when the image receptor is placed inside the patient's mouth and the source of radiation is positioned outside of the patient's mouth. The x-ray prescription for intraoral radiographs is custom fit to a patient's dental health needs. The number and type of images exposed can vary depending on the needs of the patient. The full-mouth intraoral radiographic survey is one option in choosing the necessary radiographs for a particular patient to complete the patient's oral diagnosis. A dental examination or treatment plan cannot be considered complete without current or valid radiographs; in some cases, the full-mouth survey (FMS) is the radiographic procedure of choice. The FMS is a challenging procedure to perform correctly; it requires time and meticulous attention to detail. It bears with it the responsibility of exposing the patient to the least amount of ionizing radiation to obtain the maximum diagnostic yield. Unnecessary radiographs or those of poor quality that do not have diagnostic value do not serve the patient's needs and only add to the patient's radiation burden. Regardless of which member of the dental team takes the radiographs, the same quality standards are maintained for all dental professionals.

The radiographic FMS is usually composed of 14 or more periapical projections and, where possible, four posterior bitewing projections (Fig. 9.1). The bitewing projections can be held vertically or horizontally. This text discusses a 14-periapical and a four-horizontal bitewing image technique. Some series of more than 14 periapical projections include distal maxillary molar projections, vertical bitewings, anterior bitewings, and individual radiographs using #1 size narrow anterior projections of the six maxillary and four mandibular anterior teeth.

The number of radiographs in an FMS can be modified to include extra or fewer projections, depending on the size of the patient's mouth or tooth position. In all cases, the minimum number of images that satisfies the diagnostic requirements of an FMS should be used. Film mounts and digital templates are available in various combinations of numbers and sizes of receptors. The radiographic survey should not be determined by the film mount or digital template available or by any other reason not related to dental health but strictly by the diagnostic needs of the patient. The recommended intraoral projections are listed in Table 9.1.

A periapical projection shows the entire tooth from the incisal edge or the occlusal surface to the apex of the root and 2 to 3 mm of surrounding periapical bone. This projection is necessary to diagnose normal or pathologic conditions of tooth crowns and root, bone, and tooth formation and eruption (Fig. 9.2).

The bitewing projection can be taken only if there are opposing teeth to hold the receptor in position with their occluding surfaces. This projection shows the upper and lower teeth in occlusion in one image. Only the crowns and alveolar crest of the bone of adjacent teeth are seen. It is used for detecting interproximal decay, periodontal bone loss, recurrent decay under restorations, and faulty restorations (Fig. 9.3). Bitewing projections can be taken of the anterior teeth but are usually taken in the posterior regions. Proponents of the use of vertical bitewings point out that, in this position, more root is seen and thus can be more diagnostic for root caries, receding alveolar bone levels, and in pediatric patients to see the progress of the secondary dentition.

The FMS shows all of the teeth in the mandible and maxilla, as well as the surrounding bone. Each tooth is shown at least twice in the survey; that is, the maxillary second premolar can be seen on the premolar periapical image and on the premolar bitewing projection. Some teeth may be seen in three or four views. This gives the diagnostician an opportunity to view the tooth from different radiographic angles, eliminating the possibility that an artifact could be mistaken for caries or other pathologic conditions.

Pediatric Full-Mouth Survey

Depending on the child's age and the size of the child's mouth, the composition of the FMS may vary. A report of the Selection Criteria Panel recommends that only two bitewing images be taken for the asymptomatic clinically negative pediatric patient with closed posterior contacts. For asymptomatic and clinically negative pediatric patients with open posterior contacts, no radiographs are necessary.

For patients up to 5 years old who are in need of an FMS, the operator should use the pediatric-size receptor #0 for anterior, posterior, and bitewing projections (Fig. 9.4). The FMS at this age entails 12 projections: three maxillary anterior projections, three mandibular anterior projections, four mandibular and maxillary molar projections, and two bitewing projections. Only one molar bitewing projection is taken on each side.

In the 6-year-old to 9-year-old group, the pediatric receptor (#0) or narrow adult receptor (size #1) can be used for anterior projections, because the child's arch shape at this age can still be very narrow. For posterior projections, adult size #2, narrow adult, or pediatric receptor (#0) is used, depending on the size of the arch. At this age, two posterior periapical projections in each quadrant are taken, because the 6-year molars have erupted and the dental arch has lengthened. One bitewing projection on each side is also used.

After 9 years old, the full adult series is taken, with the narrow adult receptor being used where necessary. These age

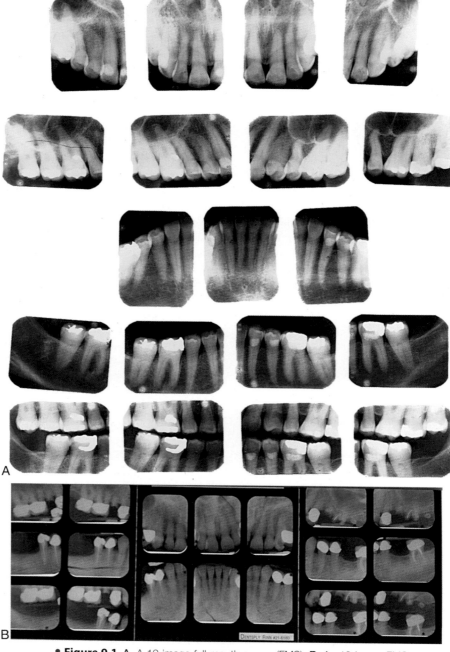

• **Figure 9.1** **A,** A 19-image full-mouth survey (FMS). **B,** An 18-image FMS.

guidelines are flexible and depend on the growth and development of the child. As a rule, it is best to use the largest receptor size that the patient can accommodate comfortably (Fig. 9.5). Keep in mind that the extraoral panoramic image can also be used with pediatric dental patients, especially to evaluate eruption patterns and growth and development.

Edentulous Series

A radiographic examination can be performed even though the patient may be wholly or partially edentulous. The absence of teeth in an area of clinical examination does not preclude the possibility of retained roots, impacted teeth, cysts, or other occult pathologic conditions that may be present in the bone. The edentulous examination may use periapical projections, occlusal projections, or a panoramic radiograph. The intraoral edentulous series is usually composed of 13 periapical projections. The bitewing images are not taken, because there are no opposing teeth to support the bitewing receptor-holding device or bitewing tabs, and only one image is taken in the maxillary central, lateral, and canine regions (Fig. 9.6). In small edentulous mouths, a survey consisting of 11 projections may suffice by use of only one mandibular periapical projection and

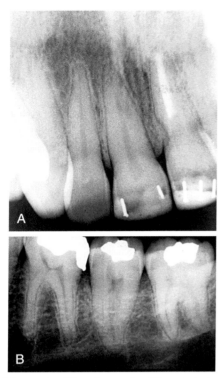

• **Figure 9.2** Anterior **(A)** and posterior (B) periapical radiographs. Note that the entire tooth and surrounding periapical bone are shown.

TABLE 9.1	The Recommended Projections of the Radiographic Survey	
Maxillary	**Mandibular**	
Central and lateral incisors	Central and lateral incisors	
Right and left canines	Right and left canines	
Right and left premolars	Right and left premolars	
Right and left molars	Right and left molars	
Bitewing		
Right and left premolars		
Right and left molars		

extension of the premolar projection anteriorly to include the canine area.

The receptors are positioned in the same way as in a regular dentulous series but with certain modifications. The crest of the edentulous ridge replaces the occlusal plane of the teeth as the plane of orientation. The receptor is positioned either ⅛ inch above (for mandibular projections) or ⅛ inch below the ridge (for maxillary projections). Because there are no teeth and there may be a great deal of ridge resorption, it may be difficult to parallel the long axis of the receptor with the long axis of the edentulous ridge. Thus, the receptor lies flatter against the palate or in the floor of the mouth. In these cases, it may be possible to support the receptor with cotton rolls to achieve parallelism

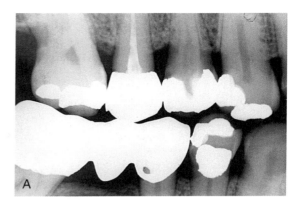

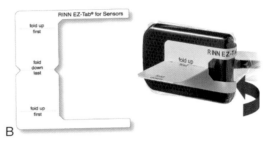

• **Figure 9.3 A,** Bitewing radiograph. Note that only the crowns, alveolar ridge, and a small part of the roots of opposing teeth are seen. **B,** Bite-wing tab for digital sensors. (Courtesy Dentsply Rinn, York, PA.)

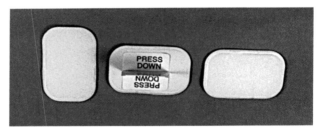

• **Figure 9.4** Size #0 pediatric film for anterior, posterior, and bitewing projections.

or, if necessary, to increase the vertical angulation and use the bisecting angle technique. The best guideline in the edentulous series is to adjust the vertical angulation so that the central ray is almost perpendicular to the receptor (similar to the angulation used for occlusal projections). Any slight foreshortening that may result will not affect the diagnosis of any intrabony conditions.

There are two possible alternatives for the edentulous periapical survey. The first is a panoramic survey (Fig. 9.7). The second is the use of an occlusal projection (Fig. 9.8), the technique of which is discussed in Chapter 10. The entire maxillary and mandibular ridges usually can be seen on their respective occlusal projections. Both the panoramic and the occlusal are survey projections; if any suspicious areas are seen, a periapical projection of the area can be done to obtain better definition for formulating a definitive diagnosis.

The criteria for judging whether a single radiograph or a FMS is diagnostically acceptable are listed in Box 9.1.

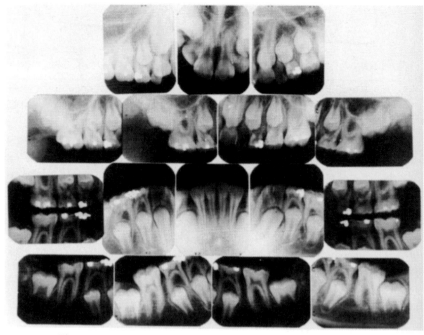

• **Figure 9.5** Pediatric full-mouth survey (FMS) of a 9-year-old patient.

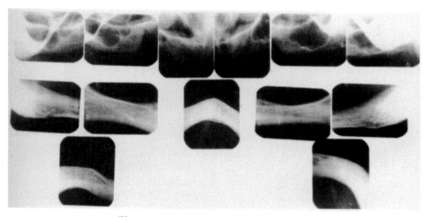

• **Figure 9.6** A 13-image edentulous survey.

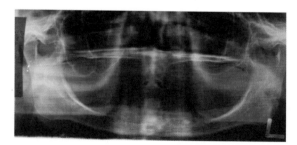

• **Figure 9.7** Edentulous panoramic survey.

If a single radiograph does not meet these criteria and cannot provide diagnostic value, it must be retaken. In an FMS, those areas and structures that do not appear on the primary image may be seen on adjacent projections in the series. Although a technically perfect FMS is ideal, retakes should not be performed unless they are necessary for proper diagnosis.

Quality Assurance

The criteria for diagnostically acceptable radiographs (as shown in Box 9.1) should be used to evaluate radiographs taken by dentists and dental professionals as part of a quality assurance program. This can be accomplished either by self-evaluation and criticism of one's own work or by peer review. In this manner, technical errors can be corrected and high-quality diagnostic radiographs will be produced. Quality assurance is discussed further in a later chapter.

Paralleling Technique

The basic principles of the paralleling technique for intraoral periapical projections is that the receptor and the long axis of the tooth being radiographed must be parallel to each other, and the central ray of the x-ray beam must be directed perpendicular to both (see Fig. 3.13). To accomplish this

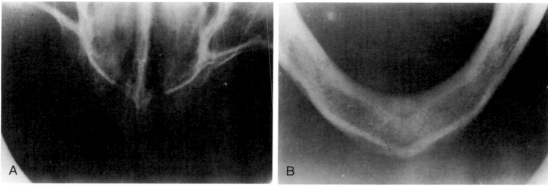

• **Figure 9.8 A,** Edentulous occlusal survey of maxilla. **B,** Edentulous occlusal survey of mandible.

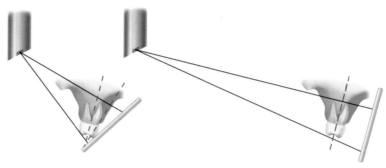

• **Figure 9.9** Bisecting 8-inch target-receptor distance (FFD) technique and paralleling 16-inch extended-cone technique. Note superimposition of zygomatic arch on apices of maxillary molar in bisecting technique. (Courtesy DENTSPLY Rinn, Elgin, IL.)

• **BOX 9.1   Criteria for Intraoral Radiographs**

1. The radiograph should show proper definition and detail and a degree of density and contrast so that all structures can be delineated easily.
2. The structures should not be distorted either by elongation or by foreshortening.
3. The radiograph should show the teeth from the occlusal or incisal edges to 2 to 3 mm beyond their apices.
4. In a full-mouth survey (FMS), the entire alveolar processes of the mandible and maxilla must be seen, as far distal as the tuberosity in the maxilla and the beginning of the ascending ramus in the mandible.
5. All interproximal surfaces of the teeth should be seen without overlapping provided that the teeth are not overlapped in the mouth.
6. The x-ray beam should be centered on the receptor so that there are no unexposed parts on the image ("collimator cutoff" or "cone cuts").
7. The radiograph should not be cracked or bent or have any other artifacts.
8. The radiograph should be processed properly.

---

parallelism, the object-receptor distance must be increased. This distance can be sizable in some areas, such as the maxillary molar projection, where the receptor may have to be held at the midline of the palate to achieve this parallelism.

The increased object-receptor distance results in loss of image sharpness, which is a problem that can be compensated for by using an increased, 16-inch, target-receptor distance (or focal-film distance [FFD]; Fig. 9.9).

The paralleling technique has often been called the long cone technique. This terminology is not as accurate in contemporary dentistry, in which the target-receptor distance may be from 12 to 16 inches because of a recessed target (in the x-ray tube head) rather than as a result of the length of the position-indicating device (PID). Other names for the paralleling technique are the extension cone paralleling (XCP) technique or right-angle technique, both of which stress two important principles of the technique.

Advantages and Disadvantages of the Paralleling Technique Compared with the Bisecting Angle Technique

When the paralleling and bisecting techniques are compared, the consensus is that dental professionals prefer the paralleling method as the technique of choice. The American Academy of Oral and Maxillofacial Radiology (AAOMR) states the following through its Parameters of Care Committee: "The paralleling technique should be used with its appropriate armamentarium, when possible, as it provides the most geometrically accurate image of the dentition." The paralleling technique produces better diagnostic images, less exposure to critical organs (such as, the thyroid gland and the lens of the eye), a smaller exit dose, and easier standardization and execution than the bisecting technique.

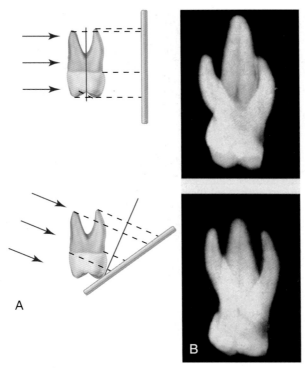

• **Figure 9.10** Radiographs of maxillary molar taken with bisecting technique **(A)** and the paralleling technique **(B)**. (Courtesy DENTSPLY Rinn, Elgin, IL.)

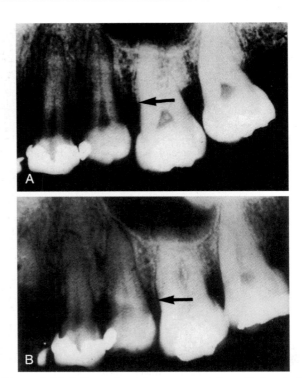

• **Figure 9.11** Radiographs of the same area taken with the paralleling technique **(A)** and the bisecting technique **(B)**. Note the difference in alveolar bone height, as indicated by *arrows*.

Advantages of the Paralleling Technique

The major advantage of the paralleling technique is that, when performed correctly, it forms an image with both linear and dimensional accuracy to support a more valid diagnosis. The key terms are dimensional accuracy and dimensional distortion.

The bisecting technique, if used properly, correctly represents the teeth linearly but produces dimensional distortion. The bisecting technique can project the images and surrounding structures on the receptor in a true linear relationship without elongation or foreshortening. The teeth and bone, however, are three-dimensional objects; and although their overall length may be recorded accurately, the relationship of one part of the tooth to another is distorted dimensionally (Fig. 9.10). Those parts of the tooth that lie farthest from the receptor, such as the buccal plate of bone and buccal roots, are foreshortened; although their lingual linear counterparts are not. A classic clinical example consists of comparing the length of the buccal roots with that of palatal roots in maxillary first molars. Clinicians who have used the bisecting technique for many years may come to believe that the buccal roots are much shorter than they really are because of dimensional distortions. One may argue that this may not be clinically important except in an initial endodontic measurement, but when this distortion is applied to periodontal evaluation of alveolar bone levels, the clinical importance becomes apparent (Fig. 9.11). In the bisecting technique, the image of the buccal bone level is figuratively added to the palatal bone height to give a distorted image. A diagnosis and treatment plan could assume the presence of adequate bone for restorations, fixed splinting, and so forth, on the basis of distorted radiographic images.

With the paralleling technique, it is possible to diagnose and evaluate caries and alveolar bone height accurately on all radiographs and not rely on the bitewing projections, as users of the bisecting technique do. It is interesting to note that bitewing projections in both techniques are paralleling projections due to the inherent parallel relationship between the receptor and the tooth in the bitewing radiographic technique.

In the bisecting technique, the radiopaque image of the zygomatic arch is often superimposed on the apices of the maxillary molars, making diagnosis difficult if not impossible. This superimposition is understandable, because the point of entry of the central ray for molar projections is along the zygomatic arch.

The paralleling technique produces no superimposition of the zygomatic arch, because the central ray, which is perpendicular to the long axis of the molars, enters below the level of the zygomatic arch. Also, in the paralleling technique, the vertical angulation of the primary beam is rarely more than plus or minus 10 degrees, compared with the vertical angulation of 40 to 50 degrees in the bisecting technique. The lack of extreme vertical angulation with the paralleling method reduces the exposure to the thyroid gland and the lens of the eye, because they no longer lie in the path of the primary beam. In addition, the 16-inch target-receptor distance (or FFD) used with the paralleling technique reduces the volume of tissue irradiated when compared with the recommended 8-inch target-receptor distance (or FFD) used in the bisecting technique (see Fig. 6.10).

The paralleling technique is easier to standardize than the bisecting technique, and serial comparison radiographs of the same area have greater validity. This is especially important in evaluating alveolar bone levels of periodontal patients at recall examinations.

If a receptor-holding device with a localizing ring (i.e., XCP instruments) is used with the paralleling technique, the patient does not have to be positioned so that the occlusal plane of the jaw being radiographed is parallel to the floor. This is especially helpful in contour chairs or when patients are treated in the supine or semi-supine position. In these instances, it is difficult to position the patient with the occlusal plane parallel to the floor.

Disadvantages of the Paralleling Technique

One of the objections most often raised about the paralleling technique is the difficulty in placement and the degree of discomfort caused by the devices used to hold the receptor parallel to the long axis of the tooth. This may present some problems for patients with small mouths or large tori, children, and patients with low palatal vaults, but the more adept an operator becomes with the technique, the less these problems are a factor. In the pediatric patient, if it is impossible to position the receptor for the paralleling method, decrease the receptor size; and then if a backup strategy is needed, use the bisecting method. At least the time element is the same, and learning the paralleling technique is as easy as or easier than learning the bisecting technique, especially when using paralleling instruments (i.e., XCP instruments).

Objections to the paralleling technique in the past focused on the "long, bulky" 16-inch PID that is used in this technique. The claim is that these PIDs were difficult to work with, especially in small operatories. This objection has no validity with the newer x-ray machines, with the extended target-receptor distance (or FFD) within the tube head as a result of a recessed target (see Fig. 3.10).

Another supposed disadvantage of the paralleling technique in the past was that with the 16-inch target-receptor distance (or FFD), longer exposure times are necessary, resulting in a greater chance of patient movement. With the use of faster-speed film and digital receptors, this is no longer true. Previously, with the use of slower film, the possibility of patient movement was greater.

Exposure Routine

Regardless of which technique (paralleling or bisecting) is used, certain basic rules must be followed for the barrier technique, infection control preparation of the patient, and radiation hygiene. Operators should develop an exposure routine to avoid mistakes that necessitate the retaking of images. Retaking a radiograph because of operator error adds unnecessarily to the patient's radiation burden.

The patient should be seated comfortably in the chair, with the back well supported and the head positioned in such a way that the jaw can be radiographed correctly. Except when paralleling instruments are used, the occlusal plane of the jaw being radiographed must be parallel to the floor when it is in the open position.

The patient should remove any nonfixed prosthetic appliances from the mouth, as well as eyeglasses and facial jewelry (i.e., in the direct path of the primary beam, such as nose or lip rings). Failure to do this would cause a superimposed radiopaque error on the image. In the case of eyeglasses and facial jewelry, any metallic component will appear radiopaque and may be superimposed on any image in which they are worn. The patient should be draped with a lead apron and thyroid collar. This is done routinely for all patients, regardless of the number of projections taken. Then, the operator turns on the x-ray machine. The infection control procedures outlined in Chapter 8 should be followed. When using film packets, the unexposed and exposed films can be placed in a cup and should be positioned outside of the operatory away from primary and scatter (secondary) radiation. Many diagnostic dental films are fogged by secondary radiation and thus made unacceptable if left in the dental operatory when other images are being exposed.

The desired number of receptors, as well as additional supplies, such as receptor-holding devices, should be brought near the operatory at this time. One of the more important general principles of taking intraoral radiographs is to have the positioned receptor in the patient's mouth for as short a time as possible. This decreases the likelihood of gagging and patient movement. The desired exposure time on the machine always should be set before the receptor is placed in the patient's mouth. Precious moments can be wasted in setting the time while the receptor is already in the patient's mouth.

While the exposure is being made from the required 6-foot distance, the operator should watch the patient. If the patient moves, the operator will be able to see the movement and avoid having to retake the image. A simple command to the patient (such as, "Please hold still") can be helpful at this time. A well-designed office permits observation from behind a suitable barrier.

After the exposure has been made, the operator removes the receptor from the patient's mouth, dries off the saliva, and places it in the exposed receptor receptacle. Some definite order should be followed for a series of radiographs. Skipping from area to area without a set pattern often results in an omitted projection when utilizing a film-based radiographic technique. A good place to start is with the maxillary central incisor projection; it is probably the easiest for the patient to tolerate. One should never start with the maxillary molar projection, because this is the projection most likely to excite the gag reflex; once the reflex is excited, the patient may gag on projections that normally could be tolerated. After starting with the maxillary central incisor projection, the maxillary canine, premolar, and molar are radiographed in that order. The opposite side of the maxilla is then radiographed. It is poor technique to radiograph left canine, right canine, left premolar, and so forth. This necessitates moving the tube head constantly from one side of the patient to the other, which is time-consuming and can result in an omitted projection.

The bitewing projections can be taken after the maxillary periapicals if the operator so chooses. It is suggested that the mandibular periapical projections should be taken in the same order as the maxillary projections. However, the ultimate choice of exposure sequence is the operator's, as long as all of the prescribed radiographs are successfully taken with the patient's comfort and time in mind.

Film Holders

The use of receptor holders is strongly recommended for a variety of reasons, including avoiding the use of the patient's (or operator's) finger to hold the receptor. In the paralleling technique, the receptor must be held in its proper position by one of a variety of receptor-holding devices all serving one purpose—to position the receptor parallel to the long axis of the tooth. Some examples of devices include hemostats, Stabes, XCPs, RAPDs, and other acceptable receptor holders (Fig. 9.12). The localizing rings on

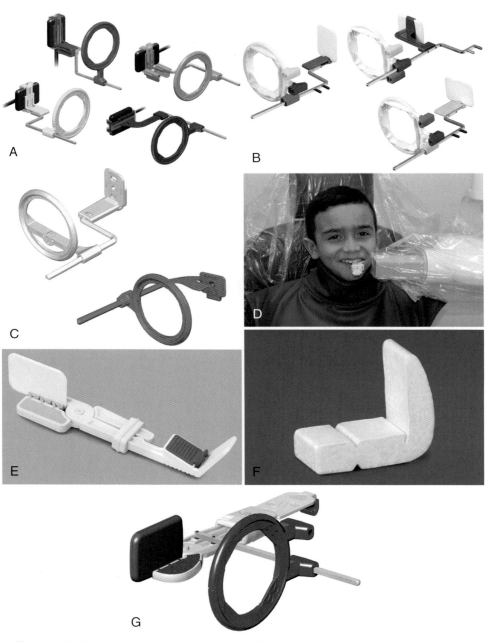

• **Figure 9.12** Beam alignment devices. **A,** Rinn XCP instruments (blue: anterior; yellow: posterior; red: bite-wing; green: endodontics). **B,** Rinn XCP-ORA devices. **C,** Rinn Flip-Ray eliminates the need for multiple devices. **D,** Snap-A-Ray intraoral film holder. **E,** Rinn Snap-A-Ray is color coded. **F,** Disposable Stabe bite block. **G,** Snap-a-Ray Bisecting option for sensor with arm and ring kit attached. (A-C, E-G Courtesy Dentsply Rinn, York, PA.)

paralleling receptor-holding devices align the PID with the receptor in both the horizontal and vertical planes, helping reduce the incidence of collimator cutoff (formerly known as *cone cutting*). The localizing rings are also a great aid with radiographic procedures performed in contour dental chairs. These chairs can make it difficult to position the patient so that the occlusal plane is parallel to the floor. However, as long as the open-ended PID can be brought into flat contact with the localizing ring, strict adherence to occlusal plane orientation is not necessary. Also, the relationship between the end of the PID and the ring can alert the operator to exposure errors before they get a chance to happen. For example, if there is spacing on the right or left of the ring, the operator should correct the horizontal angulation. In addition, if the spacing is on the top or bottom, the operator should correct the vertical angulation. Furthermore, some manufacturers have included notches on circular localizing rings to assist operators with proper placement of a rectangular PID.

Receptor holders are either disposable (e.g., Styrofoam bite blocks [Stabes]) or non-disposable (e.g., XCP) and can be used for holding films, digital sensors, or (in some cases) both films and digital sensors. Non-disposable receptor holders must be sterilized and not just disinfected. As described in Chapter 8, the choice method of sterilization is steam autoclaving. Be aware that some receptor-holding devices have parts that are not considered autoclavable.

Method

The following six factors must be considered in any periapical projection: exposure time, chair position, receptor position and placement, point of entry of the beam, vertical angulation, and horizontal angulation.

Exposure Time

Exposure time is determined by the area being radiographed, receptor speed, kilovoltage, milliamperage, and target-receptor distance (or FFD). The type of time setting controls vary depending on the manufacturer and model of the radiographic unit. Some units have up and down arrows to control the desired increase or decrease in the time setting. This type of exposure time setting control system requires that operators know the appropriate time setting for each exposure that they are taking. This can be established when the unit is calibrated; then, each time setting for the respective area being exposed is listed and posted in the operatory for the radiographer's use. It is recommended to post such a chart near the machine so that exposure times need not be committed to memory. For a majority of the newer-model x-ray units, the time can be set automatically simply by choosing an icon representing the area of exposure on the control panel (see Fig. 2.6). In any event, the timer should be set before the receptor is placed in the patient's mouth.

Chair Position: Occlusal and Sagittal Plane Orientations

The patient is positioned so that when the mouth is open and the receptor is in position, the occlusal plane of the jaw being radiographed is parallel to the floor. In the maxilla, this plane corresponds to the ala-tragus line on the face. When the maxilla is radiographed, the headrest is positioned high on the back of the patient's head, helping to position the chin downward toward the floor (Fig. 9.13). When the mandible is radiographed, the headrest is placed below the occipital protuberance (lower rear part of the human skull) in what would be the normal dental chair position (Fig. 9.14). For both upper and lower jaws, the patient's head is positioned so that the sagittal plane is perpendicular to the floor (Fig. 9.15). Note that when using paralleling

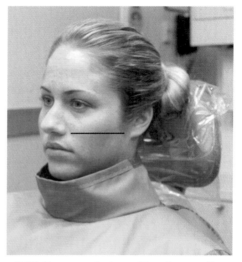

• **Figure 9.13** Proper patient position for maxillary periapical radiographs and bitewing projections. Note that the occlusal plane of maxillary teeth, or the ala-tragus line, is parallel to the floor.

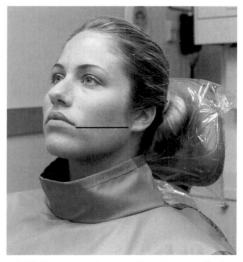

• **Figure 9.14** Proper patient position for mandibular periapical radiographs. Note that when the mouth is open, the occlusal plane of lower teeth is parallel to the floor.

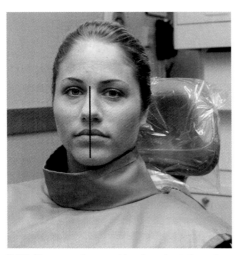

• **Figure 9.15** Proper patient position for orientation of sagittal plane of head perpendicular to the floor.

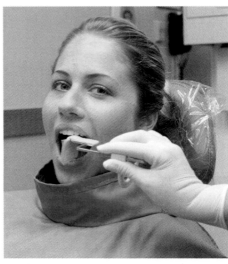

• **Figure 9.16** Placement of receptor-holding device in patient's mouth by operator. Note that the correct side of film packet faces the tube head and the mounting dot is toward the occlusal surface.

receptor-holding devices with an aiming bar and localizing ring, the position of the patient's head is not as important, such as in the case in which the holding device does not have these components.

Receptor Position

The receptor is held with its long dimension vertical for anterior projections and horizontal for posterior periapical and bitewing projections (unless vertical bitewings are being exposed). The edge of the receptor always should extend evenly either ⅛ inch below (maxillary) or ⅛ inch above (mandibular) the occlusal plane. This receptor position ensures that adequate surface area of the receptor remains at the apical areas and at the incisal or occlusal surfaces to record the image in its entirety. If a film packet is being used as the receptor of choice, it should be placed in the patient's mouth so that the mounting orientation button is toward the occlusal surface (Fig. 9.16). This helps in mounting and precludes the possibility of the dots being superimposed over the apex of a tooth, possibly creating an artifact that resembles a periapical radiolucency. One useful way of remembering the correct positioning of the film packet in the holding device is by use of the slogan "dot in the slot and the white toward me." This ensures that the operator prevents having the dot superimposed over the apex of the root and reducing the incidence of reversed films by ensuring that the front or white side of the film packet is toward the tooth and not reversed in the patient's mouth. Whichever receptor is being used, it is held in position by the patient with a receptor-holding device as opposed to the unacceptable option of the patient holding the receptor with their finger.

Point of Entry

The **point of entry** is the anatomic position on the patient's face at which the central ray of the x-ray beam is aimed. It corresponds to the middle of the receptor in the patient's

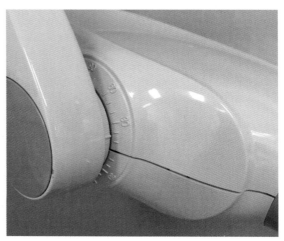

• **Figure 9.17** Vertical angulation is measured in degrees on the outside of the tubehead. (Courtesy of Dr. Kamran Azmoudeh, Santa Rosa, CA.)

mouth. The localizing ring, when used, determines the point of entry by its predetermined relationship to the receptor. The use of rectangular collimation does not change this relationship between the localizing ring, PID, and point of entry.

Vertical Angulation

In the paralleling technique, the **vertical angulation** is set to aim the central ray perpendicular to the receptor. In the bisecting technique (see Chapter 10), the vertical angulation is determined by the bisection of the angle. Vertical angulation of the x-ray beam in the paralleling technique is set by ensuring that the central ray is perpendicular to the tooth and the receptor (Fig. 9.17). When using a paralleling instrument with a localizing ring and aiming bar, the vertical angulation can be set by making sure that the

PID is parallel to the aiming bar and the open end of the rectangular or circular collimator (PID) is in equidistant close proximity to the localizing ring.

Horizontal Angulation

To achieve horizontal angulation, the central ray is directed so that it is perpendicular to the receptor in the horizontal plane. The central ray is directed through the interproximal spaces to avoid overlapping of structures. When using a holding device with a localizing ring, the operator should make sure that there is no uneven space between the end of the PID and the localizing ring on either the right or left side of the ring and PID. Furthermore, to avoid horizontal overlap, the dental professional should place the receptor parallel to the teeth in both the horizontal plane and vertical plane.

> **NOTE**
>
> The recommended paralleling technique procedure box is very detailed in terms of the preferred chair position, receptor position, point of entry, vertical angulation, and horizontal angulation. However, note the italicized recommendations for use of the extension cone paralleling (XCP) holding device for each projection listed, because the use of these instruments simplifies the exposure technique.

Text continued on p. 104

PROCEDURE 9.1 THE FULL-MOUTH SURVEY

Maxillary Central Incisors (Fig. 9.18)

Chair Position. The maxillary occlusal plane is positioned parallel to the floor and the sagittal plane of the patient's face is perpendicular to the floor.

When using paralleling receptor-holding devices with an aiming bar and localizing ring, the position of the patient's head is not as important as in the case in which the holding device does not have these components.

Receptor Position. The receptor is held vertically and positioned in the palate away from the lingual surfaces of the teeth so that the long axis of the receptor is parallel to the long axis of the teeth. The center of the receptor is positioned at the junction between the central incisors. The receptor is placed in the palate so that the entire lengths of the teeth are shown. This parallel placement of the receptor is held in position by one of the devices previously mentioned.

Point of Entry. The central ray is directed at the center of the receptor.

If a localizing ring is used, the open face of the position-indicating device (PID) contacts the ring; this determines the point of entry of the x-ray beam.

Vertical Angulation. The central ray is perpendicular to the tooth and receptor in the vertical plane.

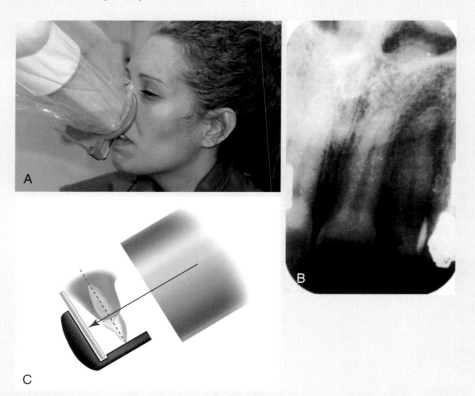

• **Figure 9.18** Maxillary central and lateral incisors. **A,** Receptor holder and position-indicating device (PID). **B,** Radiograph. **C,** Diagram.

Continued

PROCEDURE 9.1 THE FULL-MOUTH SURVEY—cont'd

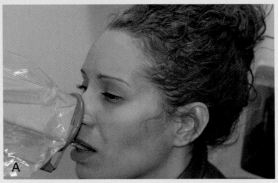

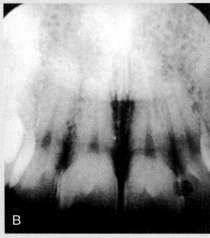

• **Figure 9.19** Right and left maxillary central and lateral incisors. **A,** Receptor-holding device and position-indicating device (PID). **B,** Radiograph.

*When using a paralleling instrument with a localizing ring and aiming bar, the vertical angulation can be set by making sure that the PID is parallel to the aiming bar and the open end of the rectangular or circular collimator (PID) is in equidistant close proximity to the localizing ring.

Horizontal Angulation. The central ray is perpendicular to the tooth and receptor in the horizontal plane (Fig. 9.19).

*When using a holding device with a localizing ring, the operator should make sure that there is no uneven space between the end of the PID and the localizing ring on either the right or left side of the ring and PID.

*To avoid horizontal overlap, the dental professional should place the receptor parallel to the teeth in both the vertical and horizontal planes.

HELPFUL HINT

When using a localizing device, make sure that it is as close to the patient's face without touching as possible. This prevents the ring position away from the receptor thereby increasing the target-receptor distance (or focal-film distance [FFD]), which would result in a thin (light) image exhibiting an application of the inverse square law.

Maxillary Canines (Fig. 9.20)

Chair Position. The maxillary occlusal plane is parallel to the floor, and the sagittal plane of the patient's face is perpendicular to the floor.

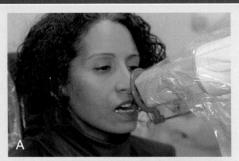

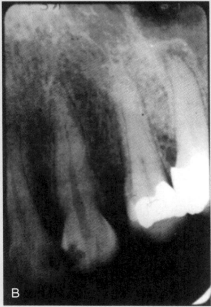

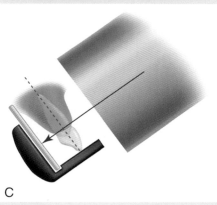

• **Figure 9.20** Maxillary canine. **A,** Receptor-holding device and position-indicating device (PID). **B,** Radiograph. **C,** Diagram.

*When using paralleling receptor-holding devices with an aiming bar and localizing ring, the position of the patient's head is not as important as in the case in which the holding device does not have these components.

Receptor Position. The receptor is held vertically, away from the lingual surface of the canine and parallel to its long axis. The center of the receptor is behind and centered on the canine and positioned in the palate so that the entire length of the canine is shown. The receptor is held in position by a holding device.

PROCEDURE 9.1   THE FULL-MOUTH SURVEY—cont'd

Point of Entry. The central ray is directed at the center of the receptor or, if a localizing ring is used, it is brought into flat contact with the open-ended PID.

*If a localizing ring is used, the open face of the PID contacts the ring; this determines the point of entry of the x-ray beam.

Vertical Angulation. The central ray is perpendicular to the receptor in the vertical plane.

*When using a paralleling instrument with a localizing ring and aiming bar, the vertical angulation can be set by making sure that the PID is parallel to the aiming bar and the open end of the rectangular or circular collimator (PID) is in equidistant close proximity to the localizing ring.

Horizontal Angulation. The central ray is perpendicular to the receptor in the horizontal plane.

*When using a holding device with a localizing ring, the operator should make sure that there is no uneven space between the end of the PID and the localizing ring on either the right or left side of the ring and PID.

*To avoid horizontal overlap, the dental professional should place the receptor parallel to the teeth in both the vertical and horizontal planes.

HELPFUL HINT

Receptor placement of the maxillary canine may be very difficult. In order to achieve parallelism, the receptor may have to be positioned across the arch, resulting in an increased object-receptor distance. Also, the operator should make sure that if a film packet is used, it is curved away from the source of radiation to accommodate the palatal arch. If the film is curved toward the radiation, the lead foil backing will be superimposed over the superior aspect of the radiograph. Furthermore, the operator must make sure that the film does not come out of the holder when it contacts the palate so as not to cut off the incisal edge.

Maxillary Premolars (Fig. 9.21)

Chair Position. The maxillary occlusal plane is parallel to the floor, and the sagittal plane of the patient's face is perpendicular to the floor.

*When using paralleling receptor-holding devices with an aiming bar and localizing ring, the position of the patient's head is not as important as in the case in which the holding device does not have these components.

Receptor Position. The receptor is held horizontally and positioned away from the lingual surfaces of the premolar so that its long axis is parallel to the long axis of the premolar. In the maxillary premolar and molar region, the receptor position may be in the middle of the palate. The center of the receptor aligns with the second premolar. The receptor is positioned in the palate so that the entire length of the teeth is shown on the receptor. The receptor is held in position by a holding device.

Point of Entry. The central ray is directed at the center of the receptor or, if a localizing ring is used, it is brought into flat contact with the open-ended PID.

*If a localizing ring is used, the open face of the PID contacts the ring; this determines the point of entry of the x-ray beam.

Vertical Angulation. The central ray is perpendicular to the receptor in the vertical plane.

*When using a paralleling instrument with a localizing ring and aiming bar, the vertical angulation can be set by

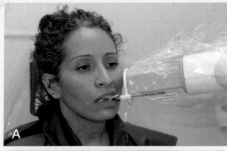

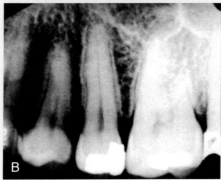

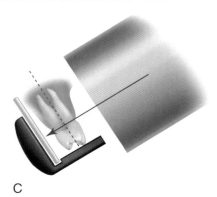

C

• **Figure 9.21** Maxillary premolars. **A,** Receptor-holding device and position-indicating device (PID). **B,** Radiograph. **C,** Diagram.

making sure that the PID is parallel to the aiming bar and the open end of the rectangular or circular collimator (PID) is in equidistant close proximity to the localizing ring.

Horizontal Angulation. The central ray is perpendicular to the receptor in the horizontal plane.

*When using a holding device with a localizing ring, the operator should make sure that there is no uneven space between the end of the PID and the localizing ring on either the right or left side of the ring and PID.

*To avoid horizontal overlap, the dental professional should place the receptor parallel to the teeth in both the vertical and horizontal planes.

HELPFUL HINT

Make sure as the arch starts to turn that the receptor remains parallel to the long axis, as well as the horizontal axis of the premolar teeth being radiographed.

Continued

PROCEDURE 9.1 THE FULL-MOUTH SURVEY—cont'd

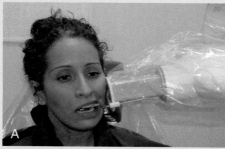

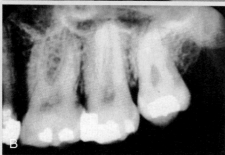

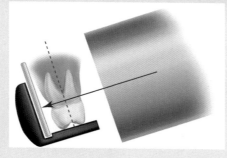

C

• **Figure 9.22** Maxillary molars. **A,** Receptor-holding device and position-indicating device (PID). **B,** Radiograph. **C,** Diagram.

Maxillary Molars (Fig. 9.22)

Chair Position. The maxillary occlusal plane is positioned parallel to the floor, and the sagittal plane of the patient's face is perpendicular to the floor.

When using paralleling receptor-holding devices with an aiming bar and localizing ring, the position of the patient's head is not as important as in the case in which the holding device does not have these components.

Receptor Position. The receptor is held horizontally and positioned away from the lingual surfaces of the molars so that the long axis of the receptor lies parallel to the long axes of the molars. The center of the receptor aligns with the middle of the second molar and the receptor is positioned in the palate so that the entire length of the teeth is shown. The receptor is held in position by a holding device.

Point of Entry. The central ray is directed at the center of the receptor or the localizing ring is brought into flat contact with the open-ended PID.

If a localizing ring is used, the open face of the PID contacts the ring; this determines the point of entry of the x-ray beam.

Vertical Angulation. The central ray is perpendicular to the receptor in the vertical plane.

When using a paralleling instrument with a localizing ring and aiming bar, the vertical angulation can be set by

making sure that the PID is parallel to the aiming bar and the open end of the rectangular or circular collimator (PID) is in equidistant close proximity to the localizing ring.

Horizontal Angulation. The central ray is perpendicular to the receptor in the horizontal plane.

When using a holding device with a localizing ring, the operator should make sure that there is no uneven space between the end of the PID and the localizing ring on either the right or left side of the ring and PID.

To avoid horizontal overlap, the dental professional should place the receptor parallel to the teeth in both the vertical and horizontal planes.

HELPFUL HINT

If you are *not* using a localizing ring, you can offset the receptor by placing the receptor distally in the bite piece and by having the center of the bite piece over the first molar.

If the mouth is unusually small or the teeth crowded, it may be necessary to use a smaller receptor, such as #0 or #1. Remember that it is the anatomic variants of the teeth and bone that dictate the receptor size that should be used.

If the operator is having difficulty placing the receptor to include the third molar region, the operator can place the receptor on the first molar when the mouth is fully open and ask the patient to close slightly, then slide the receptor onto the second molar before finally securing the receptor.

Bitewing Projections

The technique for bitewing projections is the same in the paralleling and bisecting-angle techniques except for the use of the 16-inch target-receptor distance (or FFD) used in the paralleling as opposed to the bisecting technique. Bitewing projections are always paralleled projections, no matter what technique is used for the periapical projections. The receptor is positioned by the bite piece parallel to the crowns of both upper and lower teeth, and the central ray is directed perpendicular to the receptor.

Premolar and Molar Bitewing Projections (Fig. 9.23)

Chair Position. The maxillary occlusal plane is positioned parallel to the floor, and the sagittal plane of the patient's face is perpendicular to the floor.

When using paralleling receptor-holding devices with an aiming bar and localizing ring, the position of the patient's head is not as important as in the case in which the holding device does not have these components.

Film Position. When the premolars are radiographed, the bitewing holder is placed on the occlusal surface of the second mandibular premolar. This depresses the receptor into the floor of the mouth. While the operator holds the bite piece down with one's thumb and forefinger, the patient is instructed to bite on the bite piece. The operator should be sure that the patient is biting on the back teeth and not just bringing the incisors together. If the back teeth are not moved to centric occlusion, the receptor is not secure; consequently, it may move and not be oriented correctly. The procedure for radiographing the molars is the same as that previously mentioned for the premolars except that the bite piece is centered over the occlusal surface of the second molar.

Point of Entry. The central ray is directed at the bitewing bite piece, which is held in position by the patient's teeth.

If a film holder with a localizing ring and aiming arm are used, the open end of the PID is placed against the ring.

PROCEDURE 9.1   THE FULL-MOUTH SURVEY—cont'd

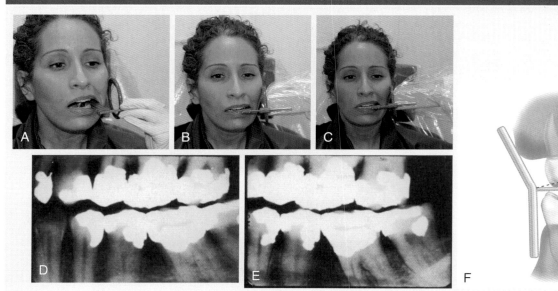

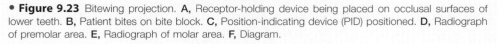

• **Figure 9.23** Bitewing projection. **A,** Receptor-holding device being placed on occlusal surfaces of lower teeth. **B,** Patient bites on bite block. **C,** Position-indicating device (PID) positioned. **D,** Radiograph of premolar area. **E,** Radiograph of molar area. **F,** Diagram.

Vertical Angulation. The central ray is perpendicular to the receptor in the horizontal plane.

When using a paralleling instrument with a localizing ring and aiming bar, the vertical angulation can be set by making sure that the PID is parallel to the aiming bar and the open end of the rectangular or circular collimator (PID) is in equidistant close proximity to the localizing ring.

Horizontal Angulation. Horizontal angulation is a critical factor in the bitewing projection; utmost attention should be paid to horizontal positioning. An overlapping image on the bitewing projection renders the image useless. The central ray should be perpendicular to the receptor in the horizontal plane and should go through the contact points of the premolars or molars.

When using a holding device with a localizing ring, the operator should make sure that there is no uneven space between the end of the PID and the localizing ring on either the right or left side of the ring and PID.

To avoid horizontal overlap, the dental professional should place the receptor parallel to the teeth in both the vertical and horizontal planes.

HELPFUL HINT

When taking bitewings without the use of a localizing ring, it helps to align the beam by having your index finger touching the bitewing tab in the buccal sulcus of the patient's mouth, using your finger as an extension of the position-indicating device (PID). You can also ask the patient to smile so that the tab is revealed.

Vertical Bitewings (Fig. 9.24)

Vertical bitewings are used when the desired area would not be seen on the image with the usual bitewing placement; this could be the case in advanced bone loss, root caries, or tooth eruption. The receptor is placed in the patient's mouth with the longer side vertically positioned. All other exposure factors remain the same. It is necessary to use the paste-on tabs and not the loops or the XCP vertical bitewing instruments with this technique. The vertical bitewing can be used in a posterior or anterior region. There are paralleling instruments available in the contemporary market that now include vertical bitewing attachments (i.e., XCP vertical bitewing instrument).

Mandibular Incisors (Fig. 9.25)

Chair Position. The patient is positioned so that when the mouth is open the mandibular occlusal plane is parallel to the floor and the sagittal plane of the patient's face is perpendicular to the floor.

When using paralleling receptor-holding devices with an aiming bar and localizing ring, the position of the patient's head is not as important as in the case in which the holding device does not have these components.

Receptor Position. The receptor is held vertically and positioned away from the lingual surfaces of the incisors so that the long axis of the receptor is parallel to the long axes of the incisors. The center of the receptor is positioned at the midline between the two mandibular central incisors so that all four incisors appear on the image. The receptor is depressed into the floor of the mouth so that the entire length of the teeth is shown. It may be necessary to displace the tongue distally and to gently depress the floor of the mouth to achieve this. The receptor is held in position by a holding device.

Point of Entry. The central ray is directed at the center of the receptor.

The localizing ring is brought into flat contact with the open-ended PID.

Vertical Angulation. The central ray is perpendicular to the receptor in the vertical plane.

When using a paralleling instrument with a localizing ring and aiming bar, the vertical angulation can be set by making sure that the PID is parallel to the aiming bar and the open end of the rectangular or circular collimator (PID) is in equidistant close proximity to the localizing ring.

Continued

PROCEDURE 9.1 THE FULL-MOUTH SURVEY—cont'd

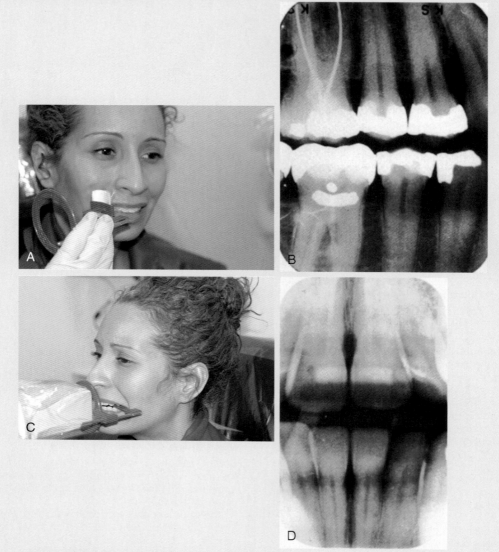

• **Figure 9.24** Vertical bitewing. **A,** Posterior receptor position. **B,** Posterior radiograph. **C,** Anterior projection position. **D,** Anterior radiograph.

Horizontal Angulation. The central ray is perpendicular to the receptor in the horizontal plane.

> **HELPFUL HINT**
>
> When taking this projection, remember that in order to achieve parallelism between the teeth and the receptor in some cases it may be necessary to position the receptor far back in the floor of the mouth at the level of the molars. You may also start out with the receptor on an angle and then bring the receptor into a parallel position slowly with the closure of the mandible. The operator may also place an opened gauze pad under the receptor to prevent it from irritating the floor of the mouth.

Mandibular Canines (Fig. 9.26)

Chair Position. The patient is positioned so that when the mouth is open the mandibular occlusal plane is parallel to the floor and the sagittal plane of the patient's face is perpendicular to the floor.

*When using paralleling receptor-holding devices with an aiming bar and localizing ring, the position of the patient's head is not as important as in the case in which the holding device does not have these components.

Receptor Position. The receptor is held vertically and positioned away from the lingual surface of the canine so that its long axis is parallel to that of the canine. The receptor is positioned so that the canine is in the center of the receptor. The receptor is depressed into the floor of the mouth so that the entire length of the tooth is shown on the image. The receptor is held in position by a holding device.

Point of Entry. The central ray is directed at the center of the receptor or the localizing ring is brought into flat contact with the open-ended PID.

Vertical Angulation. The central ray is perpendicular to the receptor in the vertical plane.

PROCEDURE 9.1   THE FULL-MOUTH SURVEY—cont'd

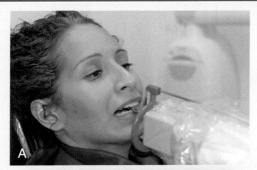

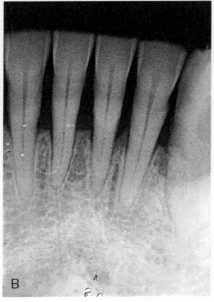

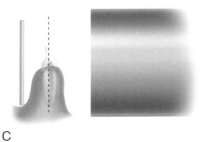

• **Figure 9.25** Mandibular incisors. **A,** Receptor-holding device and position-indicating device (PID). **B,** Radiograph. **C,** Diagram.

*When using a paralleling instrument with a localizing ring and aiming bar, the vertical angulation can be set by making sure that the PID is parallel to the aiming bar and the open end of the rectangular or circular collimator (PID) is in equidistant close proximity to the localizing ring.

Horizontal Angulation. The central ray is perpendicular to the receptor in the horizontal plane.

*When using a holding device with a localizing ring, the operator should make sure that there is no uneven space between the end of the PID and the localizing ring on either the right or left side of the ring and PID.

* To avoid horizontal overlap, the dental professional should place the receptor parallel to the teeth in both the vertical and horizontal planes.

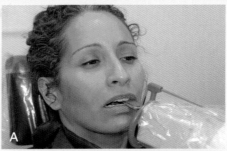

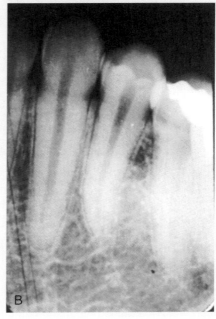

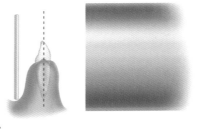

• **Figure 9.26** Mandibular canine. **A,** Receptor-holding device and position-indicating device (PID). **B,** Radiograph. **C,** Diagram.

HELPFUL HINT

Be sure that the receptor is placed below and not on top of the tongue, because it is a muscle and sometimes very difficult to displace. As it is said, "In a war with the tongue, the tongue always wins."

Mandibular Premolars (Fig. 9.27)

Chair Position. The patient is positioned so that when the mouth is open the mandibular occlusal plane is parallel to the floor and the sagittal plane of the patient's face is perpendicular to the floor.

Continued

PROCEDURE 9.1 THE FULL-MOUTH SURVEY—cont'd

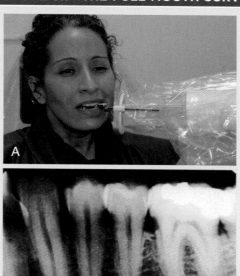

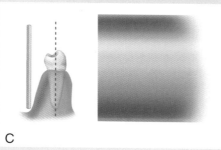

• **Figure 9.27** Mandibular premolar. **A,** Receptor-holding device and position-indicating device (PID). **B,** Radiograph. **C,** Diagram.

When using paralleling receptor-holding devices with an aiming bar and localizing ring, the position of the patient's head is not as important as in the case in which the holding device does not have these components.

Receptor Position. The receptor is held horizontally and positioned so that it is parallel to the long axis of the premolar. The object-target distance in both the mandibular premolar and molar regions is almost minimal, because the anatomy allows the receptor to be positioned very close to the tooth and still be parallel. The receptor is centered on the center of the second premolar. The receptor is depressed into the floor of the mouth so that the entire length of the teeth shows on the image. The receptor is held in position by a holding device.

Point of Entry. The central ray is directed at the center of the receptor, or if a localizing ring is used, it is brought into flat contact with the open-ended PID.

Vertical Angulation. The central ray is directed perpendicular to the receptor in the vertical plane.

Horizontal Angulation. The central ray is perpendicular to the receptor in the horizontal plane.

HELPFUL HINT

If a film packet is being used as the receptor in this instance, in a small mouth, it may be helpful to roll (not bend) the lower anterior corner of the film packet to ensure the patient's comfort.

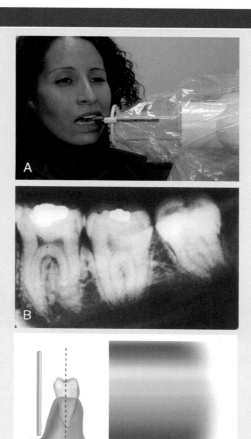

• **Figure 9.28** Mandibular molars. **A,** Receptor-holding device and position-indicating device (PID). **B,** Radiograph. **C,** Diagram

Mandibular Molars (Fig. 9.28)

Chair Position. The patient is positioned so that when the mouth is open the mandibular occlusal plane is parallel to the floor, and the sagittal plane of the patient's face is perpendicular to the floor.

Receptor Position. The receptor is held horizontally and positioned lingually to the molar so that the long axis of the receptor is parallel to the long axes of the molars. The receptor is centered behind the second molar and depressed into the floor of the mouth so that the entire length of the teeth appears on the film. The packet is held in position by a holding device.

Point of Entry. The central ray is directed at the center of the receptor or, if a localizing ring is used, it is brought into flat contact with the open-ended PID.

Vertical Angulation. The central ray is directed perpendicular to the receptor in the vertical plane.

When using a paralleling instrument with a localizing ring and aiming bar, the vertical angulation can be set by making sure that the PID is parallel to the aiming bar and the open end of the rectangular or circular collimator (PID) is in equidistant close proximity to the localizing ring.

Horizontal Angulation. The central ray is perpendicular to the receptor in the horizontal plane.

When using a holding device with a localizing ring, the operator should make sure that there is no uneven space between the end of the PID and the localizing ring on either the right or left side of the ring and PID.

PROCEDURE 9.1   THE FULL-MOUTH SURVEY—cont'd

*To avoid horizontal overlap, the dental professional should place the receptor parallel to the teeth in both the vertical and horizontal plane.

HELPFUL HINT

When positioning the receptor, make sure that the middle of the receptor is aligned with the middle of the second molar.

Common Dental Radiographic Exposure Errors

Note: Refer to the Appendix for a detailed description of each of the following exposure errors.

All of the errors mentioned and illustrated in this chapter are also possible with the bisecting technique, but the incidence differs. Although elongation and foreshortening are the most common bisecting errors, they are not as common in the paralleling technique. The most common error in the paralleling technique, even with the use of positioning devices, is in receptor placement. If the receptor and holder are not placed correctly in the patient's mouth, the paralleling technique does not work. The most common error is not placing the receptor deep enough in the floor of the mouth or high enough in the palate, thus cutting off the apices of the teeth as a result of inadequate closure.

With the use of the localizing ring, which is aligned with the center of the receptor, collimator cutoff (formerly known as *cone cutting*) can be practically eliminated.

Occlusal plane and sagittal plane orientation of the patient's head is not important if the localizing ring on the receptor-holding device is used, as long as the open end of the PID is brought into flat contact with the localizing ring.

Horizontal overlapping of the images also is eliminated with the proper use of the positioning device and localizing ring and the correct parallel placement of the receptor to the teeth in the horizontal plane.

The rest of the errors mentioned in this chapter (i.e., film reversal, overbending, crescent marks, overexposing and underexposing, double exposure, and failure to remove dental appliances) are all possible with the bisecting technique and their remedies are the same. However, film reversal, overbending of the film packet, overexposing and underexposing, and double exposure are errors that could occur with conventional (film-based) radiography but are not likely to occur with digital radiography.

An unexposed area on the radiograph occurs when the x-ray beam is not centered on the receptor. This is called collimator cutoff (formerly known as cone cutting; Fig. 9.29) and is caused by improper alignment of the x-ray beam and the receptor. Collimator cutoff can occur with both conventional and digital radiography.

Remedy. The central ray of the x-ray beam should be aligned carefully with the center of the receptor. With circular collimation, the aperture of the diaphragm allows for a beam diameter, measured at the face, of 2¾ inches (2.75 inches; 7 cm). Size #2 adult film is 1¼ × 1⅝ inches, which leaves almost ¼- to ½-inch leeway for human error in all directions. It is not sufficient to simply identify collimator cutoff; it should be analyzed to pinpoint the error and thus remedy it accordingly. For example, if it is always the distal part of a radiograph in a projection that is cut off, then the point of entry must be

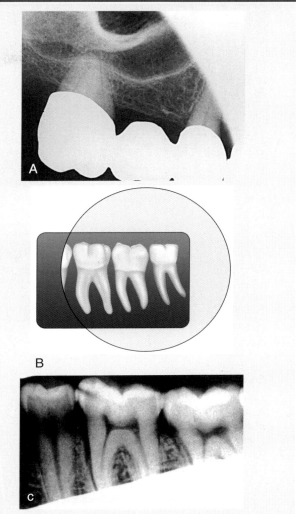

- **Figure 9.29 A,** Collimator cutoff (cone cutting). Central ray positioned too far distal. **B,** Diagram of collimator cutoff ("cone cutting"). Central ray positioned too far mesial. **C,** Cone cutting with rectangular collimation.

moved mesially. The localizing ring on a paralleling receptor-holding device aligns the beam and the receptor and aids in eliminating collimator cutoff with both circular and rectangular collimation.

Film reversal (Fig. 9.30). Film reversal was formerly referred to as the *herringbone effect*, because the herringbone pattern that was embossed on the lead foil backing was transferred to the processed reversed radiograph. The herringbone, light (thin) image results from placing the film packet backward in the patient's mouth. The x-rays are attenuated in a pattern by the lead foil before striking the film. The geometric pattern embossed by the lead foil backing distinguishes this light radiograph from other underexposure errors. The original geometric pattern was that of a herringbone; the name has survived even though the present pattern now resembles tiny adjacent boxes, a checkerboard, or even tire tracks. Because of the nature of this error, it can

Continued

PROCEDURE 9.1 THE FULL-MOUTH SURVEY—cont'd

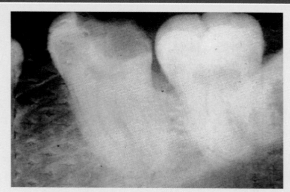

• **Figure 9.30** Film reversal. Film packet placed in mouth with the wrong side toward the tube.

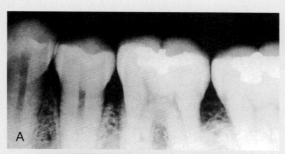

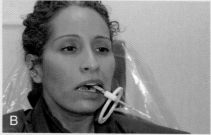

• **Figure 9.31 A,** Nondiagnostic image caused by poor film packet placement. Note that apices of teeth are not seen. **B,** Poor film placement. Note how much film is visible above occlusal plane of tooth.

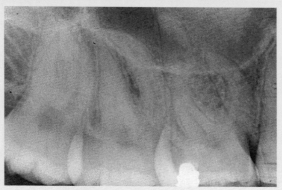

• **Figure 9.32** Overlapped images.

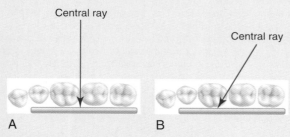

• **Figure 9.33** Proper **(A)** and improper **(B)** horizontal angulation of x-ray beam.

only occur with conventional, film-based radiography and does not occur with digital radiography.

Remedy. The front and the back of the film packet should be identified. Some manufacturers color-code or change the texture of the back of the film packet to distinguish the front side from the back side of the film packet. Operators should develop the habit of looking for these aids.

Poor receptor placement (Fig. 9.31). The receptor has been poorly positioned if the whole tooth does not show on the image. The receptor is not sufficiently placed to record the apex or biting surface of the tooth or teeth being radiographed or the tooth that should be centered is not. Poor receptor placement also occurs if the patient does not bite on both sides of the biting surface of the receptor holder. This error is known as *inadequate closure.* Furthermore, if the receptor is not positioned correctly in the patient's mouth and does not show all of the desired teeth and surrounding structures, the error exhibited is also attributed to poor receptor placement.

Poor receptor placement can occur with both conventional (film-based) and digital radiography.

Remedy. Only ⅛ inch of the receptor should project above or below the occlusal or incisal edges of the teeth. Also, the patient should adequately close on both sides of the bite piece. In addition, the receptor should be positioned correctly so that the image includes the desired teeth and their surrounding structures.

Overlapping (Figs. 9.32 and 9.33). Overlapping of the images of the teeth results if the central ray is not perpendicular to the receptor and the teeth in the horizontal plane. Another cause of horizontal overlap is when the receptor is not placed parallel to the teeth in the horizontal plane. Horizontal overlap can occur with both conventional (film-based) and digital radiography.

Remedy. Make sure that the central ray is perpendicular to the receptor in the horizontal plane. This ensures that the central ray is directed straight through the contacts instead of crossing the contacts diagonally and causing overlapping of the interproximal surfaces of the teeth. When using a holding device with a localizing ring (i.e., XCP), the operator should make sure that there is no uneven space between the end of the PID and the localizing ring on either the right or left side of the ring and PID. If the receptor is placed parallel to the teeth, the localizing ring aligns the beam perpendicular to the receptor.

Crescent marks and bent films (Figs. 9.34 and 9.35). Black crescent-shaped marks or black marks from overbending the film packet can be caused by excessive bending or excessive manipulation of the film packet, which cracks the emulsion. These marks show on the film after it is processed. In addition, if the film packet is bent but does not crack the emulsion, the tooth appears as if it had been

PROCEDURE 9.1   THE FULL-MOUTH SURVEY—cont'd

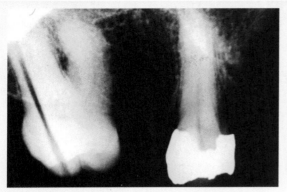

• **Figure 9.34** Black line caused by cracking of film emulsion.

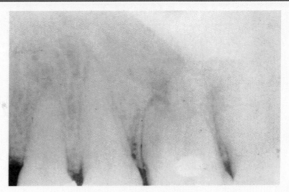

• **Figure 9.36** Underexposed radiograph.

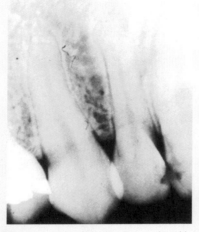

• **Figure 9.35** Result of overbending film packet. Note upper-right corner.

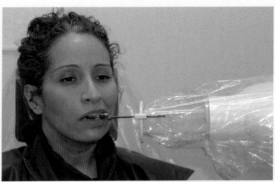

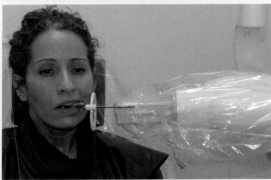

• **Figure 9.37** Light film can be caused by increased focal-film distance (FFD) without compensatory increase in exposure time. Note distance between the patient's face and position-indicating device (PID) in both photos.

stretched on the resultant image. Because of the nature of this error, it can only occur with conventional, film-based radiography and does not occur with digital radiography.

Remedy. Films can be made more pliable by rolling them slightly against one's index finger, which also may allow them to fit better in the patient's mouth. Films should not be bent to adapt to anatomic surfaces; they should be gently shaped or curved to conform to the arch. X-rays travel in straight lines; they do not turn corners to expose bent films.

Light films (Fig. 9.36). Light (thin) films without adequate density can result from underexposure or underdevelopment assuming that an improper time setting has been used. If less exposure time than is needed is set, the dental structures are not adequately penetrated, and the film does not differentiate structures of different densities. Also, the operator should avoid removing one's finger from the exposure button prematurely, because this can cause an underexposed film as well. Another radiographer's error that can cause underexposure is unwittingly increasing the target-receptor distance (or FFD) by failing to bring the open end of the PID close to the patient's face. The exposure times are calculated for a target-receptor distance (or FFD) that assumes a PID placement that is as close to the face as possible. If the PID is carelessly positioned away from the face, the inverse square law intensifies the error,

not just by the increased distance but by the square of that distance (Fig. 9.37).

Light or thin images generally occur with the use of conventional film-based radiography. Although it is possible to underexpose a digital image, the digital system has tools for rectifying this error. The resultant image can be altered by adjusting the contrast of the digital image before the image is saved.

Remedy. For preventing underexposure, the proper time settings on the machine should be set before an exposure is made. Underexposed films can also occur as a result of improper kilovoltage and milliamperage settings. However, the newer dental x-ray units have preset kilovoltage and milliamperage settings; thus, they currently are not

Continued

PROCEDURE 9.1 THE FULL-MOUTH SURVEY—cont'd

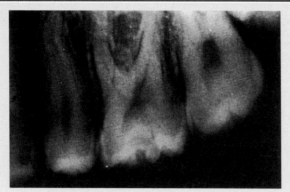

• **Figure 9.38** Overexposed radiograph.

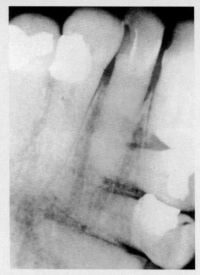

• **Figure 9.39** Double exposure on a radiograph.

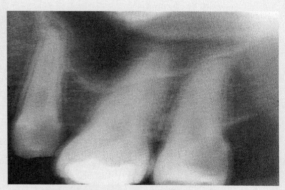

• **Figure 9.40** Blurred image caused by patient movement.

the cause of an underexposed film. For a discussion of underdevelopment, see Chapter 11.

Dark films (Fig. 9.38). Dark (dense) films are the result of overexposure or overdevelopment, the opposites of the causes of light films. The predetermined length of the target-receptor distance (or FFD) with a recessed target or the predetermined length of the PID (if the target is not recessed) prevents the possibility of a decreased target-receptor distance (or FFD) as the cause for an overexposed film. However, if the operator sets the exposure time higher than is needed for a particular projection, an overexposed film can be produced. If a film is over penetrated, it is black and no dental structures show or they are difficult to differentiate.

Dark or dense images generally occur with the use of conventional, film-based radiography. Although it is possible to overexpose a digital image, the digital system has tools for rectifying this error. The resultant image can be altered by adjusting the contrast of the digital image before the image is saved.

Remedy. To avoid overexposure, operators should check all settings on the control panel before taking an exposure. Overexposed films can also occur as a result of improper kilovoltage and milliamperage settings. However, the newer dental x-ray units have preset kilovoltage and milliamperage settings; thus, they currently are not the cause of an overexposed film. For a discussion of overdevelopment, see Chapter 11.

Double exposure (Fig. 9.39). A double exposure results from using the same film packet twice. This is a careless error and indicates lack of attention to detail. Because of the nature of this error, it can only occur with conventional film-based radiography and does not occur with digital radiography.

Remedy. After the film packet has been exposed, it should be placed in a receptacle meant for exposed films only. Exposed and unexposed films should never be kept together in the same receptacle. When barrier envelopes are used, they can be removed between exposures to easily distinguish exposed films from unexposed films.

Blurred images (Fig. 9.40). Blurred images are the result of patient, receptor, PID, or tube head movement during the exposure. Blurred images can occur with both conventional (film-based) and digital radiography. However, with the current use of fast-speed film or (especially) digital radiography, there is less of a chance for movement during exposure because of the very short exposure times utilized.

Remedy. Tube heads, PIDs, and arms should be adjusted to prevent vibration and drifting. In most states, drifting is a serious health code violation. It is also suggested to make sure that the unit arm is stabilized on a nearby wall to prevent drifting. In addition, good chairside technique by the dental professional can help to prevent receptor and patient movement.

Failure to remove dental appliances, eyeglasses (with metallic components) or facial jewelry (Figs. 9.41 and 9.42). If dental appliances or facial jewelry is not removed, the metallic portions will be superimposed on the teeth and surrounding structures.

Remedy. It should be a part of the work routine to have patients remove all dentures, nose and lip jewelry, and eyeglasses. For panoramic and extraoral projections, patients also must remove earrings, hearing aids, necklaces, hair clips, and any other metallic objects from the entire head and neck region.

Common bitewing errors (Fig. 9.43). The three most common errors seen on bitewing radiographs are overlapping, collimator cutoff, and poor receptor placement.

PROCEDURE 9.1   THE FULL-MOUTH SURVEY—cont'd

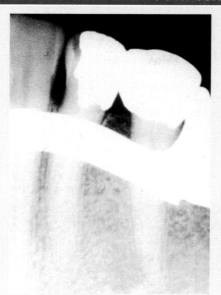

• **Figure 9.41** Patient's metal-based partial denture was not removed.

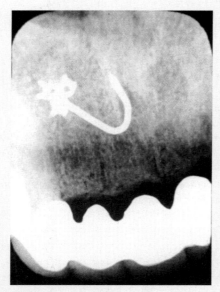

• **Figure 9.42** Facial jewelry (nose ring) was not removed.

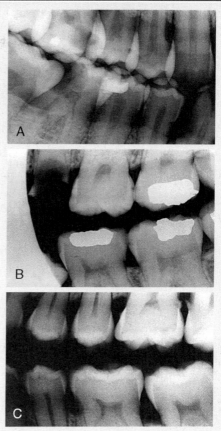

• **Figure 9.43 A,** Overlapped bitewing. **B,** Collimator cutoff on bitewing. **C,** Improper film placement on a bitewing.

Overlapping (see Fig. 9.43A). Overlapping results from improper horizontal beam alignment or improper placement of the receptor in the horizontal plane. Bitewing overlap can occur with conventional and digital radiography.

Remedy. The beam should be aligned in the horizontal plane so that it is at right angles to the receptor. Also, the receptor should be placed parallel to the teeth in the horizontal plane.

Collimator cutoff (cone cutting; see Fig. 9.43B). Collimator cutoff is failure to align the central ray with the center of the receptor. It can also occur when bitewing tabs instead of XCP instruments are being used, because the operator loses sight of the bite tab when the patient closes the mouth. This error can occur with bitewing exposures in conventional and digital radiography.

Remedy. It is recommended to use paralleling instruments (i.e., XCP devices) with localizing rings to decrease the incidence of collimator cutoff. A localizing ring can be used to help center the x-ray beam. When using bitewing tabs, the bite tab should be kept visible by asking the patient to smile while biting. If this is not possible, the operator can touch the tab with one hand while aligning the beam with the other. The central ray is then directed at the tab.

Poor receptor placement (see Fig. 9.43C). Poor receptor placement occurs with bitewing films in various ways. When the patient is allowed to bite the receptor into position after the operator has let go of the holder or when the patient bites in protrusive instead of centric relation, allowing the receptor to float free and be repositioned by the tongue. Also, inadequate closure can occur when the patient is not biting completely on both sides of the bite piece or when the patient holds the bitewing holder with the lips instead of with the teeth, which can produce an image that does not show the teeth of both arches equally represented. If all of the desired structures are not represented on the image because of improper receptor placement in the patient's mouth, this is considered a poor

Continued

PROCEDURE 9.1   THE FULL-MOUTH SURVEY—cont'd

receptor placement error as well. For example, if the operator takes a premolar bitewing and the distal surface of the canine and the first and second premolars are not shown completely, that would be considered a receptor placement error. All of these errors can occur with bitewing exposures in conventional and digital radiography.

   Remedy. The operator should not let go of the receptor holder (or bitewing tab) until the patient is biting on it in centric occlusion. The operator should make sure that the patient is biting completely on the bite piece and not using the lips to stabilize the bitewing holder in place. Also, the operator is responsible for centering the bitewing holder and receptor correctly so that all of the desired structures for that specific projection will appear on the image.

Chapter Summary

- The radiographic examination is an important part of the dental examination that stresses the need for radiographs that are diagnostically acceptable and are taken only when necessary for the patient's immediate dental health needs. The goal of dental radiography is to produce the most diagnostically acceptable radiographs for the least amount of exposure to the patient.
- A *periapical projection* shows the entire tooth from the incisal edge or the occlusal surface to the apex of the root and 2 to 3 mm of surrounding periapical bone. This projection is necessary to diagnose normal or pathologic conditions of tooth crowns and root, bone, and tooth formation and eruption (see Fig. 9.2). The *bitewing projection* shows the upper and lower teeth in occlusion in one image. Only the crowns and alveolar crest of the bone of adjacent teeth are seen. It is used for detecting interproximal decay, interproximal calculus, periodontal bone loss, recurrent decay under restorations, and faulty restorations. Vertical bitewings can be used diagnostically for root caries, bone loss of 5 mm or more, and in pediatric patients to see the growth and development of the secondary dentition.
- The basic principles of the paralleling technique for intraoral periapical projections is that the receptor and the long axis of the tooth being radiographed must be parallel to each other, and the central ray of the x-ray beam must be directed perpendicular to both. The paralleling technique is preferred when compared with the bisecting technique, because it produces better diagnostic images (dimensional accuracy), less exposure to critical organs (such as, the thyroid gland and the lens of the eye), a smaller exit dose, and easier standardization and execution. However, placement of the receptors with the paralleling technique may be difficult and uncomfortable for the patient.

- Before exposing intraoral radiographs, the operator should follow infection control procedures; exhibit radiation safety precautions, including placing the lead apron and thyroid collar on the patient and maintaining the recommended 6-foot distance standing behind an acceptable barrier when exposing radiographs; set up the receptor-holding devices; gather and place all necessary supplies near the exposure area; adjust the dental chair; ask the patient to remove any metallic objects that will be in the direct path of the primary beam; turn on the x-ray unit; and set the exposure parameters that are appropriate for the patient.
- For each exposure, the dental radiographer should place the receptor in the holding device, ensure that the receptor is placed parallel to the teeth being exposed, aim the central ray perpendicular to the teeth and receptor in both the vertical and horizontal planes, place the receptor so that all the teeth that are desired will appear on the resultant image, and direct the central ray at the center of the receptor.
- Receptor-holding devices with aiming arms and localizing rings are recommended to simplify the intraoral paralleling exposure technique and to aid the radiographer in reducing the incidence of errors, including collimator cutoff, overlapping, foreshortening, and elongation.
- The errors that could potentially occur with both conventional film-based radiography and digital radiography are collimator cutoff, horizontal overlapping, blurred images, and failure to remove metallic objects. Those errors that are related to both film-based radiography and digital radiography but are more likely to happen with conventional (film-based) radiography are underexposed (light) and overexposed (dark) images. The errors that transpire only with conventional (film-based) radiography are reversed film, double exposure, and overbending of the film packet.

Chapter Review Questions

Multiple Choice

1. A full-mouth survey (FMS):
   a. Varies in need
   b. Varies in number
   c. Is prescribed based on a patient's radiation history
   d. Can be prescribed based on the patient's immediate dental health needs
   e. All of the above

2. Interproximal caries, interproximal calculus, recurrent caries, periodontal bone loss, and the fit of metallic restorations are *best* seen on:
   a. Panoramic radiographs
   b. Bitewing radiographs
   c. Periapical radiographs
   d. Topographic occlusal radiographs
   e. Right-angle occlusal radiographs

3. Vertical bitewings can be used for viewing:
   a. Root caries
   b. Tooth eruption
   c. Advanced bone loss
   d. Bone loss of more than 5 mm
   e. All of the above

4. The advantage in using a film holder with a localizing ring is that it *primarily:*
   a. Reduces the incidence of collimator cutoff
   b. Reduces the incidence of double exposure
   c. Keeps the film in place more securely than another film holder
   d. Reduces the incidence of overlapping
   e. Under all circumstances, guarantees a more diagnostic image

5. Blurred images are a result of movement during an exposure. This error can be remedied by making sure that the white side of the film packet is toward the source of radiation.
   a. Both statements are false.
   b. Both statements are true.
   c. The first statement is true, and the second statement is false.
   d. The first statement is false, and the second statement is true.
   e. There is not enough information to answer the question.

Identify the Following Intraoral Radiographic Errors

1. This image:

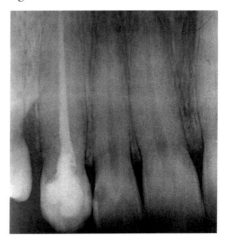

   a. Was produced by too much vertical angulation
   b. Was produced by too little vertical angulation
   c. Is known as elongation
   d. Both a and c are correct.
   e. Both b and c are correct.

2. This error can be remedied by:

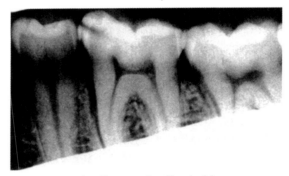

   a. Centering the film on the film holder
   b. Centering the central ray while using a cylindrical column
   c. Centering the central ray while using a rectangular column
   d. Centering the tooth on the film
   e. Making sure the developer solution contacts the entire film

3. The dark diagonal artifact on the molar in the accompanying image can be remedied by:

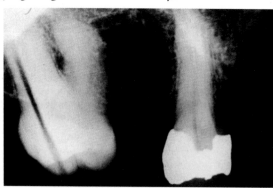

a. Avoiding excess exposure time
b. Avoiding excess film manipulation
c. Centering the central ray
d. Correcting the horizontal angulation
e. Correcting the vertical angulation

4. The associated image depicts the intraoral exposure error caused by:

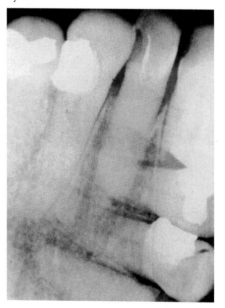

a. Using the same film packet more than once
b. Reversing a film packet
c. Using a slow-speed film
d. Tube head movement
e. Improper safelighting

5. The accompanying bitewing radiograph:

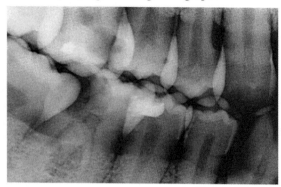

a. Is not diagnostic
b. Shows collimator cutoff
c. Shows incorrect horizontal angulation
d. Both a and b are correct.
e. Both a and c are correct.

Bibliography

American Academy of Oral and Maxillofacial Radiology: Standards of care, intraoral imaging, *AAOMR Newsletter* 25:1998.

American Dental Association Council on Scientific Affairs: An update on radiographic practices: information and recommendations, *J Am Dent Assoc* 132:234–238, 2001.

Iannucci JM, Howerton LJ: *Dental radiography: Principles and techniques*, ed 5, St Louis, MO, 2016, Elsevier Saunders.

Langland OE, Langlais RP: *Principles of dental imaging*, Baltimore, MD, 1997, Williams & Wilkins.

National Center for Health Care Technology: Dental radiology: A summary of recommendations from the Technology Assessment Forum, *J Am Dent Assoc* 103:423–425, 1981.

Stabulas JJ: Vertical bitewings, the other option, *J Prac Hyg* 11(3):46–47, 2002.

Thompson EM, Johnson ON: *Essentials of dental radiography for dental assistants and hygienists*, ed 9, Upper Saddle River, NJ, 2012, Pearson Education, Inc.

U.S. Department of Health and Human Services, Public Health Service FDA: The selection of patients for dental radiographic examinations, HHS/PHS/FDA, 88-827310-21, 1987.

White SC, Pharoah MJ: *Oral radiology: Principles and interpretation*, ed 7, St Louis, MO, 2013, Mosby.

10

Accessory Radiographic Techniques: Bisecting Technique and Occlusal Projections

EDUCATIONAL OBJECTIVES

Upon completing this chapter, the student will be able to:

1. Define the key terms listed at the beginning of the chapter.
2. Discuss the following related to the bisecting technique:
   - Know the basic principles of the bisecting technique.
   - State the indication for use of the bisecting technique as an accessory intraoral radiographic technique.
   - List and explain the advantages and disadvantages of the bisecting technique.
   - Describe the three methods of utilizing the bisecting technique.
3. List and describe the two most common errors produced with the use of incorrect vertical angulation in the bisecting technique, as well as the remedies for each.
4. Discuss the following related to occlusal film projections:
   - State the purpose and the indications for use of the occlusal exposure technique in dental intraoral radiography.
   - State the two types of occlusal projections and what each is generally used for in dental radiography.
   - List the steps involved in preparation and exposure of occlusal projections on the dental patient.
   - State the recommended vertical angulation for the maxillary and mandibular right-angle and topographic occlusal projections.

KEY TERMS

bisecting-angle technique (BAT)
dimensional distortion
imaginary bisecting line

occlusal receptor
occlusal projection
receptor plane

right-angle occlusal projection
topographic occlusal projection

Introduction

An accessory technique in dental radiography is employed when there is a specific indication for its utilization. This indication for use is usually based on the patient's individual dental health needs, anatomic constraints, the need for further radiographic evaluation, or a deviation from the usual course of radiographic examination. This chapter discusses the use of, principles of, and information gathered from the bisecting-angle and occlusal radiographic techniques in dental radiography.

Bisecting Technique

Another method for taking intraoral periapical radiographs is the bisecting-angle technique (BAT). In the bisecting technique, the receptor is placed as close to the tooth as possible. Because of the anatomy of the mouth, the long axis of the tooth is not parallel in most areas to the plane of the receptor with this placement. The vertical angulation of the tube head is directed so that the central ray is perpendicular to an imaginary line that bisects the angle formed by the long axis of the tooth and the plane of the receptor (see Fig. 3.14). With this receptor placement, the object-receptor distance is minimal. No compensation for image enlargement is necessary; therefore, the technique usually calls for an 8-inch target-receptor distance (or focal-film distance [FFD]). Although a "short cone" is used, this is not the determining factor in the technique. Bite pieces without localizing rings and aiming arms should be used in this method.

Before listing the (supposed) advantages of the bisecting technique, we must note again that the consensus of opinion among dental professionals and the American Academy of

Oral and Maxillofacial Radiology (AAOMR) regarding the standard of care for intraoral periapical radiography is the paralleling technique. The bisecting technique should be considered an ancillary or accessory method that can be used in special circumstances when it is not possible to use the paralleling technique. Basically, if the dental radiographer cannot position the receptor parallel to the teeth because of anatomic constraints or any other feasible reason, the bisecting technique is recommended as a substitute method for exposing the desired intraoral images. It is in this context that the bisecting technique is presented in this textbook.

Advantages of the Bisecting-Angle Technique

The bisecting technique is said to be easier to perform than the paralleling technique. For patients with small mouths, children, and patients with low palatal vaults, paralleling devices may be extremely difficult to use. The BAT is currently used with simple receptor-holding devices and, in the past, with the patient's finger as a holding device for the receptor. It is no longer acceptable for the patient to hold the receptor with the finger, because this practice unnecessarily exposes the patient's finger to radiation.

Because the receptor is held close to the tooth, it is acceptable to use an 8-inch target-receptor distance (or FFD) with the bisecting technique as opposed to the 12- to 16-inch target-receptor distance used with the paralleling technique. Shorter exposure times can be used in the bisecting technique because of the shorter target-receptor distance (or FFD) and the use of faster-speed film and digital sensors; hence, there is less of a chance for patient movement.

Disadvantages of the Bisecting-Angle Technique

The major disadvantage of the bisecting technique is that the image projected is dimensionally distorted. **Dimensional distortion** is a variation in the true size and shape of the structure being radiographed and is inherent in the use of the bisecting technique, as discussed in Chapter 9.

The bisecting technique is difficult to perform with the patient in a contour chair or in the supine or semi-supine position. With the newer dental chairs, it is very hard to place the patient in the correct position so that the occlusal plane of the jaw being radiographed is parallel to the floor and all vertical angulations used in the bisecting technique are measured from this line. Other disadvantages of the bisecting technique are related to the use of an 8-inch target-receptor distance (or FFD). The 8-inch target-receptor distance (or FFD), when compared with the extended 16-inch target-receptor distance (or FFD), causes greater image enlargement and distortion (see Fig. 3.8). There is also more tissue volume exposed with an 8-inch target-receptor distance (or FFD) than with a 16-inch target-receptor distance (or FFD; see Chapter 6). If the patient's finger is used to support the receptor, as is common in this method, then the patient's finger and hand

are unacceptably exposed to primary radiation. A bite piece should always be used instead of the patient's finger.

Method

In this technique, the receptor is held as close to the tooth as possible without bending the receptor. The long axis of the receptor therefore is not parallel to the long axis of the tooth. An **imaginary bisecting line** is drawn to bisect the angle formed by the long axis of the tooth and the plane of the receptor. The central ray of the x-ray beam is directed perpendicular to this bisecting line; this determines the vertical angulation of the x-ray beam (see Fig. 3.14). For the maxillary teeth, positive angulation (position-indicating device [PID] pointing down) is used; for mandibular teeth, negative angulation (PID pointing up) is used. At zero-degree angulations, the PID is parallel to the floor; this becomes the reference point from which vertical angulations are measured. Therefore, it is crucial to have the occlusal plane of the jaw being radiographed positioned parallel to the floor for predetermined angulations to be valid.

> **NOTE**
>
> There are basically three bisecting methods that can be used, two of which are outlined in Procedure 10.1. These two methods for vertical angulation involve using predetermined vertical angles or using the operator's subjective placement of the central ray perpendicular to the imaginary bisector. Both of these methods are dependent on the patient's occlusal plane being positioned properly (parallel to the floor). The third method is more simplified, not dependent on the occlusal plane orientation of the patient, and can leave less room for human error if utilized properly. The procedural steps for this method are:
>
> 1. Place the receptor in a simple receptor-holding device, such as an XCP bite piece (without the aiming bar or localizing ring) or a Stabe.
> 2. Place the receptor as close to the teeth being radiographed as possible.
> 3. Set the central ray (PID) so that it is perpendicular to the receptor.
> 4. Check the vertical angle setting on the yolk of the x-ray unit.
> 5. Divide that noted vertical angle in half.
> 6. Reset the vertical angulation at that half-way setting.
> 7. Expose the projection.
>   For example, the operator is exposing a mandibular central/lateral incisor radiograph and sets the central ray (PID) so that it is perpendicular to the receptor (Step 3). The operator notes that it is at a −20-degree angle (Step 4) and then divides that noted vertical angle in half (Step 5). Finally, the operator resets the adjusted angulation to −10 degrees (Step 6). Using this principle of the bisecting technique, which involves aiming the central ray at the imaginary bisector in a more concrete, objective way, makes it easier to standardize from one operator to the next.

Occlusal Projections

Occlusal projections are used to localize objects and pathologic conditions in the buccolingual dimension and

Text continued on p. 115

PROCEDURE 10.1   THE FULL-MOUTH BISECTING SERIES

Note: This procedure can be applied to conventional or digital radiography.

Maxillary Central and Lateral Incisors (Left or Right or Midline; Figs. 10.1 and 10.2)

Chair Position. The maxillary occlusal plane is positioned parallel to the floor, and the sagittal plane of the patient's face is perpendicular to the floor.

Point of Entry. For the maxillary central/lateral projection, the central ray is directed just below the midpoint of the nares (the nostrils) and aimed at the center of the receptor (see Fig. 10.1). For the maxillary right and maxillary left central and lateral incisors projection, the center of the receptor is placed between the central incisors, and the central ray is directed just below the tip of the nose (see Fig. 10.2).

Vertical Angulation. Can be preset at +50 degrees or aimed perpendicular to the imaginary bisector in the vertical plane.

Horizontal Angulation. The central ray is aimed perpendicular to the receptor in the horizontal plane. To avoid horizontal overlap, the dental professional should be sure to place the receptor parallel to the teeth in the horizontal plane.

> ### HELPFUL HINT
> Make sure that the occlusal plane is kept parallel to the floor in the event that the patient changes position in the chair.

Maxillary Canines (Fig. 10.3)

Chair Position. The maxillary occlusal plane is positioned parallel to the floor, and the sagittal plane of the patient's face is perpendicular to the floor.

Receptor Position. The receptor is held vertically and extends ⅛ inch below the tip of the canine. The canine is in the center of the receptor, which is held firmly against the lingual surface of the canine.

Point of Entry. The central ray is directed at the base of the lateral nasal groove, aimed at the center of the receptor.

Vertical Angulation. Can be preset at +50 degrees or aimed perpendicular to the imaginary bisector in the vertical plane.

Horizontal Angulation. The central ray is perpendicular to the receptor in the horizontal plane. To avoid horizontal

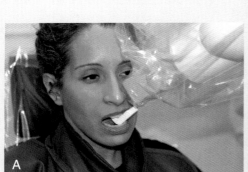
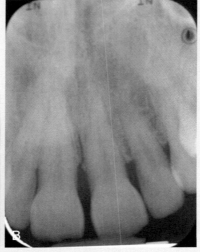
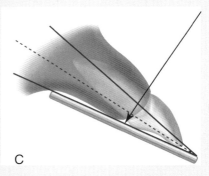

• **Figure 10.1** Maxillary central and lateral incisors. **A,** Receptor and position-indicating device (PID). **B,** Radiograph. **C,** Diagram.

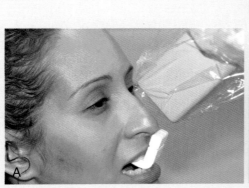
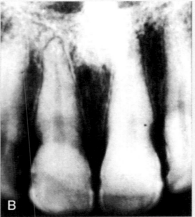

• **Figure 10.2** Right and left central and lateral incisors. **A,** Receptor packet and position-indicating device (PID). **B,** Radiograph.

Continued

PROCEDURE 10.1   THE FULL-MOUTH BISECTING SERIES—cont'd

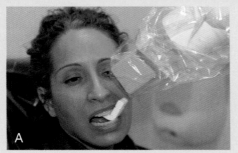

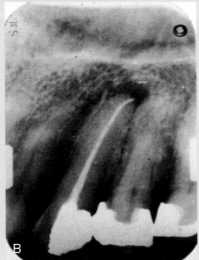

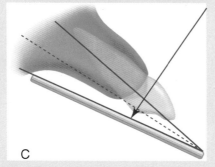

• **Figure 10.3** Maxillary canines. **A,** Receptor and position-indicating device (PID). **B,** Radiograph. **C,** Diagram.

overlap, the dental professional should be sure to place the receptor parallel to the teeth in the horizontal plane.

NOTE

When a film packet is used for this projection, try to avoid bending the film packet in a small mouth to prevent overbending (crescent-shaped marks). It is important to remember that fast-speed films (i.e., F-speed film) are more sensitive to the consequences of excessive manipulation.

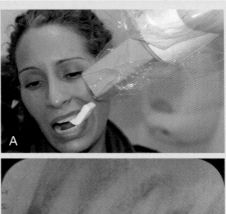

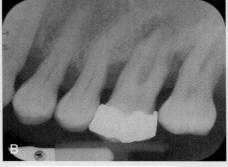

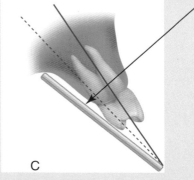

• **Figure 10.4** Maxillary premolars. **A,** Receptor and position-indicating device (PID). **B,** Radiograph. **C,** Diagram.

Maxillary Premolars (Fig. 10.4)

Chair Position. The maxillary occlusal plane is positioned parallel to the floor, and the sagittal plane of the patient's face is perpendicular to the floor.

Receptor Position. The receptor is held horizontally and extends ⅛ inch below the occlusal surfaces of the teeth. The second premolar is in the center of the receptor. The receptor is held in position against the lingual surfaces. If a film packet is being used, the operator should avoid shaping the packet to the arch to the point of bending the film enough to actually crack the emulsion.

Point of Entry. The central ray is directed at the most anterior part of the cheekbone, aimed at the center of the receptor.

PROCEDURE 10.1   THE FULL-MOUTH BISECTING SERIES—cont'd

Vertical Angulation. Can be preset at +40 degrees or aimed perpendicular to the imaginary bisector in the vertical plane.

Horizontal Angulation. The central ray is perpendicular to the receptor in the horizontal plane and is directed through the interproximal spaces. To avoid horizontal overlap, the dental professional should be sure to place the receptor parallel to the teeth in the horizontal plane.

> **HELPFUL HINT**
>
> Make sure that the anterior part of the receptor is positioned behind the center of the canine to include the distal part of the canine in the premolar projection.

Maxillary Molars (Fig. 10.5)

Chair Position. The maxillary occlusal plane is positioned parallel to the floor, and the sagittal plane of the patient's face is perpendicular to the floor.

Receptor Position. The receptor is held horizontally and extends ⅛ inch evenly below the occlusal surfaces of the teeth. The second molar is in the center of the receptor. The receptor is held against the lingual surfaces of the teeth.

Point of Entry. The central ray is directed through the zygomatic arch at the center of the receptor. The distal curvature of the open-ended collimator should not be distal to the outer canthus (corner) of the eye.

Vertical Angulation. Can be preset at +30 degrees or aimed perpendicular to the imaginary bisector in the vertical plane.

Horizontal Angulation. The central ray is perpendicular to the receptor in the horizontal plane and is directed through the interproximal spaces. To avoid horizontal overlap, the dental professional should place the receptor parallel to the teeth in the horizontal plane.

> **HELPFUL HINT**
>
> Make sure that the middle of the receptor in the horizontal position is at the center of the second molar.

Mandibular Incisors (Fig. 10.6)

Chair Position. The patient is positioned so that when the mouth is open, the mandibular occlusal plane is parallel to the floor, and the sagittal plane of the patient's face is perpendicular to the floor.

Receptor Position. The receptor is held vertically so that it extends ⅛ inch above the incisal edges of the incisors. The midpoint of this ⅛-inch border should be between the central incisors. All four lower incisors are shown on one image. The receptor is held against the lingual surfaces of the incisors.

Point of Entry. The central ray is directed at the depression in the face just above the chin (mental groove), aimed at the center of the receptor.

Vertical Angulation. Can be preset at –20 degrees or aimed perpendicular to the imaginary bisector in the vertical plane.

Horizontal Angulation. The central ray is perpendicular to the receptor in the horizontal plane. To avoid horizontal

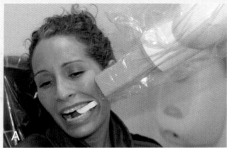
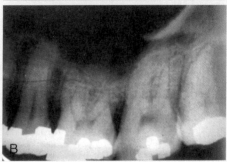
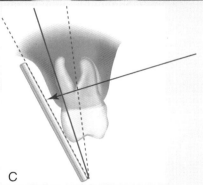

• **Figure 10.5** Maxillary molars. **A,** Receptor and position-indicating device (PID). **B,** Radiograph. **C,** Diagram.

overlap, the dental professional should place the receptor parallel to the teeth in the horizontal plane.

> **HELPFUL HINT**
>
> In some small and crowded arch shapes, it may be necessary to use a smaller-sized receptor (#1 receptor) for a lower anterior projection.

Mandibular Canines (Fig. 10.7)

Chair Position. The patient is positioned so that when the mouth is open, the mandibular occlusal plane is parallel to the floor, and the sagittal plane of the patient's face is perpendicular to the floor.

Receptor Position. The receptor is held vertically and extends ⅛ inch above the tip of the canine, which is at the center of the receptor. The receptor is held against the lingual surface of the canine.

Continued

PROCEDURE 10.1 THE FULL-MOUTH BISECTING SERIES—cont'd

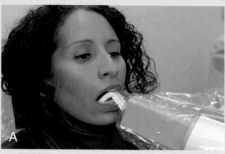

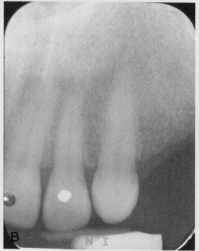

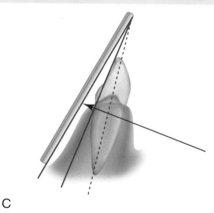

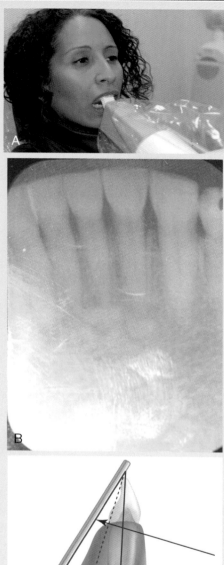

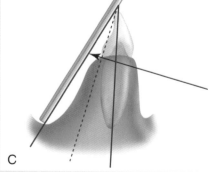

• **Figure 10.6** Mandibular incisors. **A,** Receptor and position-indicating device (PID). **B,** Radiograph. **C,** Diagram.

Point of Entry. The central ray is directed at the root of the canine, aimed at the middle of the receptor.

Vertical Angulation. Can be preset at −20 degrees or aimed perpendicular to the imaginary bisector in the vertical plane.

Horizontal Angulation. The central ray is perpendicular to the receptor in the horizontal plane. To avoid horizontal overlap, the dental professional should place the receptor parallel to the teeth in the horizontal plane.

• **Figure 10.7** Mandibular canines. **A,** Receptor and position-indicating device (PID). **B,** Radiograph. **C,** Diagram.

> **NOTE**
>
> In the canine area, it may be necessary to use one or two extra size #1 receptors to cover the canine area completely.

Mandibular Premolars (Fig. 10.8)

Chair Position. The patient is positioned so that when the mouth is open, the mandibular occlusal plane is parallel to the floor, and the sagittal plane of the patient's face is perpendicular to the floor.

PROCEDURE 10.1   THE FULL-MOUTH BISECTING SERIES—cont'd

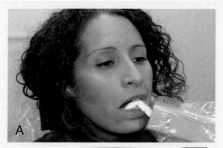

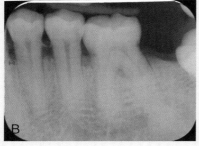

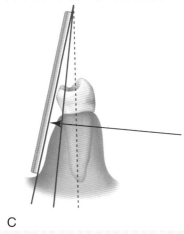

• **Figure 10.8** Mandibular premolars. **A,** Receptor and position-indicating device (PID). **B,** Radiograph. **C,** Diagram.

Receptor Position. The receptor is held horizontally and extends ⅛ inch above the occlusal surfaces of the teeth. The second premolar is in the center of the receptor. The receptor is held against the lingual surfaces of the teeth.

Point of Entry. The central ray is directed at the mental foramen, aimed at the center of the receptor.

Vertical Angulation. Can be preset at −15 degrees or aimed perpendicular to the imaginary bisector in the vertical plane.

Horizontal Angulation. The central ray is perpendicular to the receptor in the horizontal plane. To avoid horizontal overlap, the dental professional should place the receptor parallel to the teeth in the horizontal plane.

NOTE

It may be necessary to bend the inferior anterior corner of the receptor (if a film packet is being used) to follow the curve of the arch.

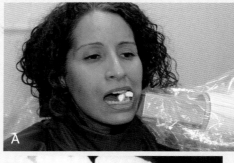

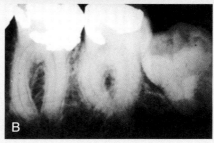

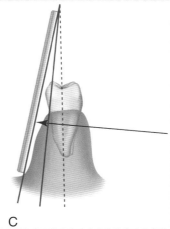

• **Figure 10.9** Mandibular molars. **A,** Receptor and position-indicating device (PID). **B,** Radiograph. **C,** Diagram.

Mandibular Molars (Fig. 10.9)

Chair Position. The patient is positioned so that when the mouth is open, the mandibular occlusal plane is parallel to the floor, and the sagittal plane of the patient's face is perpendicular to the floor.

Receptor Position. The receptor is held horizontally and extends ⅛ inch above the occlusal surfaces of the molars. The second molar is in the middle of the receptor. The receptor is held against the lingual surface of the molars. Because of the anatomy of the area, the receptor is almost parallel to the long axis of the tooth; consequently, most molar periapical projections exposed with the bisecting technique are really paralleled projections.

Point of Entry. The central ray is directed at the roots of the molars, aimed at the center of the receptor.

Vertical Angulation. Can be preset at −5 degrees or aimed perpendicular to the imaginary bisector in the vertical plane.

Continued

PROCEDURE 10.1 THE FULL-MOUTH BISECTING SERIES—cont'd

Horizontal Angulation. The central ray is perpendicular to the receptor in the horizontal plane. To avoid horizontal overlap, the dental professional should place the receptor parallel to the teeth in the horizontal plane.

Bitewings

The technique for the bitewing projection is the same as in the paralleling method, because both call for the receptor and the teeth to be parallel and the x-ray beam to be perpendicular (at right angles) to both.

> **HELPFUL HINT**
>
> When inserting the receptor in the patient's mouth, it is advised to use a finger from your other hand to depress the floor of the mouth if needed.

> **HELPFUL HINT**
>
> Make sure that the patient closes in centric and not protrusive relation when biting on the bitewing receptor-holding device or bitewing tab.

COMMON ERRORS 10.1

Bisecting Technique

Note: Refer to the Appendix for a detailed description of each of the following exposure errors.

The following text presents the most common errors seen in the bisecting technique. Recognition and correction of occasional errors in technique are important. Not all patients are cooperative or have mouths that are anatomically easy to radiograph. Remember that images retaken because of poor technique add unnecessarily to the patient's radiation burden. See Chapter 9 for a discussion of other chairside errors. The following errors, elongation and foreshortening, can occur with both conventional (film-based) and digital radiography.

Elongation (Fig. 10.10). Elongation, or lengthening of the image, can be caused by *inadequate vertical angulation,* improper occlusal plane orientation because of patient positioning, or poor receptor placement.

Remedy. The receptor and the central ray must be in the correct relationship. In the bisecting-angle technique (BAT), the vertical angulation should be increased to correct elongation. The occlusal plane of the jaw being radiographed should be parallel to the floor. Patients may tend to move after a few exposures or lift their heads to watch the operator or observe their surroundings. Their movements disorient the occlusal plane. Check the patient's head position before taking each exposure.

Foreshortening (Fig. 10.11). Foreshortening (the shortening of the image) is not as common an error as elongation. It can be caused by *excessive vertical angulation* or poor occlusal plane orientation.

Remedy. In the BAT, the vertical angulation should be decreased to overcome errors of foreshortening.

Sagittal plane orientation (Fig. 10.12). When the periapical radiographs show the occlusal surfaces of the teeth, the patient's head has tipped away from the proper sagittal plane. This is accompanied by elongation of the image.

Remedy. The operator should make sure that the patient does not tip their head away from the tube head as it is brought into approximation with the facial skin.

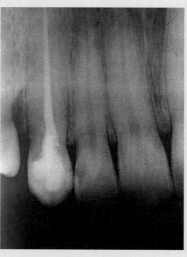

• **Figure 10.10** Elongated image.

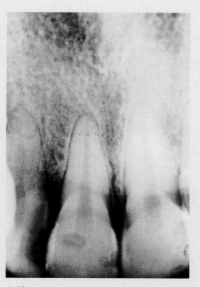

• **Figure 10.11** Foreshortened image.

COMMON ERRORS 10.1—cont'd

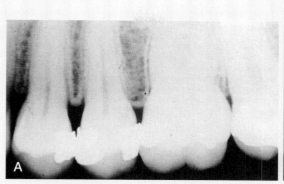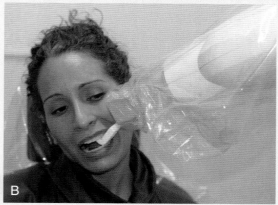

• **Figure 10.12 A,** Elongated and distorted radiograph caused by poor sagittal plane orientation of the patient's head. **B,** Poor sagittal plane orientation.

• **BOX 10.1   Use of Occlusal Projections**

Clinical examples of the use of occlusal projections include the following:
- To locate retained roots of extracted teeth
- To locate supernumerary (extra), unerupted, or impacted teeth
- To locate foreign bodies in the maxilla or the mandible
- To locate salivary stones in the floor of the mouth and in the submandibular duct and gland (mandibular right-angle projection)
- To locate and evaluate the extent (i.e., buccal bone expansion) of intraosseous lesions (e.g., cysts, tumors, malignancies) in the maxilla or mandible
- To evaluate the boundaries of the maxillary sinus (maxillary occlusal projection)
- To evaluate fractures of the maxilla or mandible
- To aid in the examination of patients who cannot open their mouths more than a few millimeters
- To examine the area of a cleft palate (maxillary occlusal projection)
- To evaluate changes in the size and shape of the maxilla or mandible
- To evaluate teeth for vertical fractures that cannot be seen on periapical radiographs due to superimposition of normal tooth structure
- To examine the depth (buccolingual perspective) of periapical lesions

---

to visualize areas that would not be seen on periapical and bitewing projections because of insufficient field size. The right-angle occlusal technique is used for localizing structures and lesions in the (extreme) buccolingual dimension; the topographic occlusal technique is used to view larger structures and pathologic areas. Occlusal receptors can also be used when proper placement of periapical receptors is not possible in children or handicapped patients (Box 10.1; see Chapter 18).

Right-Angle Projection

With right-angle occlusal projections (also known as the *90-degree* or *cross-sectional projection*) the central ray is directed at an angle of 90 degrees to the receptor. This technique would be used, for example, to locate an object such as an impacted tooth in the third dimension. It has been mentioned that dental radiographs picture a three-dimensional subject in a two-dimensional plane, usually vertical and horizontal. The radiographs do not indicate depth. In the example of the impacted tooth, one might know from a conventional radiograph the impaction's mesiodistal location and its vertical height from the crest of the alveolar ridge, but we would not know its depth in the bone in a buccolingual dimension. One way to determine whether an impacted mandibular molar lies buccal or lingual to the alveolar ridge is to take a radiograph from another direction. In this example, it would be an occlusal radiograph, with the central ray coming from underneath the mandible, directed at a right angle to a receptor placed on the occlusal surface of the mandibular teeth.

Topographic Projections

The angulation of the topographic occlusal projection may vary from 35 to 75 degrees, depending on the anatomic area and arch being radiographed. Because the occlusal receptor is larger than the size of the intraoral receptor, it can record areas that would not be seen on the smaller receptor. The extreme vertical angulations are necessary to compensate for the lack of parallelism between the object and the receptor. This is a modification of the BAT.

Occlusal Receptor

The occlusal receptor (size #4) is $2\frac{1}{2} \times 3$ inches. When it is a film packet, it can be supplied with either single- or double-packet films (Fig. 10.13) and is available in various

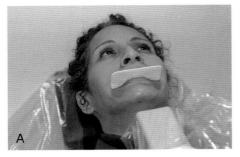

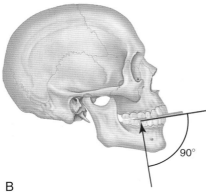

• **Figure 10.13** Front and back of moisture-proof dental film packet. (Courtesy Carestream Health, Inc., Rochester, NY.)

film speeds, including F speed. Phosphor plates for indirect digital radiography systems are also available in the #4 size for occlusal radiography. These #4 size receptors are sometimes called *sandwich receptors,* because they are positioned in the patient's mouth with the teeth closed on the receptor, resembling the position for biting on a sandwich. The #2 size receptor can be used for pediatric occlusal projections if the #4 size cannot be accommodated. When film packets are used, the occlusal film is processed in the same way as other intraoral films. The exposure time setting used for occlusal projections is equivalent to that which is used for the maxillary molar intraoral periapical projection.

Mandibular Occlusal Technique

In the mandibular occlusal technique, the receptor is placed in the patient's mouth on the occlusal surfaces of the lower teeth. If a #4 size film packet is being used, the front (white side) of the packet should be facing the mandible on the occlusal surfaces of the lower teeth. The film is placed horizontally (with the longer side extending from right to left) as long as it can be accommodated in that direction and as far posterior on the mandible as possible. The patient is directed to bite gently on the receptor. For the right-angle projection, the central ray of the x-ray beam is directed from under the mandible so that it is perpendicular to the center of the film packet at a 90-degree angle to the receptor (Figs. 10.14 and 10.15). The back of the chair is lowered and the patient's chin is tilted up so that the PID can be positioned below the mandible. For the topographic view of the mandible, the central ray is directed at a point just above the mental eminence at a vertical angulation of 35 to 45 degrees (Figs. 10.16 and 10.17).

Maxillary Occlusal Technique

In an anterior topographic occlusal view of the maxilla, the receptor is placed in the patient's mouth on the occlusal surfaces of the maxillary teeth. When the patient is ready, the patient is instructed to close lightly (gently) on the receptor. If a film packet is being used, the packet is placed with the front of the film packet facing the palate and the

• **Figure 10.14** A, Receptor placement and position-indicating device (PID) position for mandibular right-angle occlusal projection. Note that the central ray is directed at 90 degrees to center of film packet. **B,** Diagram.

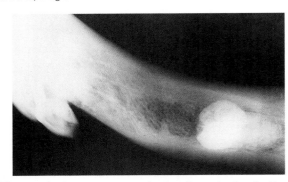

• **Figure 10.15** Right-angle occlusal radiograph of patient's mandibular posterior area. Note buccal and lingual cortex of bone and central position of the impaction.

long dimension of the packet running across the mouth (unless the patient cannot accommodate it in that position, in which case it should be placed with the long end running from anterior to posterior). The receptor is positioned as far posterior as possible so that the posterior edge of the film packet touches the ascending ramus of the mandible. With the patient's head positioned so that the **receptor plane** is parallel to the floor, the central ray is directed at a 65 to 75 degree vertical angulation aimed at the bridge of the nose (point of entry; Figs. 10.18 and 10.19). In the right-angle occlusal view of the maxilla, the receptor is placed in the same position as the maxillary topographic projection, but the central ray is directed perpendicular to the center of the film packet. To do this, the PID must be positioned above the patient's head at about the hairline. The vertical angulation is 90 degrees (Figs. 10.20 and 10.21). When using rectangular collimation with any of these occlusal

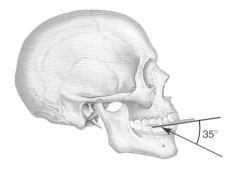

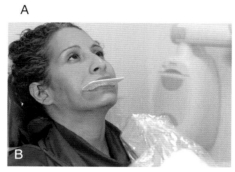

• **Figure 10.16 A,** Topographic mandibular occlusal projection. **B,** Diagram.

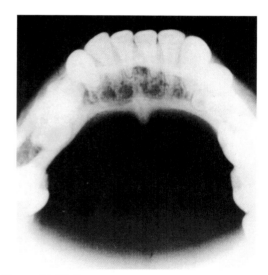

• **Figure 10.17** Topographic occlusal projection of mandible.

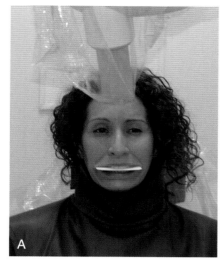

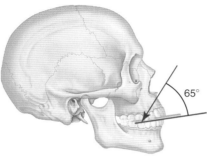

• **Figure 10.18 A,** Receptor placement and position-indicating device (PID) position for topographic occlusal view of maxilla. Note that the central ray is directed at 65 to 75 degrees to the bridge of the nose. **B,** Diagram.

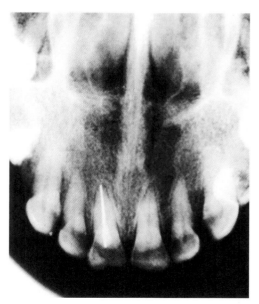

• **Figure 10.19** Occlusal radiograph of the maxilla, topographic view.

projections, make sure that there is at least a 5-inch distance from the end of the rectangular column to the point of entry. This ensures a larger beam diameter, which is needed to expose a larger area and receptor size.

The posterior occlusal topographic view can be considered a topographic view of the maxillary sinus and surrounding structures. The receptor is positioned on either the left or the right side of the patient's mouth, from the midline, laterally with the long side running anteroposteriorly. The central ray is directed to a point just above the apices of the premolars at a vertical angulation of approximately 65 degrees (Figs. 10.22 and 10.23).

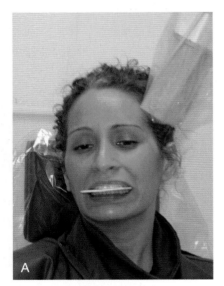

• **Figure 10.20 A,** Receptor placement and position-indicating device (PID) position for a right-angle occlusal view of the maxilla. Note that the central ray is directed at 90 degrees to the receptor. **B,** Diagram.

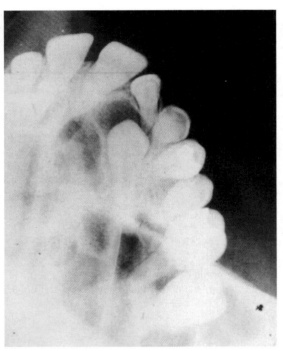

• **Figure 10.21** Right-angle occlusal projection of the maxilla showing the palatal relationship of the impacted canine.

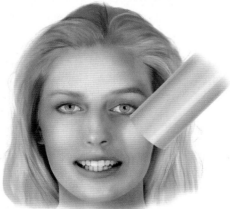

• **Figure 10.22 A,** Posterior topographic occlusal projection. **B,** Diagram. The point of entry corresponds to the apices of the premolars; vertical angulation is approximately 65 degrees.

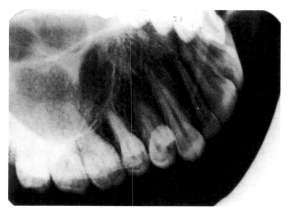

• **Figure 10.23** Topographic occlusal radiograph of the maxillary sinus.

Chapter Summary

- An accessory dental radiographic technique is employed when there is a specific indication for its use. This indication for use is usually based on the patient's anatomic constraints, dental health needs, need for further radiographic evaluation, or a cause for a deviation from the usual course of radiographic examination.
- The bisecting technique is considered an accessory technique, because it is employed only when the paralleling technique cannot be used to expose periapical radiographs. This usually occurs when it is not possible to place the receptor parallel to the teeth due to a patient's anatomic constraints or for another valid reason.
- The two basic principles of the bisecting technique are that the receptor is placed as close to the tooth as possible and the central ray is aimed perpendicular to the imaginary bisector that divides the angle formed by the tooth and the receptor in half.
- The most important advantage of the bisecting technique is that the receptor placement is easy to achieve and is also more comfortable for the patient once it is in place. The greatest disadvantage of the bisecting technique is that the resultant images are dimensionally distorted.
- There are basically three methods for exposing bisecting periapical radiographs. The first method consists of using predetermined vertical angles, the second uses the basic

principles of the bisecting technique, and the third is a more standardized way of using the basic concepts of the technique.
- Occlusal projections are used to localize structures in the buccolingual dimension and to visualize areas that would not be seen on periapical and bitewing projections because of insufficient field size. They are used to visualize salivary stones in the submandibular gland, cleft palate, buccal bone expansion, impacted teeth, and other conditions of the teeth and bones in the buccolingual dimension.
- The occlusal receptor is the #4 size receptor. It is placed on the occlusal surfaces of either the maxillary or mandibular teeth. The film is usually held with the longer side positioned from the right to the left unless the posterior teeth are being exposed or the patient cannot accommodate the receptor in the horizontal position. In this case, the receptor is positioned with the longer side in the anteroposterior position.
- There are two types of occlusal projections: (1) the topographic projection and (2) the right-angle projection (also known as the *90-degree* or *cross-sectional projection*) used to view different perspectives of the buccolingual dimension.

Chapter Review Questions

Multiple Choice

1. In the bisecting angle technique, the central ray is positioned:
   a. Perpendicular to the receptor
   b. Perpendicular to the tooth
   c. Perpendicular to the bisector between the tooth and the receptor
   d. Parallel to the bisector between the tooth and the receptor
   e. Parallel to the receptor

2. The bisecting technique is utilized when:
   a. The insurance company requests that the images be taken with that technique
   b. When the patient cannot open the mouth at all
   c. When the receptor cannot be held parallel to the tooth because of anatomic constraints
   d. When it is required to see dimensional accuracy on the dental image
   e. When paralleling receptor-holding devices are used

3. The two errors that are caused by incorrect vertical angulation and are very common with the bisecting technique are known as:
   a. Overlapping and reversed image
   b. Collimator cutoff and overlapping
   c. Collimator cutoff and elongation
   d. Foreshortening and elongation
   e. Foreshortening and overlapping
4. The occlusal radiograph utilized for viewing a salivary stone in the submandibular gland is (indicate all that apply):
   a. The mandibular right-angle projection
   b. The mandibular topographic projection
   c. The mandibular 90-degree projection
   d. The maxillary topographic projection
   e. The maxillary right-angle projection
5. Occlusal film packets are:
   a. A #4 size film packet
   b. Held flat on the biting surfaces of the teeth
   c. Nicknamed "the sandwich receptor"
   d. Used to project the buccolingual dimension
   e. All are correct

Case-Based Critical Thinking Exercise

A patient presents with redness and swelling in the floor of the mouth. The area is sensitive upon palpation, and the patient reports decreased salivary flow, especially after eating. A panoramic radiograph shows a superimposed radiopacity in the mandibular region.

1. What should the next step be in identifying this radiopacity?
   a. Expose a periapical projection in the area of the lesion.
   b. Expose an anterior vertical bitewing in the area of interest.
   c. Expose another panoramic radiograph to make sure that the radiopacity seen was not an artifact on the previous projection taken.
   d. Expose a mandibular topographic occlusal projection.
   e. Expose a mandibular right-angle occlusal projection.
2. What dimension of the oral cavity should be projected in order to show this radiopacity without superimposition?
   a. The mesial-distal dimension
   b. The buccolingual dimension
   c. The incisal-apical dimension
   d. The occlusal-apical dimension
   e. The vertical dimension
3. Considering the signs, symptoms, and radiographic finding, what could this finding potentially be identified as?
   a. A calculus deposit
   b. An extra tooth (supernumerary tooth)
   c. An amalgam restoration
   d. a salivary stone in the submandibular gland
   e. a salivary stone in the parotid gland

Radiographic Interpretation

1. This image:

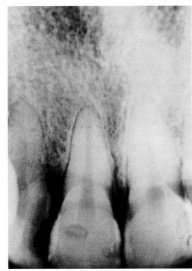

   a. Was produced by too much vertical angulation
   b. Was produced by too little vertical angulation
   c. Is known as foreshortening
   d. Both a and c are correct.
   e. Both b and c are correct.
2. The following diagram shows the relationship of the tooth, receptor, and central ray for the:

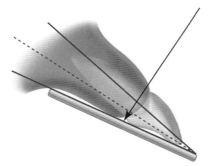

   a. Maxillary right-angle occlusal technique
   b. Mandibular topographic occlusal technique
   c. Paralleling technique
   d. Bisecting technique
   e. Maxillary topographic occlusal technique

3. The following diagram shows the relationship of the central ray and the receptor for the:

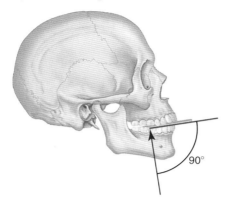

a. Maxillary right-angle occlusal technique
b. Mandibular topographic occlusal technique
c. Paralleling technique
d. Bisecting technique
e. Mandibular right-angle occlusal technique

Bibliography

Iannucci JM, Howerton LJ: *Dental radiography: Principles and techniques*, ed 5, St Louis, MO, 2016, Elsevier Saunders.

Langland OE, Langlais RP: *Principles of dental imaging*, Baltimore, MD, 1997, Williams & Wilkins.

Thompson EM, Johnson ON: *Essentials of dental radiography for dental assistants and hygienists*, ed 9, Upper Saddle River, NJ, 2012, Pearson Education, Inc.

White SC, Pharoah MJ: *Oral radiology: Principles and interpretation*, ed 7, St Louis, MO, 2013, Mosby.

11
Film Processing Techniques

EDUCATIONAL OBJECTIVES

Upon completing this chapter, the student will be able to:

1. Define the key terms listed at the beginning of the chapter.
2. Explain the steps in manually processing dental film.
3. Describe the following related to the design and requirements of the darkroom:
   - Describe what a darkroom is used for and what the components of an acceptable darkroom are.
   - Know the types of lighting that are in a darkroom.
   - Explain what a safelight is and what the *coin test* is used for.
   - Discuss the plumbing of the darkroom.
   - Discuss the contents of the darkroom, including processing tanks, solutions, replenishing solutions, timer and thermometer, film hangers, and dryers.
   - Discuss the sequence for manual and automatic processing and the roles of the developer, fixer, and water in both methods.
4. Explain and discuss the development process, including:
   - Define the term *latent image,* and discuss how it is different from the visible image in dental film processing.
   - Describe the procedures for manual and automatic processing.
5. Describe the time-temperature development method, and compare it to the sight development method.
6. Explain the indication for use of *rapid processing,* and state what the components of this method are.
7. State the importance of the care and maintenance of the darkroom and automatic processors and how they are included in a quality assurance program in dental facilities.
8. Discuss the environmental concerns that are associated with film processing.
9. Know what automatic processing is, as well as describe the steps involved in automatic processing.
10. Know the common processing errors for manual and automatic processing and how to remedy each error.

KEY TERMS

automatic processing	film roller	safelight
clear film	fixer	sight development
coin test	generators	stop bath
dark image	latent image	thermometer
darkroom	light leak	thermostatic valve
daylight loader	light-tight	thin image
dense image	manual processing	time-temperature technique
developer	overdeveloped	torn emulsion
developer cutoff	rapid processing	underdeveloped film
drying rack	reference film	visible image
electrostatic artifact	replenisher	water bath
film hanger	reticulation	wet reading

Introduction

Although the use of digital radiographic techniques are on the rise in dental facilities, conventional film-based radiography is still being used. While film processing is slowly becoming a technique of the past, the basic knowledge and understanding of film processing is still required in a thorough study of dental radiography. The fundamental familiarity with the manual and automatic film processing techniques continues to be included in dental radiology education. This chapter discusses manual and automatic processing, the components of a darkroom, the fundamentals of processing, common processing errors, film processing quality assurance, and environmental concerns in dental film processing.

Manual Processing

The processing of exposed x-ray film (either manually or automatically) is an important step in the radiographic chain of events. It is at this point that a visible image is produced, from which a diagnosis can be made. The x-rays that have penetrated the hard and soft tissue in the patient's mouth have created a latent image on the exposed x-ray film. The processing of this film converts the latent image to a visible diagnostic image.

Manual processing can occur inside or outside of the darkroom. In the darkroom, manual processing is performed with the required armamentaria, including manual processing tanks, processing solutions, proper lighting, film-holding hangers, a thermometer, and other needed equipment. It should be noted that with increased use of digital radiography, the need for a darkroom has become less necessary (see Chapter 15).

The darkroom is a room in the dental office set aside for radiographic processing. In addition to processing film, the dental professional must keep the darkroom clean, change solutions regularly, keep accurate records of processed radiographs, and maintain a quality assurance program. It is important to realize that the processing of films is vital in the production of the diagnostic radiograph. Errors in the darkroom can easily ruin what would otherwise have been diagnostic radiographs, making it necessary to retake the films with the resultant loss of time and increased radiation exposure to the patient. It is important to remember that every film that requires retaking doubles the patient's radiation exposure for that film. An acceptable chairside radiographic technique must be coupled with an equally acceptable processing technique. The importance of eliminating darkroom errors should be uppermost in the minds of dental professionals.

Design and Requirements of the Darkroom

The essential requirements and components of a darkroom that is used for manual processing are that it should be light-tight and have safelight and white light illumination, processing tanks, a thermostatically controlled supply of water, thermometer, timer, film hangers, drying racks, and storage space.

Location and Size

The darkroom should be a space unto itself, located near the rooms in which the x-ray units are placed. The darkroom should be a minimum of 16 square feet (4 × 4), allowing enough room for one person to work comfortably. The factors that should be considered in determining the space needed are (1) the volume of radiographs to be processed; (2) the number of dental professionals handling the processing; (3) the type of processing to be done (manual, automatic,

or both); and (4) the space required for duplicating, drying, and storage.

The walls of the darkroom should be a light color that reflects the safelighting; darkroom walls do not have to be black. The surfaces of the walls and floor should be of materials that are resistant to staining and can be cleaned of the processing solutions that inevitably spill or splash onto them.

The darkroom must be completely light-tight so that when the safelight is on, it is the only illumination in the darkroom. Because x-ray film is sensitive to white light, any light leaks can fog the film. A fogged film is less diagnostic and in some cases may be useless. The easiest way to check for light leaks is to stand in the darkroom in complete darkness; any leaks around the door or in other areas will be apparent and should be corrected. The darkroom door should have an inside lock so that the door cannot be opened from the outside while films are being processed. There are also darkrooms with solid revolving doors to prohibit light from entering the room during processing as well.

It is advised that the darkroom should be well ventilated to exhaust the moisture from the drying films or the heat, if a dryer is used, and maintain comfortable working conditions. Keeping the darkroom at a reasonable temperature makes it easier to maintain desired processing solution temperatures. Another consideration to maintain film quality is to avoid storing unexposed film in the darkroom cabinets, because at high temperatures (greater than 90° F) the films can experience film fog.

Lighting

A well-designed darkroom has five different light sources: (1) an illuminating safelight, (2) an overhead white light, (3) a viewing safelight, (4) an x-ray viewbox, and (5) an outside warning light.

Illuminating Safelight

When film packets are opened, film is attached to hangers, or film is being processed, safelight conditions must be maintained. As mentioned, white light darkens x-ray film. Safelight is any illumination that does not affect the x-ray film (Fig. 11.1). It is a low-intensity light composed of long wavelengths from the orange/red range of the spectrum.

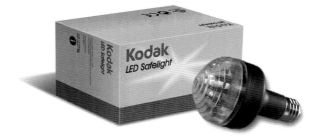

• **Figure 11.1** A variety of safelights are available for use in the darkroom including safelights now available in LED format for intraoral and extraoral films. (Courtesy Carestream Health, Rochester, NY.)

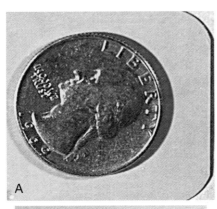

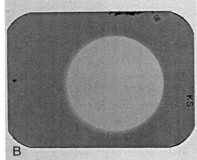

• **Figure 11.2** Coin test for safelighting. **A,** Coin placed on unexposed film. **B,** Processed radiograph showing an outline of the coin, indicating that the safelight is not safe.

As shown in Chapter 4 in the discussion of intensifying screens, x-ray films are more sensitive to the blue/green region of the light spectrum, where the wavelengths are relatively short. The determining factors are the sensitivity of the x-ray film to the type of light used and the position and intensity of the light source. Usually, a $7\frac{1}{2}$- to 10-W bulb with a yellow filter (e.g., Kodak yellow Morlite M-2) placed 3 to 4 feet from the work surface is used for working with intraoral film. If extraoral screen film is used, a Kodak GBX-2 Safelight Filter with a 15-W bulb is needed because of the film's increased sensitivity to light. This filter also can be used for intraoral film. If both intraoral and extraoral film is being processed, an extraoral safelight (e.g., Kodak GBX-2) is recommended, because it will be safe for both intraoral and extraoral film processing.

A simple and reliable way to check a safelight is by the coin test, in which a coin is placed on an unwrapped, unexposed piece of dental film on a flat surface under safelight conditions. After 3 minutes of exposure to the safelight, the film is developed. If the film shows an outline of the coin, the light is not safe; the uncovered part of the film should have been as unaffected as the part covered by the coin (Fig. 11.2).

Cell Phones

The recent increase in the use of cell phones has produced another possible source of light that could fog or completely expose and ruin the film. When the cell phone is on, it produces light that affects the film. This is more likely to happen with extraoral and panoramic film, because they are more sensitive to light and have a larger film surface area. However, the newer cell phones have a brighter light and are apt to expose intraoral and extraoral films. Therefore, it is advised that cell phones should not be on or actually used in the darkroom.

Overhead White Light

The only requirement for overhead white light is that it must provide adequate illumination for the size of the room. The switch for this light should be placed either outside of the darkroom or in a position inside of the darkroom where it cannot be bumped accidentally and turned on, potentially exposing films to white light illumination.

Viewing Safelight

Some dental offices use wet readings or rapid processing techniques especially for emergencies and working films. In these cases, it is convenient to have a viewing safelight mounted on the wall behind the processing tanks. Then, films can be removed from the fixer after 3 minutes and checked by safelight to see if they have cleared enough for washing and reading.

X-Ray Viewbox

The ability to read wet films in the darkroom is a great convenience. A proper interpretation of the radiographs can be made more adequately by having an acceptable viewing mechanism in the darkroom. If there is adequate space in the darkroom, it should have a viewbox to allow for proper viewing of the radiographs after they are processed.

Outside Warning Light

This light should be wired so that when the safelight is on in the darkroom, the warning light is on outside the darkroom. This alerts members of the office staff to the presence of a colleague who is processing film inside the darkroom and helps to prevent entry into the darkroom when safelight precautions are in effect.

Plumbing

The darkroom should have intake lines of hot and cold water with an adequate drainage line. There should be a thermostatic valve controlling intake to maintain constant temperatures of the solutions. The disposal line should be made of materials that resist the action of the processing chemicals. If automatic processors are used, the flow rate of the incoming water should be considered in planning darkroom plumbing. Automatic processors have individual requirements for flow rates of water, which should be a factor in darkroom planning and choosing an automatic processor.

A sink with a gooseneck faucet is extremely convenient for tank cleaning and solution changing. This is often overlooked in darkroom planning; dental personnel will realize that oversight the first time they carry processing

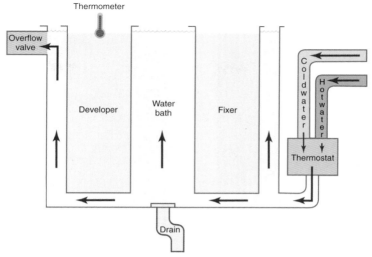

• **Figure 11.3** Typical processing tanks in a dental office.

tanks to the nearest sink for cleaning and replenishing. The gooseneck faucet is essential because a normal-size faucet neck does not allow enough room to place the tanks under the faucet for cleaning.

Contents

Processing Tanks

Most dental offices have processing units that contain either 1- or 2-gallon developer and fixer insert tanks suspended in a tank of running water (Fig. 11.3). The unit should be made of stainless steel, and the water bath should have a thermostatically controlled flow valve to keep the solutions at the desired temperature. Each tank is equipped with a lid that should be kept on at all times. The cover protects developing films from accidental exposure to white light and prevents oxidation and evaporation of the processing solutions.

Solutions

Table 11.1 lists the main ingredients of the developer and fixer solutions and their functions. The developer and fixer solutions used for manual processing are usually supplied as liquid concentrate that must be diluted. Extra amounts of prepared solutions should be stored in either dark bottles or opaque plastic containers away from heat and light sources.

Under normal working conditions, developer and fixing solutions should be changed at a minimum of every 2 to 3 weeks. A normal workload is considered to be 30 intraoral films per day. If an office exceeds 30 intraoral films per day and/or processes many panoramic films, solutions should be changed more often. The chemical solutions lose strength when exposed to air and should be replaced even if normal workload maximums have not been met. Remember that film development is a chemical reaction: Every time the developer and fixer solutions affect a film emulsion, the solutions become weakened. Consequently, in a busy office, solutions may have to be changed more frequently. Weak

TABLE 11.1	Chemicals for Development Process
Ingredient	**Function**
Developer	
Elon or Metol and hydroquinone (developing agent)	Reduces the energized silver bromide crystals to silver
Sodium sulfite (preservative)	Prevents oxidation of developer
Sodium carbonate (activator)	Provides alkaline medium and softens gelatin to allow developing agents to reach silver bromide crystals
Potassium bromide (restrainer)	Controls activity of developing agents and prevents chemical fog
Fixer	
Sodium thiosulfate (clearing solution)	Removes undeveloped or unexposed silver bromide crystals from the emulsion
Sodium sulfite (preservative)	Prevents the decomposition of the thiosulfate clearing agent
Potassium aluminum sulfate (hardener)	Shrinks and hardens gelatin
Acetic acid (acidifier)	Maintains acid medium

developer and fixing solutions do not bring out the optimum image on the film and thus do not provide the maximum diagnostic information for the radiation exposure.

Replenishing

Developer and fixer solutions should be replenished daily. Commercially prepared replenishment solutions are available, but it is usually easier to use the standard developer

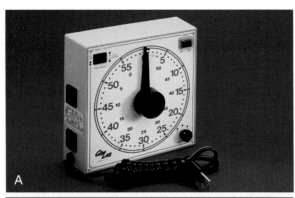

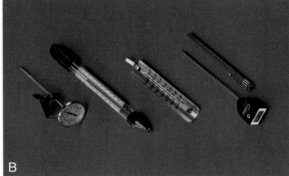

• **Figure 11.4** Darkroom timer **(A)** and thermometer **(B)**. Both are essential parts of the time-temperature technique. (Courtesy Flow Dental, Deer Park, NY.)

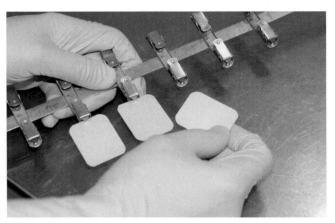

• **Figure 11.5** Placing film on hangers in the darkroom under safe-light conditions.

and fixer solutions to fill the tanks. Approximately 8 oz of replenishment are required each day for the developer and fixer solutions. Commercial replenishers include manufacturer's instructions. The **replenisher** is added directly to the existing solutions in their respective tanks to bring them to the proper fluid levels. The levels of solutions always should be kept at the top of the tank to ensure that all immersed films are completely covered with solution. Water should never be added to the solutions to bring them to tank-top level; this dilutes the strength of the chemicals.

Timer and Thermometer

A darkroom is not complete without a timing device and a thermometer (Fig. 11.4). Even with the most modern radiographic equipment, optimum results will not be produced without time and temperature control in the darkroom. The timer is used to determine the length of time the films stay in the developer solution. This is solely dependent on the temperature of the developer. To determine the temperature of the developer, a **thermometer** must be suspended in the developer solution. Each day, it may take some time for equalization of temperatures between the water tank and the developer tank. For this reason, the temperature of the developer bath is read, not the temperature of the water entering the surrounding water tank. These charts may vary slightly from manufacturer to manufacturer. A time-temperature chart like the following chart should be referenced when manually processing films.

Manual Processing: Time and Temperature Chart

80° F   2½ minutes in the developer
75° F   3 minutes in the developer
70° F   4 minutes in the developer (optimum)
68° F   4½ minutes in the developer
60° F   6 minutes in the developer

Film Hangers

Film hangers come in various sizes and contain clips for 2 to 20 films. In all cases, the films should be unwrapped and attached to the clips (Fig. 11.5). It is important that the film not be touched with *contaminated* gloves or ungloved hands. The working surface on which the hanger is loaded should be clean and dry to prevent film staining. Film hangers should be labeled to avoid mix-ups. Hangers with defective clips should be discarded, because a defective clip can scratch films on adjacent hangers in the solution. Defective clips may also lead to lost films in the solutions.

Dryer

After films have been washed for 20 to 30 minutes, they are ready for drying. This can be accomplished with the use of an x-ray dryer or simply by hanging them on towel racks in the darkroom and letting the films air dry. In either method, the films should not touch one another or they will stick together; separating them will tear the emulsion. Drying racks should be in a clean area.

The Development Process

Explanation and Discussion

Latent Image

Radiographs after having been exposed are said to contain a *latent image*. The silver halide on the radiographic emulsion is energized by the x-ray beam. The pattern of the energized silver halide crystals depends on the densities of the objects being radiographed. For instance, the silver halide crystals on the film that lie behind a metallic restoration receive almost no radiation, because the density of the metal absorbs

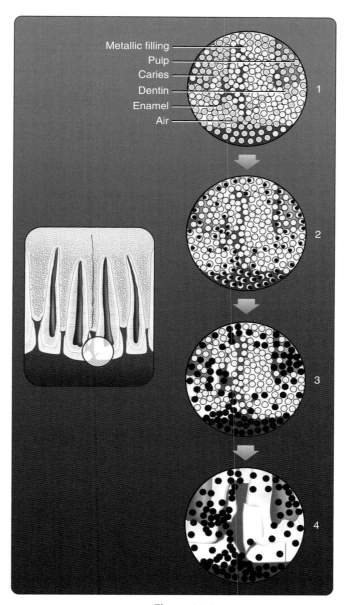

Metallic filling
Pulp
Caries
Dentin
Enamel
Air

1 Latent image; energized crystals are shaded gray

2 Start of development; energized crystals are precipitated as free silver (black areas)

3 Development complete; completely energized silver precipitated as black areas

4 Fixer removes unaffected crystals, leaving black, white, and gray areas

• **Figure 11.6** X-ray film development.

all the x-ray energy. Silver halide crystals on the film that correspond to an area (such as, the pulp of the tooth or a cavity) receive more radiation energy, because these areas are less dense and absorb little x-ray energy.

Developing

Exposed dental film packets should be processed as soon as possible. In the darkroom under safelight conditions, the x-ray films are removed from the packets and placed on film racks. The developer is the first solution into which these film racks are placed. The **developer** has a pH above 7 and thus is a "basic" solution as compared with the "acidic" fixing solution. The developer softens the gelatin and allows the solution to chemically reduce the energized silver halide crystals by precipitating silver on the film base.

This precipitation corresponds to the black (radiolucent) areas on the radiograph. An area of less density, such as the pulp, allows greater penetration of x-rays; therefore, more x-rays reach that part of the film. The silver halide crystals are more greatly energized, and more silver precipitates to give a black, or radiolucent, outline to the pulp chamber when compared to the dense areas that correspond to the radiopaque areas on the radiographic image (Fig. 11.6).

This is a chemical reaction. The optimum precipitation of silver for the amount of x-ray energy delivered to the object takes place in a specified amount of time with the developing solution at a certain temperature. This is the basis and importance of the **time-temperature technique**.

If films are left in the developing solution too long, more silver precipitates than was intended, and dense and

PROCEDURE 11.1   MANUAL PROCESSING

1. Lock the darkroom door from the inside, and label the film hanger.
2. Stir the solutions to equalize the temperature and the chemical distribution of the processing solutions. Use a different utensil for stirring each solution to prevent cross-contamination of the solutions. Check the levels of solutions and replenish if necessary.
3. Check the temperature of the developing solution and set the timer. Refer to the time-temperature chart, which should be accessible when processing, and set the time for the desired interval.
4. Turn off the white light, and turn on the safelight.
5. Put on gloves and open the film packets while dropping the films on a clean working surface if barrier envelopes were not used while exposing the films. If barrier envelopes were used while exposing the films, then clean, dry, ungloved hands may be used to handle the films. When applicable, discard contaminated film packets and/or barrier wraps, remove gloves, and load the film hangers. Work carefully, avoiding finger marks or film scratches. Be sure that the film is securely fastened to film hanger clips.
6. Immerse the film hanger in the developer solution and activate the timer. After immersing the film, immediately raise and lower the hanger slowly a few times so that the film surfaces are covered totally by solution.
7. Remove the film rack from the developer when the timer sounds (under safelight conditions).
8. Rinse thoroughly for 20 seconds in the water bath (under safelight conditions).
9. Place the film rack in the fixer solution. Gently agitate the rack up and down immediately after the initial placement. Films should remain in the fixer for a minimum of 10 minutes (approximately twice the developer time) for permanent fixation but may be removed after 3 or 4 minutes for use as a wet reading. After fixing, with the tank lids firmly in place, normal lighting can be resumed in the darkroom. Safelighting is not needed after the timer signals that fixation is complete and films are moved from the fixer to the water bath.
10. Place the films in the running water bath for 20 minutes.
11. Dry the films. Remove the films from the water bath and suspend them from rack holders or place them in a film dryer to dry.

HELPFUL HINT

While the film is in the developer, it is preferable for you to remain in the darkroom. If necessary, you can leave the darkroom, but be sure to check that the tank lids are securely in place before you leave.

PROCEDURE 11.2   AUTOMATIC PROCESSING

1. If there is no daylight loader on the automatic processor, lock the darkroom door, and make sure to keep a record of the name of the patient whose films are to be processed.
2. Turn on the processor or switch from the standby to the ready mode.
3. Turn off the white light, and turn on the safelight.
4. Put on gloves and open the film packets while dropping the films on a clean working surface on the automatic processor if barrier envelopes were not used while exposing the films. If barrier envelopes were used while exposing the films, then clean, dry, ungloved hands may be used to handle the films. When applicable, discard contaminated film and/or barrier wraps, remove gloves, and load the film into the processor. Be sure that the films are aligned with the film tracks and that they are not put in so quickly as to produce overlapping of the films during processing.
5. Retrieve the dried films, and place them in a mount.

HELPFUL HINT

When loading film into the automatic processor, it is a good idea to alternate tracks to avoid the films overlapping and sticking together.

less dense structures lose their distinctions. A completely overdeveloped film results when all the silver is precipitated by the developer and the film is totally black.

Crystals of silver halide that have received small amounts of radiation have correspondingly less silver precipitated and appear gray. The silver halide that was not energized by radiation, such as the area on the film behind a gold crown, precipitates no silver and appears white, or radiopaque, on the x-ray film.

Rinsing (Stop Bath)

The main purpose of this step is to rinse the film to remove the developer from the film so that the development process stops. This step is similar to photographic developing of the past when a chemical stop bath was used to stop the developing and also remove the "basic" developer so that it does not contaminate the "acidic" fixer.

In dental radiography, this is usually accomplished by agitating the film hanger in a water bath for about 20 seconds. Safelight conditions must be maintained when the films are transferred from the developer to the wash tank and then to the fixing solution.

Fixing

The acidic fixing solution (fixer) removes the unexposed and undeveloped (unaffected) silver halide crystals from the film emulsion and rehardens the emulsion, which has softened during the development process. For permanent fixation, the film is kept in the fixing solution for a minimum of 10 minutes. However, films may be removed from the fixing solution after 3 minutes for viewing. This procedure is known as the wet reading and is useful when films are needed immediately. For example, a wet reading of a film would be used to check that all of the root tip has been removed in an extraction before dismissing the patient. As previously mentioned, a film is ready for a wet reading if it has cleared enough for washing and reading. Operators should always check for clearance or the lack of murkiness under safelight conditions.

Because all films should be made part of the patient's permanent record (archival), they should be returned to the fixing solution to complete the required 10 minutes. Films not fixed properly fade and turn brown in a short time. Excessive fixing (i.e., 2–3 days) can completely remove the image from the film.

Washing and Drying

The film is washed for about 20 minutes in the water tank to completely remove the fixing solution from the emulsion. The film is then dried in a clean, dust-free area. Be aware that excessive washing that continues for 24 to 48 hours will remove the image from the film and should be avoided.

Time-Temperature Versus Sight Development

The best way to manually process dental x-ray films is by the time-temperature development method, as described in this chapter. This scientific method produces optimum information on the film. Even so, many dental offices develop x-ray films by using sight development. The usual technique is to immerse the film hanger in the developer, removing it at frequent intervals to hold it up to the safelight, until fillings or root shapes are visible. At that point, the films are washed and placed in the fixer. This is obviously an inexact, unacceptable technique. Sight development is ultimately unfair to the patient, because it does not provide the maximum diagnostic information for the radiation exposure. The time-temperature method, performed either manually or by automatic processors, is the most acceptable and standardized way to process dental radiographs.

Rapid Processing

Rapid processing of dental radiographs is done with the use of higher-solution temperatures, concentrated solutions, agitation of the film, or a combination of these. It is sometimes called *hot processing,* which is a term that refers to the temperature of the solutions. Rapid processing does not require an increase in radiation to the patient, but the images produced by this technique are not comparable in density and definition to films processed by standard methods. The use of rapid processing is clinically indicated when time is more important than exacting detail of the

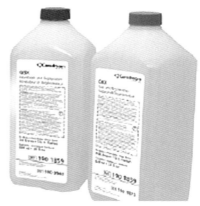

• **Figure 11.7** Concentrated solutions of film developer and fixer. (Courtesy Carestream Health, Inc, Rochester, NY.)

image. For example, it may be used when a patient has just had an extraction and a radiograph is taken to make sure that no debris is left in the socket before suturing. Working or operative endodontic radiographs can also be processed with this method. Rapid processing can be helpful with endodontic working films and postoperative films in oral surgery when a high degree of definition is not essential. It should not be used for routine processing of films.

The use of regular-strength developing solutions at 92° F with agitation of the film can produce acceptable diagnostic images in less than 1 minute (20 seconds developing, 3 seconds washing, and 30 seconds fixing). Concentrated processing solutions are also available that can be used at room temperature. The increased chemical activity of these solutions makes the rapid processing possible. Some of these solutions use a two-bath technique—developer and fixer; others use a single-bath technique, or monobath, that contains the developer and the fixer (Fig. 11.7).

Extraoral and Panoramic Films

Extraoral and panoramic films are processed in the same manner as intraoral films, using the time-temperature technique with the same solutions. As mentioned, the only precaution that must be taken is to check safelight intensity. Those extraoral films that are used in combination with intensifying screens (screen films) are more sensitive to light than nonscreen films. Darkroom illumination that may be safe for intraoral films may adversely affect screen films. The safety of the light can be checked by using the coin test discussed earlier in this chapter.

Care and Maintenance of the Darkroom

Darkroom maintenance is a means of ensuring quality control. Maintenance should be likened to our regard for sterility to avoid contamination and subsequent infection. Contaminants in the darkroom or other errors resulting from sloppy techniques may ruin diagnostic radiographs and require retaking of films, which leads to an unnecessary increase in the patient's radiation burden.

Cleanliness

The working surface, where film packets are opened and the films are placed on hangers, always should be clean and dry. Developer, fixer, and water produce the most common stains. Drying films should not be placed above the working surface without a surface protector under them. If the working surface is made of Formica, it can be cleaned easily with a mild detergent. Film hangers should be clean and dry when films are loaded. Hangers used for wet readings are the most likely ones to be insufficiently washed and can contain residual fixer that can stain the next film. Hangers should be washed after each use and clean, and dry hangers should always be used.

Processing tanks should be cleaned thoroughly when solutions are changed. This includes not only the insert tanks that hold the developer and fixer, but also the water reservoir. The water tank may accumulate sludge and algae, especially under the metallic lip and in the overflow tube. Operators can use a bland detergent or preferably one of the tank cleaners made specifically for this purpose. It is in this routine tank cleaning that one can appreciate a deep sink and a gooseneck faucet in the darkroom.

Solutions

Solutions should be brought to the optimal temperature at the beginning of the working day and kept at that temperature by the thermostatic control on the mixing valve.

Tanks should be kept full by the use of replenishers rather than by the addition of water, because water dilutes the concentration and weakens the solutions. If the tanks are not kept full, the films or portions of the films on the top clips of the film rack may not be immersed fully in solution and will not be developed (Fig. 11.8).

As mentioned earlier, both the developer and fixer solutions should be changed at least every 2 to 3 weeks. In practices with heavy film volume, it may be necessary to change solutions as often as once a week. Processed films should always be compared with a reference film (Fig. 11.9) of desired density and contrast that is kept posted on

the darkroom viewbox. When the processed films start to show a thin image, the solutions should be changed even if it is before the scheduled change date.

The lids of the processing tanks always should be closed when the tanks are not in use to prevent oxidation and weakening of the solutions.

Record Keeping

Two types of records are important in the darkroom. The first is the supply inventory, including the date of the next scheduled solution change. It is helpful to post the date of the next scheduled solution change in a prominent place.

Film identifications are the second important type of records in the darkroom; accurate records are essential to processing radiographs. The patient's name, chart number (if applicable), the number of films, the number or letter of the hanger on which the films were placed, and the date should be recorded. This eliminates the likelihood of lost films or mixed radiographs.

Environmental Concerns

Dental professionals must be aware of and comply with a growing number of environmental laws that regulate the management of waste materials. It is our professional responsibility to be aware of these federal and local regulations as they apply to our office and to comply.

Dental radiology generates the following three types of waste: (1) solid waste, (2) x-ray processing solution effluent, and (3) medical waste. Solid waste is the x-ray film packaging, including the lead foil but not the outside packet wrapping. The effluent is the liquid waste coming from the x-ray processing chemicals. The medical waste consists of only the intraoral dental packets that have been contaminated by blood or blood components and saliva.

The federal statute that regulates discarded material is the Resource Recovery Act of 1976. Professionals who create hazardous wastes are referred to in this statute as generators. Most dental offices in the United States would be classified as "conditionally exempt small-quantity

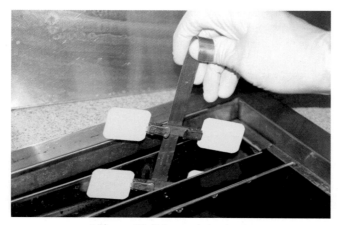

• **Figure 11.8** Low solution levels.

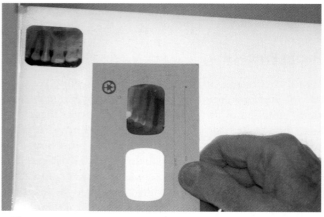

• **Figure 11.9** Processed film being compared with a reference film.

generators," because the small amount of hazardous waste that they generate is exempt from federal regulations. State and local laws vary, and exemption from federal regulation does not mean automatic exemption from local laws. Under most local laws, the hazardous waste must be removed by a certified carrier (in red bags) in the same way that used gauze pads or cotton rolls are removed. Large dental clinics and dental schools, because of their volume, may be classified as "small-quantity generators" and may be subject to federal regulation.

Silver

There are two sources of silver retrieval in the dental office. In the category of solid waste are the old, no longer needed, or unusable processed radiographs. The second source is the exhausted fixer solution, which falls under the effluent category.

Silver can be recovered from the processed radiographs by ashing the film above the melting point of silver. Ashing is an environmentally sound practice and is preferred to ordinary disposal. Discarded film is generally not a regulated waste. The discharge of fixer processing solution effluent into a sewer system or a septic tank is not recommended and in many localities is prohibited by law, depending on the concentration of silver in the effluent. The concentration depends on the volume of films processed. Chemical precipitation or electrolysis can retrieve residual silver from the fixer and the wash water. There is no residual silver in developer solution; thus, it can be discharged into the sewage system (Fig. 11.10). Exhausted silver solutions can be removed by a certified carrier.

Throwing the lead foil inserts of film packets in regular trash is not environmentally sound; although there is very little lead in each packet, the total amount of lead entering the environment because of the discarding is significant. There are cardboard holding boxes for collecting and shipping the foil to qualified disposal facilities.

Medical waste must be removed by a certified carrier in the same manner as for disposal of used gauze pads, cotton rolls, and so on.

Automatic Processing

Automatic dental x-ray film processing is currently more popular than manual processing in dental facilities that are still using conventional film for radiographic exposures. The major advantage of automatic processing is the maintenance of standardized procedure; these units provide solutions of proper strength, correct temperature, and regulated processing time. In short, they provide automated time-temperature processing. Other advantages of the units are the time saved and the increased volume of films that can be processed when compared with the manual method. These units also require maintenance and a quality-control program.

The typical automatic processor has three solutions—developer, fixer, and water—and have a built-in drying chamber (Fig. 11.11). The wash between developer and

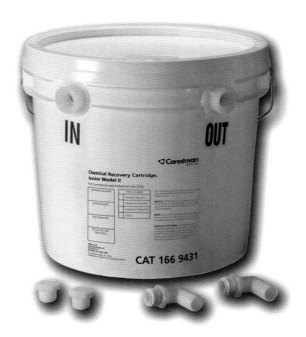

• **Figure 11.10** Cartridges allow for recovery of silver from photographic solutions. (Courtesy Carestream Health, Inc, Rochester, NY.)

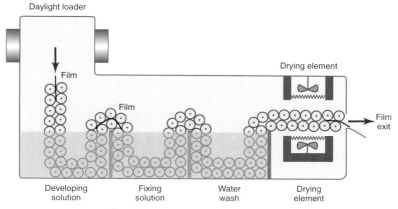

• **Figure 11.11** Automatic film processor.

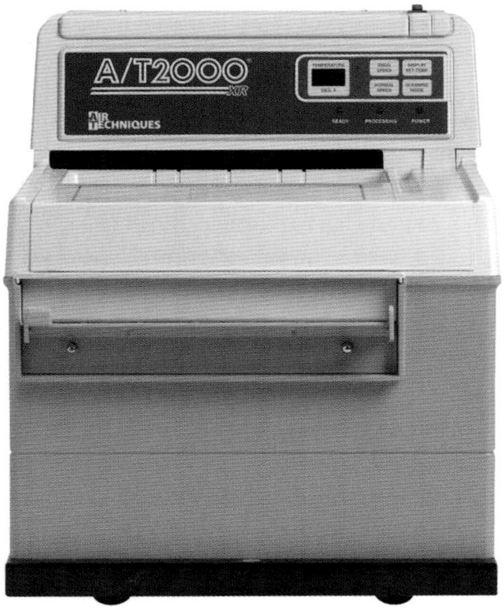

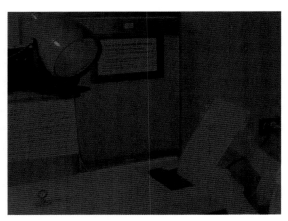

• **Figure 11.13** Film being inserted into an automatic processor in the darkroom under safelight conditions. (From Langlais RP, Miller CS: *Exercises in Oral Radiology and Interpretation,* ed 5, St Louis, 2017, Elsevier.)

• **Figure 11.12** Automatic processor that could accommodate panoramic-sized film. (Courtesy Air Techniques, Inc., Melville, NY.)

fixer solution is eliminated in most automatic processors. A transport system of either rollers or tracks driven by gears, belts, or chains moves the film from solution to solution and then into the drying chamber. Finished film is produced in 4 to 7 minutes; some units have the capacity to process even faster by elevating the temperature of the solutions.

Automatic processors vary in the size of film that they can accept, their safelight and plumbing requirements, and the option of automatic replenishment. Freestanding units are not connected to water and waste lines and may be kept in the operatory, as films are fed into the unit through a **daylight loader**.

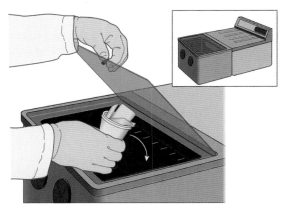

• **Figure 11.14** Daylight loader of an automatic processor being loaded outside the darkroom. (From Langlais RP, Miller CS: *Exercises in Oral Radiology and Interpretation,* ed 5, St Louis, 2017, Elsevier.)

Size of Film

Some units accept only periapical and bitewing size film (#0, #1, #2, and #3; Fig. 11.12), whereas others can accommodate all sizes, including 8 × 10-, 5 × 12-, or 6 × 12-inch panoramic film (see Fig. 11.12).

Safelight

Some processors must be located in the darkroom, because safelight procedures are required for opening and inserting the film into the automatic processor (Fig. 11.13). Units with daylight loaders do not have to be in the darkroom, because they have light-tight baffles into which the hands are placed while opening the film packet and inserting the film into the rollers (Fig. 11.14). The problems of infection control with daylight loaders were discussed previously in Chapter 8.

Plumbing

If there is a constant flow of water in the wash chamber, plumbing is required to bring in the water and a waste line

for recapturing the fixer to remove the silver. This arrangement can be more desirable than a freestanding chamber, in which the water level may drop and constant change is necessary.

Automatic Replenishment

More sophisticated processors maintain solution concentration and levels by automatic replenishment. Each time a piece of film is fed into the unit, a few drops of fixer and developer are added automatically to the baths to maintain solution strength.

Care and Maintenance

Automatic processors require daily or weekly cleaning, depending on the volume of films processed. The **film rollers** should be cleaned at the beginning of the day by running an extraoral size film or clean-up film that is designed to clean through the rollers. This removes any residual debris or dirt from the rollers. The rollers should be removed weekly from the processor and soaked in a water bath for about 20 minutes.

Solution levels should be checked at the beginning of every day and replenished when necessary. Quality-assurance checks are also necessary. The processors are only as good as the care that their operators give them.

Technique remains important and cannot be neglected just because the machine runs automatically. Films should not be fed into the rollers too quickly. Operators should maintain at least a 10-second interval between films on the same track. This prevents overlapping of films in processing and failure of chemicals to reach overlapped portions of the film. Carelessness in feeding the films too quickly may lead to the films overlapping in the automatic processor.

Quality assurance for processing is also discussed in a later chapter.

Duplicate Radiographs

After the exposure to light in the duplicating device, duplicate radiographs (see Chapter 4) are processed in the same manner, either manually or automatically, as other films are processed.

Text continued on p. 138

COMMON ERROR 11.1   THE DARKROOM (see also the Appendix)

Fogged Film (Fig. 11.15). A fogged film has an overall gray appearance because of diminished contrast. This can be caused by light leaks in the darkroom, cell phone light exposure, improper safelighting, or improper film storage, as well as exposure to scatter (secondary) radiation.

Remedy. Safelight conditions can be checked with a coin test (see Fig. 11.2). All doors should be checked for possible leaks, unexposed and exposed film should be kept away from scatter radiation, cell phones should be off or not brought into the darkroom, and old film should be used first.

> **NOTE**
>
> It is important to store films according to their expiration dates. We recommend the FIFO method. FIFO stands for first-in, first-out, meaning that the films that will expire first should be stored in the front of the storage area so that they are used first and do not expire before they are used.

Underdeveloped Film: Thin Image (Fig. 11.16). Underdeveloped film is light (thin) in appearance and does not contain all possible diagnostic information. This results when the optimum amount of silver has not been precipitated because of weak or cold developing solutions or insufficient developing time. This type of film is identical to the thin image produced by such chairside technique errors as incorrect time setting or increased focal film distance (underexposed image).

Remedy. The developer and fixing solutions should be changed every 2 to 3 weeks, and the time-temperature method should be used. That is, the temperature of the developer should be checked before films are immersed in the solution, and the timer should be set for the appropriate time. This error can also occur with sight developing and can be avoided by using the time-temperature processing technique. Daily quality assurance checks should be performed to determine solution strength.

Overdeveloped Film: Dense Image (Fig. 11.17). Overdeveloped film may vary from dark to totally black depending on the degree of overdevelopment. This type of film is of no diagnostic value. A dense image, or dark image, results when too much silver has been precipitated on the film base; in the case of the totally black film, all the silver from the silver bromide has been precipitated. This error can be caused by hot developing solutions or prolonged developing time. As mentioned with light films, chairside errors—including setting the exposure time incorrectly—can produce an overexposed image that is similar in appearance to an overdeveloped film.

Remedy. The time-temperature method of processing should always be used. The timer should have a bell or buzzer that rings when the developing time has elapsed. This enables the dental professional to leave the darkroom while the films are being processed. Without the bell, the dental professional may be distracted by other duties and forget to remove the

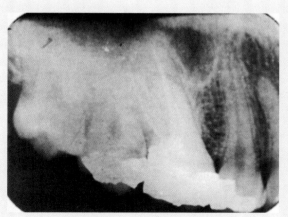

• **Figure 11.15** Maxillary molar radiograph that has been fogged. Note lack of definition and contrast.

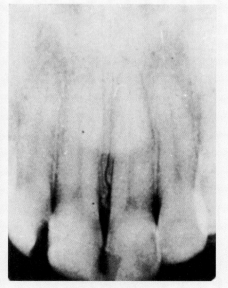

• **Figure 11.16** Underdeveloped film.

Continued

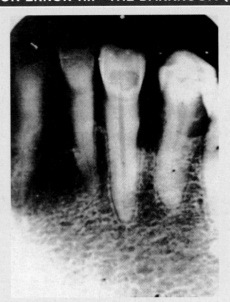

• **Figure 11.17** Overdeveloped film.

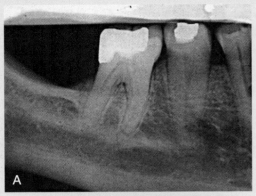

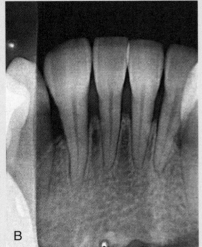

• **Figure 11.18** Radiographs with developer cutoff.

films from the developer at the proper time. This error can also occur with sight developing and can be avoided by using the time-temperature processing technique. Operators should perform daily quality assurance checks on solution strength as well.

Developer Cutoff (Fig. 11.18). Films with developer cutoff show a straight radiopaque border on what was the upper edge of the top film on the processing hanger. This is an undeveloped area of the film. When the solutions are allowed to deplete in the processing tanks, the films on the top positions on the racks may not be covered by solution when the racks are placed in the tanks. This error should be differentiated from collimator cutoff with a circular column, which results in a curved radiopaque border. In collimator cutoff, the film portion is unexposed; in developer cutoff, the film portion is undeveloped. However, developer cutoff is similar in appearance to collimator cutoff with a rectangular column; it is recommended for operators to retrace their steps when trying to investigate if the error was caused during exposure or processing.

Remedy. One should always make sure that processing tanks are full. If the levels of solutions have dropped, water should not be added; this only dilutes the solution and results in underdeveloped films. Proper replenisher solutions should be added to maintain the desired level.

Clear Films (Fig. 11.19). Films are clear because the entire emulsion has been washed off. This occurs when films are left in the fixer or running water baths for 24 to 48 hours. Clear films due to a processing error are identical in appearance, but not in cause, to unexposed film that is developed and processed. With unexposed film, the fixer removes all the unaffected silver bromide crystals. Clear films can also result if a film is placed in the fixer solution before the developing solution.

Remedy. Films should never be left in water baths overnight. Processing should be complete before one leaves the office. Films should not be left in the fixer overnight or for prolonged periods beyond the recommended 10 minutes; the fixer will lighten and ultimately remove the image. Do not place exposed films in the fixer before the developer.

• **Figure 11.19** Clear film can result from excessive washing or fixing or an unexposed film.

Stained Films (Fig. 11.20). If the working surface in the darkroom is wet and dirty, films can be stained either before or after processing. Stains caused by the developing solution are dark; and if they are caused by the fixer solution, they are light.

Remedy. Darkroom work surfaces *must* be kept clean and dry.

Discolored Films (Fig. 11.21). Films that have not had adequate fixation (approximately twice the developing time)

COMMON ERROR 11.1 THE DARKROOM (see also the Appendix)—cont'd

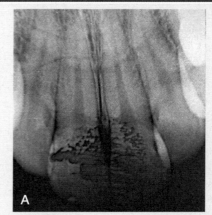

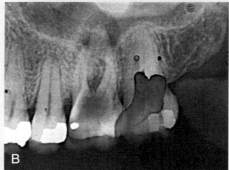

• **Figure 11.20** Stained radiographs.

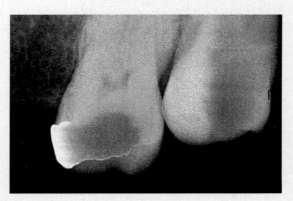

• **Figure 11.21** Insufficient fixing results in a partially discolored film.

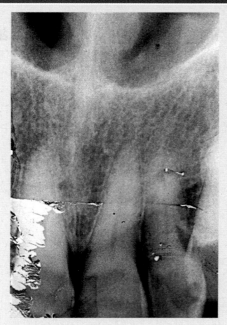

• **Figure 11.22** Radiograph with torn emulsion.

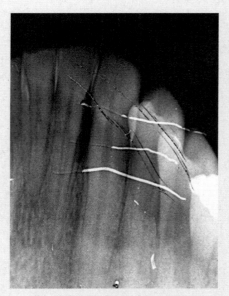

• **Figure 11.23** Scratched radiograph.

turn brown after a period and are useless as part of the patient's permanent record. A radiograph should have an archival life of at least 7 years.

Remedy. All films must have adequate fixation time (10 minutes). All wet readings should be returned to the fixing solution after the patient has been treated for optimum fixing.

Torn Emulsion (Fig. 11.22). If films that are drying are allowed to touch and overlap, they stick together, leading to a torn emulsion. When one separates the films by tearing them apart, the emulsions are usually torn off the film base in the overlapped area, rendering the film useless for diagnosis.

Remedy. Film racks should be checked to ensure that drying films from different racks are not touching. If there are films stuck together, it is recommended to wet those films with water and gently separate them from each other.

Scratched Films (Fig. 11.23). A radiopaque line on a film is usually an artifact caused by scratching the emulsion on the film base in film processing. Most often, it is the result of putting a second film rack into a tank that already contains a film rack. It also can be caused by fingernails scratching the film while it is being unpacked and placed on a rack, or it can be scratched by a broken clip on a film rack.

Remedy. When film racks are put into the processing solution, care should be taken to avoid touching those already immersed. Any film racks should be discarded if they have sharp edges or broken clips that could scratch other films.

Continued

COMMON ERROR 11.1   THE DARKROOM (see also the Appendix)—cont'd

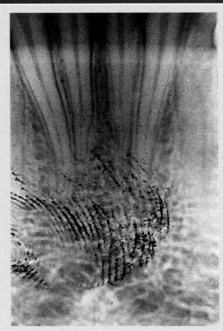

• **Figure 11.24** Fluoride artifact. Operator's fingertip, contaminated by fluoride, touched film during stripping and placing of film on hanger.

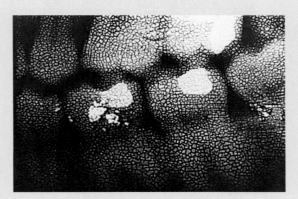

• **Figure 11.25** Reticulation.

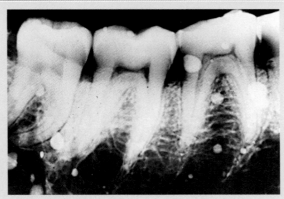

• **Figure 11.26** Artifact caused by air bubbles trapped on the film, preventing processing solution from touching film in the area.

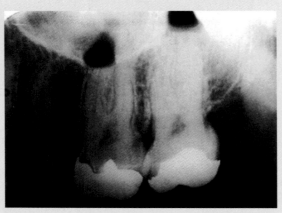

• **Figure 11.27** Periapical radiograph with static marks.

Lost Film In Tanks. If films are not firmly clipped onto the hangers, they may fall off in any of the three processing baths. A lost film could necessitate a retake.

Remedy. All films should be checked to see that they are clipped securely to the hangers before processing.

Fluoride Artifacts (Fig. 11.24). Some fluorides, especially stannous fluoride, produce black marks on radiographs.

Remedy. After working with fluoride, the dental professional should wash hands thoroughly with an appropriate cleanser or change gloves before handling films in the darkroom.

Reticulation (Fig. 11.25). If film is developed at an elevated temperature and then placed in a cold water bath (or vice versa), the sudden change in temperature causes the swollen emulsion to shrink rapidly and give the image a wrinkled appearance called reticulation.

Remedy. Sharp contrasts in temperatures between processing and the water bath should be avoided.

Air Bubbles (Fig. 11.26). If air bubbles are trapped on the film as it is placed in the processing solutions, the chemicals cannot affect the emulsion in that area.

Remedy. The film hangers always should be gently raised and lowered when they are placed in the processing solutions to coat the films with solution. Aggressive agitation can cause air bubbles to stick to the films.

Static Marks (Fig. 11.27). Static electricity can be produced when intraoral film packets are opened forcefully in the darkroom. This is not a common occurrence with intraoral films. The same effect occurs much more often on extraoral films. With these films, static electricity may result when the piece of film is removed from a full box; the sliding of the film out of the tightly packed box may produce static electricity. Static electricity also may be produced during loading and unloading of cassettes in panoramic machines as the film is slid in or out between the intensifying screens. In addition, walking around a carpeted office may produce static electricity. If the dental professional does not touch a conductive object before unwrapping the film, electrostatic artifacts may result on the film. Static electricity occurs most often on cold, dry days.

Remedy. Operators should ground themselves by touching any conductive object in the darkroom before handling film and should avoid friction of any kind against the film that will produce static electricity especially on cold, dry days.

COMMON ERROR 11.1   THE DARKROOM (see also the Appendix)—cont'd

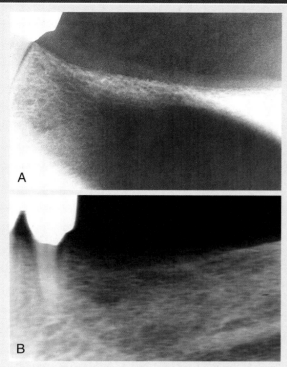

A

B

• **Figure 11.28 A,** Artifact caused by a light leak in the daylight loader, resembling a large pathologic area in bone. **B,** Normal radiograph of the same area.

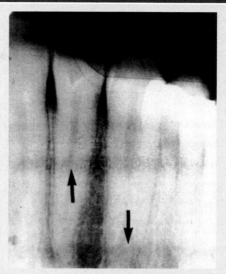

• **Figure 11.29** Bands of stain *(arrows)* from dirty rollers of an automatic processor.

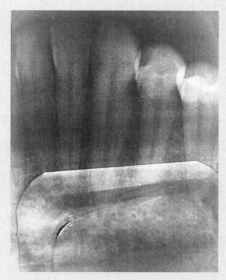

• **Figure 11.30** Overlapped films during automatic processing.

Automatic Processing

Daylight Loaders: Light Leaks (Fig. 11.28). Film fog, a ruined film, or unusual artifacts can be caused by removing one's hands from the baffle (see Fig. 11.14) before the film has entered the processor.

Remedy. The operator's hands must be kept on the film until it has been completely taken up by the rollers. The material that makes up the baffle should fit tightly around the hands. Rips and tears should be repaired immediately and stretched elastic replaced. It is a good idea to remove wristwatches and bracelets, because they tend to tear the baffle material.

Dirty Rollers (Fig. 11.29). If the rollers are not cleaned periodically, radiolucent bands or white chalky debris will appear on the finished film.

Remedy. Rollers should be cleaned periodically by removing and soaking them in accordance with the manufacturer's recommendations. A piece of extraoral or cleaning film should be run through at the beginning of every work day to clean the rollers.

Overlapped Films (Fig. 11.30). If the films are fed into the processor too quickly, they overlap, and the processing solutions cannot reach the emulsion.

Remedy. The operator should wait 10 seconds before putting the next film into each processing track. If there are films stuck together, it is recommended to wet those films with water and gently separate them from each other. In this case, however, there still may be areas on the films that were not processed properly, and gently separating the films will just avoid tearing the emulsion.

Chapter Review Questions

Multiple Choice

1. If a safelight is adequate, the coin test will:
   a. Show an outline of the coin
   b. Be blurred
   c. Not show an outline of the coin
   d. Show a completely black film
   e. None of the above
2. The chemicals in the developing solution used to reduce the energized silver halide crystals to silver is:
   a. Hydroquinone and sodium carbonate
   b. Sodium thiosulfate and Metol
   c. Sodium carbonate and Elon
   d. Elon or Metol and hydroquinone
   e. Sodium sulfite and sodium thiosulfate
3. A clear radiograph can result from:
   a. Prolonged fixing
   b. Prolonged time in the water bath
   c. No exposure
   d. Not turning on the radiographic unit
   e. All of the above
4. In manual and automatic processing:
   a. Fixing follows developing
   b. Fixing comes before developing
   c. Developing follows fixing
   d. Drying is never necessary
   e. Complete fixing is never necessary
5. If the temperature of the processing solutions is slightly above normal, radiographs of desired density may be best obtained by:
   a. Increasing the developing time
   b. Increasing the exposure time
   c. Increasing the fixing time
   d. Decreasing the developing time
   e. Increasing the fixing time

Case-Based Critical Thinking Exercise

A patient presents to your dental facility for radiographs. The facility employs conventional film-based radiography and the manual method of processing films. Three of the radiographs taken reveal processing errors. Answer the following questions accordingly:

1. The processing error shown at the superior border on this radiograph can be remedied by:

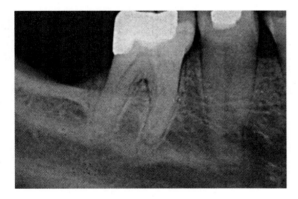

   a. Not exposing the film to cell phone light
   b. Making sure that the films do not stick together
   c. Checking the safelight regularly
   d. Making sure that the whole film is immersed in the developing solution
   e. Not exposing the film to white light

2. The dark stain on the accompanying radiograph is as a result of:

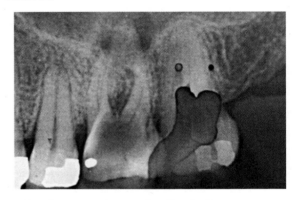

   a. Developer contacting the film before processing
   b. Air bubbles contacting the film
   c. Contaminated fixer solution
   d. Water splashing on the film
   e. Fixer contacting the film before processing

3. The operator did not pay attention to the different temperatures of the processing solutions while manually processing. The accompanying image resulted from this error and is best known as:

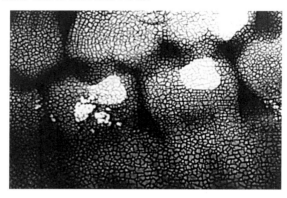

a. Static electricity
b. Overdeveloping
c. Hot processing
d. Reversed processing
e. Reticulation

Bibliography

Alcox RW, Jameson WR: Rapid dental x-ray film processor for selected procedures, *J Am Dent Assoc* 8:517–519, 1969.

Beideman RL, Johnson ON, Alcox RW: A study to develop a rating system and evaluate dental radiographs submitted to a third party carrier, *J Am Dent Assoc* 93:1010–1013, 1976.

Eastman Kodak Co: *Quality assurance in dental radiography*, 1989. Rochester, NY: Health Science Division.

Eastman Kodak Co: *Waste management guidelines*, 1994. Rochester, NY: Health Science Division.

Langland OE, Langlais RP: *Principles of dental imaging*, Baltimore, MD, 1997, Williams & Wilkins.

National Council on Radiation Protection and Measurements: NCRP Report No. 145, Radiation in Dentistry, 2004.

Stabulas-Savage J, Kwan J, Phelan J: The effects of cell phone light on dental radiographic film, *Research* 1:838, 2014.

Suleiman OH, Spelic DC, Conway B, et al: Radiographic trends of dental offices and dental schools, *J Am Dent Assoc* 130:1104–1110, 1999.

Swanson RL, Roethel FJ, Bauer H: Reuse of lead from dental X-rays, *N Y State Dent J* 65:34–36, 1999.

Thompson EM, Johnson ON: *Essentials of dental radiography for dental assistants and hygienists*, ed 9, Upper Saddle River, NJ, 2012, Pearson Education, Inc.

White SC, Pharoah MJ: *Oral radiology: Principles and interpretation*, ed 7, St Louis, MO, 2013, Mosby.

12

Panoramic Radiography

EDUCATIONAL OBJECTIVES

Upon completing this chapter, the student will be able to:

1. Define the key terms listed at the beginning of the chapter.
2. Discuss the purpose of panoramic radiography.
3. Know the significance of the slit beam in panoramic radiography.
4. Explain the basics of panoramic radiography, including the importance of a focal trough or image layer.
5. Describe concepts related to pantomograms:
   - Describe how a panoramic image is produced.
   - List the positioning requirements for panoramic images.
   - Define *ghost image,* and explain its role in panoramic radiography.
6. List the advantages and disadvantages of panoramic imaging.
7. Discuss the main indications for use of a panoramic radiograph, and describe the interpretation of the images produced.
8. Know the cause, appearance, and remedy for technique errors in panoramic radiography.
9. Discuss the common contemporary artifacts that can be found on panoramic images.

KEY TERMS

ala-tragus line	image layer	pantomogram
centers of rotation	laminogram	point of rotation
focal trough	midsagittal plane	slit beam
Frankfort plane	panoramic image	tomogram
ghost image	Panorex	tomography

Introduction

Panoramic dental x-ray units have become commonplace in dental offices, and the panoramic radiograph is considered to be an essential element in radiographic diagnosis. Therefore, dental professionals should be familiar with panoramic x-ray machines, technique, and interpretation. As shown in this chapter, the panoramic radiograph is not meant to replace intraoral periapical and bitewing images but rather to complement them in the diagnostic process. The term *panorama* means "an unobstructed view of a region in any direction;" thus, a **panoramic image** shows the mandible and maxilla on one radiograph from condyle to condyle.

Panoramic radiography was introduced into the US dental market in 1959 by the S. S. White Corporation as their **Panorex** unit. The design of this unit was based mainly on the work of Dr. Y. V. Paatero, a Finnish dentist, and was published in 1949. The panoramic radiographic technique makes use of a slit beam and curved or flat-surface rotational tomography. The term **slit beam** refers to the width, usually 1 to 2 mm, of the beam that is produced by the collimator (Fig. 12.1). This chapter discusses the use of conventional and digital panoramic radiography, as well as the basic concepts, patient positioning, and errors involved with this type of extraoral radiography.

The Basics of Panoramic Radiography

Tomography is a radiographic technique that allows radiographing in one plane of an object while blurring or eliminating images from structures in other planes. *Tomo* is the Greek word for "section," and sections or radiographic slices of the object are seen. These projections also could be called **laminograms,** from the word *lamina* (layer), because this is a layered radiographic technique. Tomography is used extensively in medicine and is the basis for computed tomography (CT) and magnetic resonance imaging (MRI), both of which are discussed in Chapter 16.

A **tomogram** is made by moving the x-ray source and the image receptor in opposite directions in a fixed relationship through one or a series of rotation points while the patient remains stationary (Fig. 12.2). The plane of the object that is not blurred on the radiograph is called the "plane of acceptable detail" or **focal trough**. It is also called the **image**

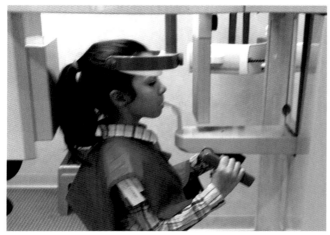

• **Figure 12.1** Slit beam collimator. Only the part of the receptor that is in back of the narrow beam is exposed. (From Bird DL, Robinson DS: *Modern Dental Assisting,* ed 12, St Louis, 2018, Elsevier.)

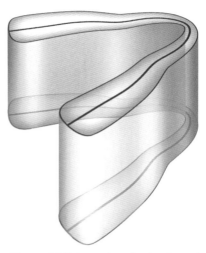

• **Figure 12.3** Image layer, or focal trough.

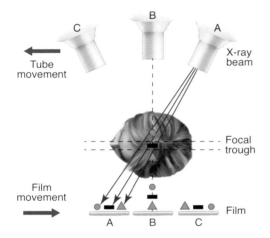

• **Figure 12.2** Principles of tomography. Note that only objects in the focal trough (square) project onto the same area of the image and are not blurred out.

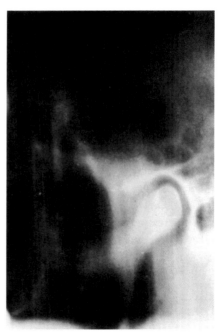

• **Figure 12.4** Tomogram of the temporomandibular joint (TMJ). Note the clarity of the condyle and the blurring of the rest of the image.

layer (Fig. 12.3). The image layer is an invisible area that is located in the space between the source of radiation and the image receptor. The shape of the image layer varies. Clinically, this concept is very important, because many of the errors in technique that are discussed later in this chapter are caused by improper patient positioning, the result of which is not having the desired area in the image layer. The **points of rotation** around which the tube head travels can be either inside or outside of the focal trough. The width or thickness of the focal trough is governed by many factors, including the angle of movement of the x-ray beam, the width of the x-ray beam, and the size of the focal spot. Any object that lies in the focal plane is shown clearly, and objects above and below it appear blurred. By varying the focal-object distance—the distance between the tube head and the patient—on a tomographic series, different focal troughs or "cuts" can be achieved. A tomographic series is usually composed of multiple cuts, 0.5 cm apart,

with the number of cuts varying according to the thickness of the object (Fig. 12.4).

Some tomographic units are made combined with a panoramic unit specifically for use in the head and neck region. These units enable dentists to do tomography in their own offices. Indications for dental office tomography include implant planning, temporomandibular joint (TMJ) tomography, and diagnosis of pathologic lesions. The majority of these tomographic units are computer-driven (Fig. 12.5). This means that the computer controls the motion of the tube head and receptor and other exposure parameters based on choices and information entered by the operator. In some of these computer-directed units, the imaging system is still a film screen combination. In these

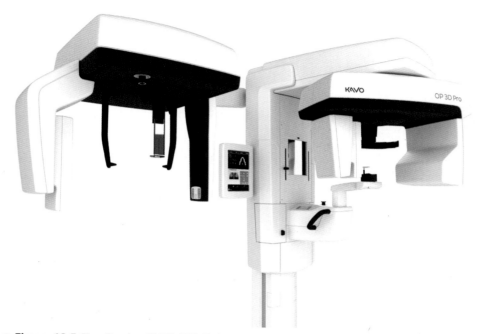

• **Figure 12.5** The Gendex GXDP 700 Series is a 3-in-1 system that provides digital panoramic, cephalometric, and 3D radiography. (Courtesy KaVo Kerr, Orange, CA.)

systems, the computer does not produce or store images as in digital imaging; it simply directs the patient exposure, after which the film is processed to produce the diagnostic image.

Pantomogram

A panoramic radiograph of the maxilla and the mandible produced by using tomography is also called a **pantomogram**. The pantomogram is a curved-surface tomogram (Fig. 12.6), in contrast to the plane surface or straight-line tomogram illustrated in Fig. 12.2. In common usage, the term *panoramic radiograph* is usually substituted for *pantomogram*. The term *Panorex* should never be used as a substitute for a *panoramic radiograph* unless the Panorex unit is being used. It is not a generic term but rather the manufacturer's name for the first panoramic unit introduced in the dental market.

> **NOTE**
>
> Dental professionals often use the term *Panorex* to describe the panoramic radiographic technique, although it is actually the name of the manufacturer that originated the first panoramic unit. Calling a panoramic radiograph a Panorex is like calling a facial tissue a Kleenex and is not the actual terminology that should be appropriately utilized in dental radiography.

Digital Radiography

Digital imaging is widely used in dental radiography for intraoral periapical and bitewing projections, as well as for digital panoramic imaging. Digital radiography is discussed in detail in Chapter 15, in which the basic principles of

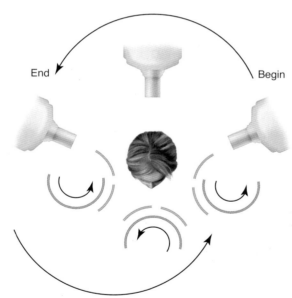

• **Figure 12.6** Rotational tomography. Note the slit opening in the receptor carrier and that the receptor and the tube travel around the patient in opposite directions.

intraoral digital imaging are shown to apply to panoramic digital radiography. Basically, a digital complementary metal oxide semiconductor (CMOS), charged-coupled device (CCD), or phosphor storage plate (PSP) sensor approximately the size of the slit beam collimating device is in the carrier instead of a film-screen combination. As the carrier moves around the patient, the electronic impulses are sent back to the computer, and an image is generated. The digital panoramic image can be altered in the same way as the digital intraoral image—the operator can change various image qualities, including contrast, density, and magnification.

Advantages and Disadvantages: Panoramic Radiography

Like any technique, panoramic radiography has its advantages and disadvantages when compared with conventional intraoral techniques. The panoramic unit is expensive (approximately four times the cost of a regular x-ray unit). The standard x-ray unit is still necessary even in an office with a panoramic unit.

There are many pantomographic units available on the market today. They differ primarily in the number and locations of the centers of rotation, the choice of a fixed or adjustable focal trough, and the type and shape of the receptor transport mechanism. All conventional panoramic units use intensifying screens, with a film size of either $5\frac{1}{2}$ or $6\frac{1}{2}$ inches. Design differences in both conventional and digital panoramic units include head-positioning devices, manual or automatic setting controls, bite blocks, kilovoltage and milliamperage range, standing or sitting patient positioning, and wall-mounted or freestanding units. Some more advanced units offer the option of being able to do other extraoral projections, cross-sectional tomography, or digital panoramic imaging. Each manufacturer's machine has its own technique for operation, which can be learned easily from the instruction manual (Figs. 12.7 and 12.8). However, there are certain positioning requirements that are common to all units, which are discussed in Procedure Box 12.1.

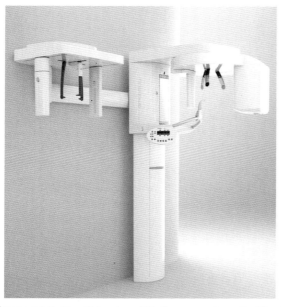

• **Figure 12.7** The Orthophos XG 5 panoramic unit. (Courtesy Dentsply Sirona, Charlotte, NC.)

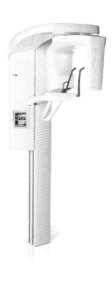

• **Figure 12.8** PM 2002 CC Proline panoramic machine. (Courtesy Planmeca, Inc., Roselle, IL.)

PROCEDURE 12.1 COMMON POSITIONING REQUIREMENTS FOR PANORAMIC UNITS

1. Midsagittal plane: The midsagittal plane should be perpendicular to the floor (Fig. 12.9).
2. Frankfort plane: The Frankfort plane is the imaginary line connecting the floor of the orbit and the external auditory meatus. In most units, this plane should be parallel to the floor (Fig. 12.10). Some units may use the ala-tragus line (imaginary line connecting the lower border of the *ala* of the nose to the upper border of the *tragus* of the ear) for patient positioning.
3. Bite block position: The anterior teeth should be positioned in the proper groove in the bite block (Fig. 12.11) and not forward or posterior to the groove (Figs. 12.12 and 12.13). If the patient is edentulous, then some other type of extraoral positioner should be used (Fig. 12.14).
4. Chin position: The chin should not be angled up or down (Figs. 12.15 and 12.16).

5. Head position: The head-positioning devices should be firm to prevent tipping or rotating during the exposure and loss of proper midsagittal plane orientation (Fig. 12.17).
6. Patient stabilization: The patient must not move during the exposure or a blurred image will result.
7. Tongue position: The patient should place and maintain the tongue against the roof of the mouth.
8. Posture: The patient should keep the spine erect and avoid slumping during panoramic exposure.
9. Lead apron: A double-sided lead (or lead substitute) apron is used without a thyroid collar, because the collar will block the primary beam (Fig. 12.18). In addition, the lead apron should be positioned below the level of the clavicles during exposure.

Continued

PROCEDURE 12.1 COMMON POSITIONING REQUIREMENTS FOR PANORAMIC UNITS—cont'd

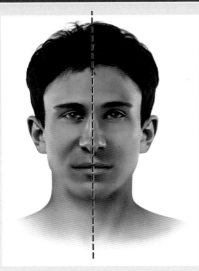

• **Figure 12.9** Midsagittal plane.

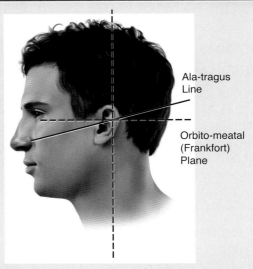

Ala-tragus Line

Orbito-meatal (Frankfort) Plane

• **Figure 12.10** Anatomic horizontal positioning planes.

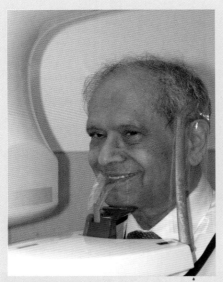

• **Figure 12.11** Patient positioned with anterior teeth in placement groove.

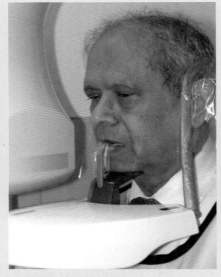

• **Figure 12.12** Patient positioned with anterior teeth forward of the groove in the bite block.

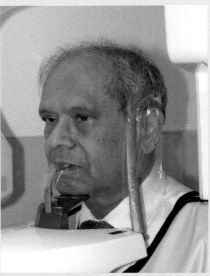

• **Figure 12.13** Patient positioned with anterior teeth posterior to the groove.

NOTE

Patient posture is very important. Without correct posture positioning, the structure to be radiographed may not be in or remain in the plane of focus (focal trough) and will appear blurred on the panoramic radiograph.

PROCEDURE 12.1 COMMON POSITIONING REQUIREMENTS FOR PANORAMIC UNITS—cont'd

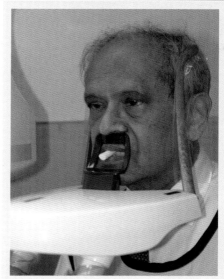

• **Figure 12.14** Positioning of the edentulous patient.

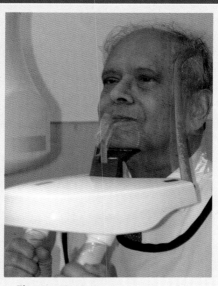

• **Figure 12.15** Patient positioned incorrectly with the chin up.

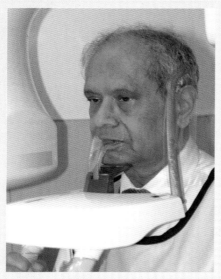

• **Figure 12.16** Patient positioned incorrectly with the chin down.

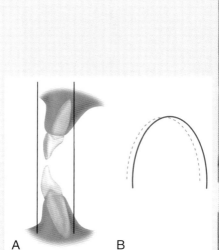

A   B

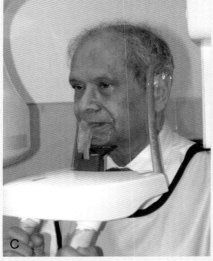

C

• **Figure 12.17** **A,** Anterior teeth positioned correctly. **B,** Broken line is focal plane, and unbroken line is mandibular arch, showing that neither side is in the focal plane. **C,** Patient positioned with head rotated.

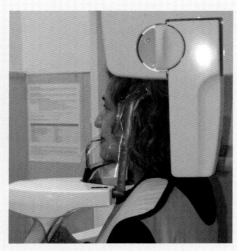

• **Figure 12.18** Patient with lead apron in place. Note that there is no thyroid collar used.

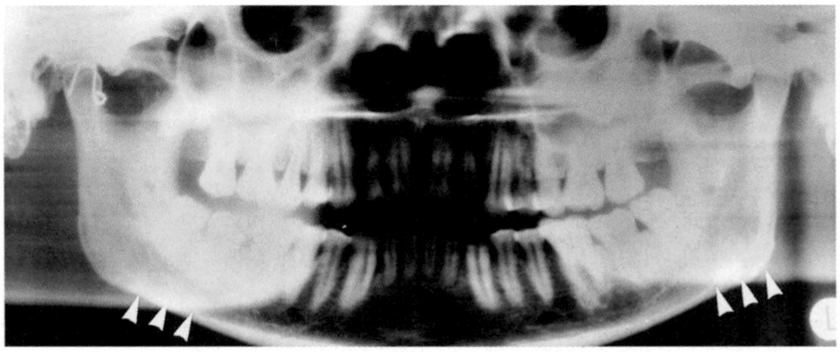

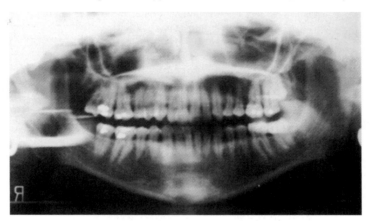

• **Figure 12.19** Ghost images of the opposite sides of the mandible, outlined by the *arrows*.

• **Figure 12.20** Radiopaque markings caused by the patient's earring. Note the ghost image and the sharp image.

Panoramic Image

The panoramic image shows the entire dentition and supporting bone from condyle to condyle on one image. However, the image does not have the same definition seen on an intraoral periapical or bitewing projection. This factor is inherent in the pantomographic process. These images also have a significant amount of horizontal distortion but less vertical distortion.

All objects in the field of the x-ray beam, even those out of the plane of focus, are projected onto the receptor, but most are not seen. The objects that have the greatest density (e.g., bone or metal objects) and are out of the plane of acceptable detail (focal trough) are shown in two places on the panoramic image. One place is the intended image or the usable image, and the other is referred to as the **ghost image** (Fig. 12.19). The ghost image always has less sharpness and is seen at a point higher on the radiograph than the desired image. The ghost image is always reversed; that is, the left appears on the right and vice versa. This can be best illustrated by an image in which the patient did not remove large earrings (Fig. 12.20).

Some panoramic units can be used to take tomograms of the TMJ (Fig. 12.21). To accomplish this, the unit must have an adjustable focal plane. The plane is set for the position of the condyle instead of the usual focal plane, which is through the body of the mandible. By stopping the rotation and rewinding the receptor carrier, an open view and a closed view can be taken on each side with one receptor producing four images (R-closed position, R-open position, L-closed position, and L-open position).

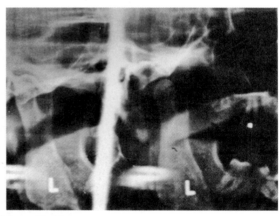

• **Figure 12.21** Pantomography of the temporomandibular joint (TMJ) done using a panoramic unit with an adjustable focal trough. The focal trough is set for the plane of the condyles instead of the body of the mandible.

Advantages
Size of the Field

Field size is one of the major advantages of panoramic radiography. The full-mouth series is composed of radiographs of the entire mouth but only of the teeth, alveolar ridges, and part of the supporting bone. Panoramic radiography covers an area that includes all of the mandible from condyle to condyle and the maxillary regions extending superiorly to the maxillary sinus and nasal cavity (Figs. 12.22 and 12.23). Areas of the mandible—such as the condyles, inferior border, angle, ascending ramus, and coronoid process, as well as the entire maxillary arch, which are not visualized on

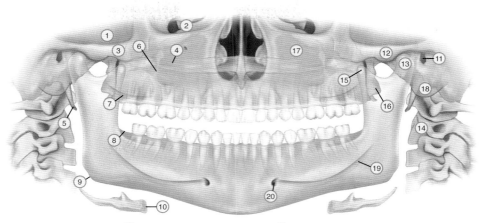

① Middle Cranial Fossa	⑪ Glenoid Fossa
② Orbit	⑫ Articular Eminence
③ Zygomatic Arch	⑬ Mandibular Condyle
④ Palate	⑭ Vertebra
⑤ Styloid Process	⑮ Coronoid Process
⑥ Septa in Maxillary Sinus	⑯ Pterygoid Plates
⑦ Maxillary Tuberosity	⑰ Maxillary Sinus
⑧ External Oblique Ridge	⑱ Ear Lobe
⑨ Angle of Mandible	⑲ Mandibular Canal
⑩ Hyoid Bone	⑳ Mental Foramen

• **Figure 12.22** Panoramic radiograph and tracing showing numbered anatomic landmarks. (Courtesy KaVo Dental/GENDEX Imaging, Lake Zurich, IL.)

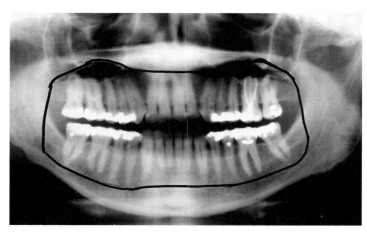

• **Figure 12.23** Panoramic radiograph with tracing of the area seen on a full-mouth survey *(outlined)*.

intraoral surveys—are seen routinely on panoramic images. Lesions that might be undetected on intraoral surveys may be seen in the enlarged field size of the panoramic image.

A contemporary indication for the use of panoramic images has been reported. Some patients who are at risk for cerebrovascular accidents because of the presence of atherosclerotic plaque in their carotid arteries can be identified in the dental office by appropriate evaluation of their panoramic images for calcifications. Most panoramic images show the area adjacent to or below the intervertebral space between C3 and C4, which is the location of the carotid arteries that might show evidence of calcifications (Fig. 12.24). Panoramic radiographs should not be taken solely to screen for carotid artery atherosclerotic plaque. However, their presence should be evaluated on every patient who has

a pantomogram taken. It is your professional obligation to do this, and patients should be referred to a physician regardless of their symptoms. If a finding is observed on a radiograph that was not the primary purpose of the exposure, this finding is considered to be an *incidental finding,* and the appropriate referral is made based on the image produced.

Quality Control

In maintaining quality control, good chairside technique is essential so that the undistorted complete image is seen. Full visualization of all the teeth and surrounding bone, including the third molar area, is of prime importance. This is more easily done with a panoramic unit than an intraoral full-mouth series, because the technique, although not simple, is not as demanding as intraoral radiography.

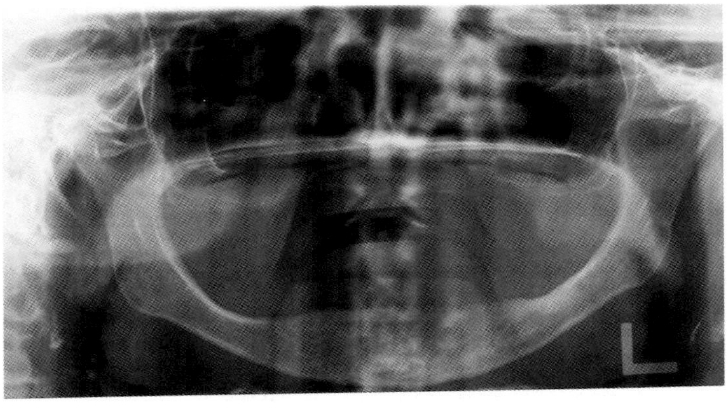

• **Figure 12.24** Panoramic radiograph showing calcifications in the left carotid arteries distal and inferior to the angle of the mandible. (Courtesy Dr. Laurie Carter.)

There are fewer retakes, and quality control is easier to maintain. Quality control for processing of conventional panoramic films is discussed in Chapter 11.

Simplicity

Panoramic procedures, as mentioned, are relatively simple to perform. With minimal training and strict attention to detail, any member of the dental team can become proficient in taking these projections.

Patient Cooperation

Because panoramic radiography is an extraoral procedure, it requires a minimum of patient cooperation in comparison with intraoral techniques. Receptors are not placed in the patient's mouth. The patient is asked to bite on a bite piece and is only required to sit or stand still for 12 to 22 seconds of exposure. When applicable, most units can be operated without radiation to demonstrate to an apprehensive patient what the procedure will be like.

Panoramic radiography practically eliminates problems with intractable gaggers, patients with trismus, and fearful or uncooperative adults or children.

Time

Less time is required for a panoramic radiographic examination than an intraoral survey. The most skilled operator requires at least 15 to 20 minutes to expose an intraoral survey; panoramic radiographs can be taken in less than 5 minutes.

Dose

There seems to be general agreement that the radiation dose to the patient is less than that in intraoral radiography. The conventional panoramic dose is about equivalent to that received from four bitewing projections. This dose can be reduced even further by using digital panoramic units.

Disadvantages

Image Quality

Panoramic radiographs inherently show magnification, geometric distortion, and poor definition. Compared with an intraoral radiograph, the panoramic image does not give comparable definition. In addition to the tomographic process, other factors that tend to degrade the images as compared with intraoral images are (1) external placement of the receptor with resulting increased object-receptor distance, (2) the use of intensifying screens (in conventional panoramic radiography), and (3) faster film with large grain size (in conventional panoramic radiography).

Many diagnostic problems in dentistry require a high degree of radiographic definition. Early detection of conditions (such as, interproximal caries, disruption of the lamina dura, loss of crestal alveolar bone, and a thickened periodontal membrane) all require the maximum of radiographic definition. Because of these factors, panoramic images have very limited value in the diagnosis of periodontal disease and the detection of caries and early periapical lesions. These are common diagnostic problems for practitioners, and the panoramic radiographic technique is lacking in these areas. If a panoramic image is used instead of a full-mouth series, it must be augmented with bitewings and selected periapical projections where indicated.

Focal Trough (Image Layer)

Areas that lie outside (either in front of or behind) the focal trough may be seen poorly or not at all. The focal trough or plane of acceptable detail is not as wide as either the mandible or maxilla, and only structures or changes that lie within the trough are visualized clearly. Pantomographic units that have adjustable focal troughs have far greater diagnostic capabilities than those that do not, but the cost is greater.

Overlap

Pantomographic units have a tendency to produce overlapping images, particularly in the premolar area.

Superimposition

Often, superimposition of the spinal column shows up on the anterior portion of the pantomogram. If the patient is positioned properly, this should not happen. However, not all patients are in perfect physical condition, and some have physical problems that make proper positioning difficult.

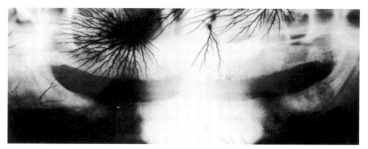

• **Figure 12.25** Panoramic radiograph showing static marks.

The anterior teeth and periapical bone are the most difficult to interpret on pantomograms.

Distortion

The amount of vertical and horizontal distortion varies from one part of the image to another, resulting in an uneven magnification of the image. Therefore, structures, spaces, and distances may appear larger than they actually are. This is a critical factor, because some dentists use panoramic radiographs for bone evaluation and case planning involving implant patients.

Overuse

Overuse is one of the prime concerns regarding patient exposure. The ease and convenience in obtaining the panoramic image might lead to careless substitution for other projections that would yield better results. The panoramic radiograph might be taken instead of a periapical projection of an area.

Cost

Panoramic units are not inexpensive, but they are a great aid to a practice. Costs vary depending on the manufacturer and design. It is very desirable to have a panoramic unit in a dental office and, if not, to have a pathway for referrals.

Indications

The main indication for panoramic radiography is attaining a larger field size than is possible with periapical and bitewing radiography. Clinical situations in which a panoramic unit is useful and helpful include detecting large areas of pathologic conditions, visualizing impacted teeth, jaw fractures, patients who cannot or will not open their mouths, evaluating tooth development and eruption patterns and timing for both the permanent and deciduous dentition, TMJ problems, foreign bodies, and implant evaluation.

Interpretation

Because there is a larger field size, it follows that it will be necessary to be able to identify more anatomic structures not seen on an intraoral survey. There will be some structures that will be seen on both. The new structures are (see

Fig. 12.22) the middle cranial fossa, orbit, styloid process septa in the maxillary sinus, palate, pterygomaxillary fissure, angle of the mandible, hyoid bone, TMJ, vertebra, coronoid process, pterygoid plate, the entire maxillary sinus, tonsillar tissue, ear lobe, mandibular foramen, and mandibular canal.

Technique

Procedure 12.2 presents the general rules of technique for preparing and positioning the patient for panoramic radiography. These rules are valid for all units, but some slight technique changes may be necessary for individual units, depending on the manufacturer's specific instructions.

> **NOTE**
>
> Always follow the manufacturer's manual regarding which anatomic line is to be used for positioning the patient. For example, the ala-tragus line is tilted slightly down, about 5 degrees, from a parallel line to the floor, or the Frankfort plane is parallel to the floor.

Processing

Conventional panoramic films are processed with regular dental solutions either by hand processing or automatically if the processor can accommodate the panoramic size film. The time-temperature method is used with the same fixation and washing times as with intraoral films. The film used in panoramic radiography, as in other extraoral projections, is especially sensitive to excessive safelighting or exposure to cell phone light and may be fogged or completely ruined. One should make sure that the film-screen combination used is compatible with the intensity and type of safelight used.

One of the most common artifacts seen on conventional panoramic films is caused in the darkroom by static electricity. Multiple black linear streaks resembling tree branches without leaves appear on the radiograph (Fig. 12.25). This artifact can be caused by pulling a piece of film quickly and forcefully out of a tightly packed full box of film or when loading or unloading film between the intensifying screens of a cassette. Static electricity is produced most often on cold, dry days.

Text continued on p. 154

PROCEDURE 12.2 RULES AND TECHNIQUES FOR PREPARING AND POSITIONING THE PATIENT FOR PANORAMIC RADIOGRAPHY

1. Explain the procedure to the patient, pointing out the importance of not moving during the procedure. Point out the movement of the receptor and tube around the patient's head and the possibility that the receptor may touch the shoulder or ear gently during the exposure rotation.
2. Follow infection control procedures for panoramic imaging, including making sure that equipment barriers and personal protective infection control equipment are in place.
3. Have the patient remove a jacket or any other bulky piece of clothing that might interfere with movement of the machine.
4. Ask the patient to remove any dentures, eyeglasses, earrings, nose rings, necklaces, hearing aids, hairpins, and other metallic objects in the entire head and neck region to avoid their appearance on the panoramic image.
5. Seat or stand the patient in the most erect position possible so that the spinal column is straight. Instruct the patient to hold the support handles on the unit, take one step forward, and keep the feet together.
6. Align the patient's head so that the midsagittal plane is perpendicular to the floor.
7. Place the patient's chin on the chin rest. Secure the head-positioning devices to prevent head movement.
8. Drape the front and back of the patient with the lead apron. Do not use a thyroid collar or a bib chain, because it would be superimposed on the image.
9. Place a cotton roll or a bite stick, if the unit has one, between the patient's upper and lower incisors.
10. Have the patient close the lips and place the flat portion of the tongue against the roof of the mouth. In addition, instruct the patient to swallow and hold this position. These instructions help to prevent the formation of an airspace that is represented as a radiolucent area above the apices of the maxillary teeth.
11. Properly set the exposure factors.
12. Instruct the patient not to move during the exposure.
13. Press the exposure button and keep your finger on the exposure button for the length of the appropriate exposure time.

Panoramic Exposure Errors

Patient Positioned Too Far Forward (Fig. 12.26). If the patient is positioned in front of the focal plane, the upper and lower anterior teeth appear blurred and narrow. The spinal column is superimposed on the ramus, and the premolars are overlapped.

Remedy. The patient's teeth or edentulous ridges must be in the proper position in the anteroposterior plane. Check the position of the teeth on the bite block and the position of the patient's chin on the rest.

Patient Positioned Too Far Back (Fig. 12.27). If the patient is positioned in back of the focal plane, the maxillary and mandibular anterior teeth appear blurred and widened. Increased ghosting of the mandible also appears.

Remedy. The patient's teeth or ridges must be in the proper position on the bite block. Check the position of the chin rest and the chin for the correct distance in the posterior-anterior plane.

Patient's Head Tilted Up (Fig. 12.28). If the patient's head is tilted up, the forehead is too far back and the chin too far forward. This position causes the maxillary incisors to be out of focus, and the radiopaque hard palate is superimposed over the apices of the maxillary teeth. The condyles may be off the image.

Remedy. The reference lines on the patient's face, the Frankfort plane or the ala-tragus line, should be aligned parallel to the floor.

Patient's Head Tilted Down (Fig. 12.29). If the patient's head is tilted down, then the chin is back and the forehead is forward. This position causes the mandibular incisors to be blurred. The radiopaque image of the hyoid bone is superimposed on the anterior part of the mandible. The superior portions of the condyles may be cut off the image, and the premolars are overlapped.

Remedy. The reference lines on the patient's face, the Frankfort plane or the ala-tragus line, should be aligned parallel to the floor.

Patient Movement during Exposure (Fig. 12.30). If the patient moves anytime during the exposure, the part of the image that was being exposed at that time will appear blurred. This effect differs from that in intraoral radiography, in which patient movement blurs the entire image.

Remedy. Talk to the patient during the exposure, reminding the patient not to move.

Large Radiolucent Area below the Palate (Fig. 12.31). If the patient does not hold the flat part of the tongue against the roof of the mouth, a radiolucent pharyngeal air space artifact is created that produces a dark shadow on the radiograph, obliterating the apices of the maxillary teeth.

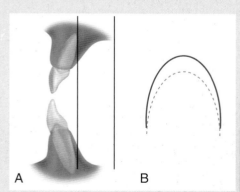
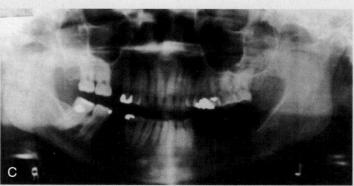

• **Figure 12.26** Patient positioned too far forward. Anterior teeth appear blurred and narrow. Spinal column is superimposed on the ramus, and premolars are overlapped. **A,** Anterior teeth forward of the focal plane. **B,** Dental arch *(solid line)* anterior to focal plane *(broken line).* **C,** Radiograph.

PROCEDURE 12.2   RULES AND TECHNIQUES FOR PREPARING AND POSITIONING THE PATIENT FOR PANORAMIC RADIOGRAPHY—cont'd

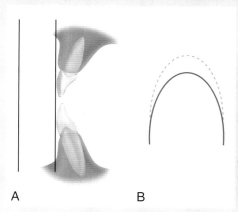
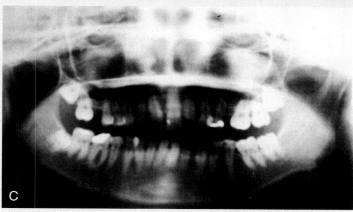

• **Figure 12.27** Patient positioned too far back. Upper and lower anterior teeth appear blurred and widened. **A,** Anterior teeth positioned behind the focal plane. **B,** Dental arch *(solid line)* posterior to focal plane *(broken line).* **C,** Radiograph.

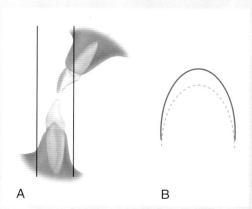
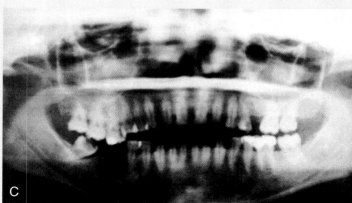

• **Figure 12.28** Patient's head tilted up. Hard palate (radiopaque band) image is superimposed on apices of upper teeth. **A,** Roots of maxillary incisors outside of focal plane. **B,** Mandibular arch *(unbroken line)* in focal trough. Maxillary arch *(broken line)* positioned in back of focal plane. **C,** Radiograph.

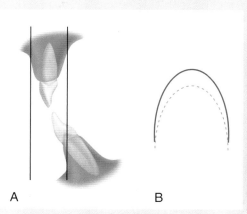
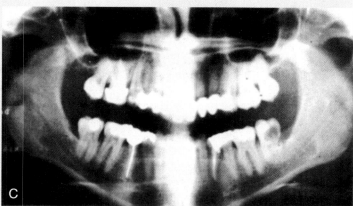

• **Figure 12.29** Patient's head is tilted down. Lower incisors are blurred and image of the hyoid bone is superimposed on the mandible. **A,** Roots of mandibular teeth outside of focal plane. **B,** Maxillary arch *(unbroken line)* positioned in focal plane. Mandibular arch *(broken line)* positioned in back of focal plane. **C,** Radiograph.

Continued

PROCEDURE 12.2   RULES AND TECHNIQUES FOR PREPARING AND POSITIONING THE PATIENT FOR PANORAMIC RADIOGRAPHY—cont'd

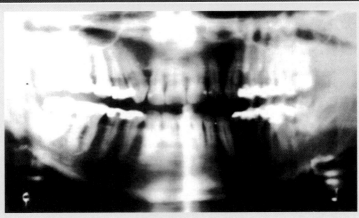

• **Figure 12.30** Patient movement during exposure. Note the blurred and sharp areas.

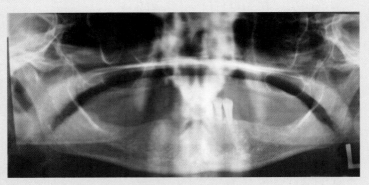

• **Figure 12.31** Tongue not against roof of the patient's mouth. Note the large radiolucent band superimposed over apices of the maxillary teeth.

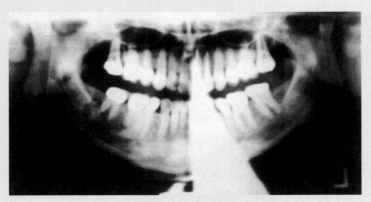

• **Figure 12.32** Patient slouching. Note superimposition of triangular radiopacity, representing the spinal column and not a lead apron.

Remedy. Remind patients during the exposure to keep the tongue against the roof of the mouth.

Patient Does Not Sit or Stand Erect (Fig. 12.32). If the patient slumps while standing or sitting, the spinal column causes a triangular radiopacity to be superimposed on the anterior teeth.

Remedy. Keep the patient's spine erect in the positioning process. In the seated position, the operator can place a cushion or support in the small of the patient's back to help the patient sit upright.

Failure to Remove Metal Objects from the Face, Head, Neck, and Mouth (Fig. 12.33). Metal objects (such as, dentures with metallic components, jewelry, eyeglasses, or other metallic objects), if not removed, cause ghosting on the opposite, superior side of the image and may obscure structures, making the image undiagnostic.

Remedy. Remove all metallic objects from the patient's mouth, head, and neck regions.

Lead Apron Placed Too High on the Patient (Fig. 12.34). The lead apron cannot be placed on the patient

PROCEDURE 12.2   RULES AND TECHNIQUES FOR PREPARING AND POSITIONING THE PATIENT FOR PANORAMIC RADIOGRAPHY—cont'd

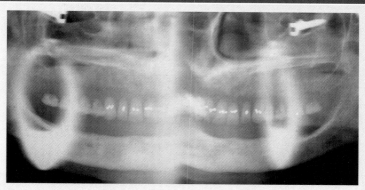

• **Figure 12.33** Failure to remove metal earrings, maxillary denture, and eyeglasses from patient's face. Note ghosting effect of the metal.

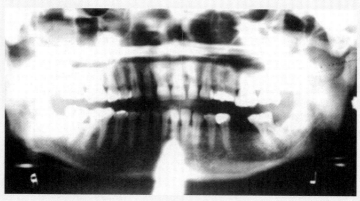

• **Figure 12.34** Placement of the lead apron too high on the patient's neck.

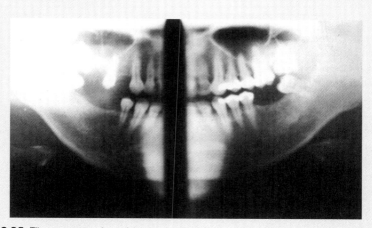

• **Figure 12.35** Film cassette slowed because of patient contact. Note radiolucent band where the overexposure took place.

above the level of the clavicles, because it will create a large radiopacity on the image.

Remedy. Keep the lead apron low on the patient, never use a thyroid collar, and remember to fasten both sides of the back of the double-sided lead apron evenly when taking a panoramic radiograph.

Film Cassette Slowing Down Because of Patient Contact (Fig. 12.35). If the panoramic unit is slowed down or stopped for an instant during the exposure travel around the patient, dark vertical bands will appear on the image as a result of the localized overexposure.

Remedy. Position the patient carefully. With large-framed patients, the operator should run the machine first without radiation to acquaint the patient with the procedure and to check on the patient's position, ensuring that the patient does not contact the rotating panoramic unit.

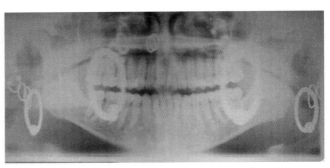

• **Figure 12.36** Panoramic film fogging because of exposure from cell-phone light.

• **Figure 12.37** Ghosting of various piercings on a panoramic radiograph.

Contemporary Panoramic Imaging Artifacts

There have been new findings evident in dental panoramic imaging that reflect changes in society over time. Although we may interpret these findings as "artifacts," they could simply be images that we cannot readily identify.

One of these artifacts that accurately reflects today's lifestyle is cell phone fogging on panoramic images. Panoramic conventional film is much more sensitive to light than intraoral film, and it takes longer for the entire panoramic film to be fed into an automatic film processor. Although it may seem unlikely, when the operator exposes the panoramic film to the light emitted from a cell phone, the film becomes fogged and, therefore, is not acceptable for diagnostic use (Fig. 12.36).

There are several fashion trends that are common today, which are visible more often on panoramic dental images. Common among these are facial jewelry. These items should be removed before dental radiographic exposure when possible. If they are metallic in composition, they could be superimposed over images that need to be observed and/or they could cause ghosting on panoramic radiographs, interfering with the diagnostic capability of the image. In some instances, the patient is unable to remove the piercings because, in keeping with contemporary body piercing procedures, they were soldered into place permanently. The artifacts will be visible, along with the ghosting caused by these objects, which appear more superior, reversed, and with less definition than the actual images (Fig. 12.37).

Images that involve medical consideration and surgical intervention can also be seen on panoramic radiographs. These images may include carotid stents, aneurysm clamps, and hearing aids (Figs. 12.38, 12.39, and 12.40).

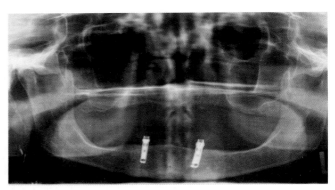

• **Figure 12.38** Carotid artery stents on patient's right side on a panoramic radiograph.

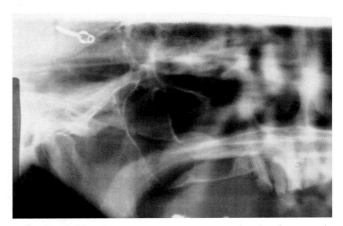

• **Figure 12.39** Aneurysm clamp seen on upper border of panoramic radiograph, on patient's right side.

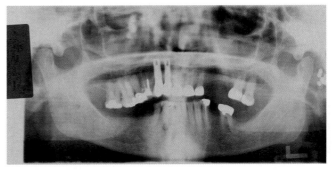

• **Figure 12.40** Hearing aid in patient's left ear on a panoramic radiograph.

Chapter Summary

- Panoramic radiography was introduced into the U.S. dental market in 1959 by the S. S. White Corporation. The Panorex was the first panoramic radiographic unit invented and used in extraoral radiography.
- Panoramic radiography is based on the principles of tomography, which is a radiographic technique that allows radiographing in one plane of an object while blurring or eliminating images from structures in other planes.
- The plane of the object that is not blurred on the radiograph is called the "plane of acceptable detail" or **focal trough**. It is also called the **image layer** and is an invisible area that is located in the space between the source of radiation and the image receptor. Many panoramic technique errors are caused by improper patient positioning, the result of which is not having the desired area in the image layer. Common positioning requirements for panoramic units include midsagittal plane orientation, Frankfort horizontal or ala-tragus plane orientation, bite-block positioning, chin position, head position, patient stabilization, tongue position, posture, and placement of the lead apron.
- In panoramic imaging, objects that have the greatest density (e.g., metal objects) and are out of the plane of acceptable detail (focal trough) are shown in two places on the panoramic image. One place is the usable image,

and the other is referred to as the *ghost image*. The ghost image is always reversed, has less sharpness, and is seen at a point higher on the radiograph than the desired image.
- The advantages of panoramic radiography include: the field size, quality control, simplicity, patient cooperation, minimal set-up and exposure time, and no significant increase in radiation dose as compared with intraoral radiography, especially in the case of digital panoramic radiography.
- The disadvantages of panoramic radiography include issues with image quality; limitations of the focal trough (image layer); inherent overlapping, especially in the premolar regions; superimposition of structures, such as the spinal column; a certain amount of vertical and horizontal distortion; overuse of panoramic radiographs; and the cost of panoramic units.
- The primary indication for use of a panoramic radiograph is when a larger field size is warranted for dental purposes. These situations include visualizing impacted teeth, large pathologies, jaw fractures, tooth development, and other conditions.
- Panoramic exposure errors are mostly due to improper patient positioning but can include static electricity artifacts, movement during exposure, failure to remove metallic objects, and incorrect lead apron placement as well.

Chapter Review Questions

Multiple Choice

1. Radiopaque superimposed images result from:
   a. The patient's failure to place the tongue to the palate
   b. The patient's failure to stay in one position during exposure
   c. The patient's failure to remove metallic objects
   d. The patient's failure to lift the chin
   e. The operator's failure to avoid static electricity
2. Panoramic radiographs can be used to detect:
   a. Periodontal disease
   b. Incipient periapical lesions
   c. Impacted third molars
   d. Incipient interproximal caries
   e. Incipient widened periodontal ligament
3. If the lead apron is placed too high on the patient during panoramic exposure:
   a. It will create a large RL artifact on the image
   b. It will create a large RO artifact on the maxilla only

   c. It will create a large RL artifact on the maxilla only
   d. It will create a large RO artifact on the image
   e. It will not create an artifact on the image
4. The anatomic landmarks that are more visible on panoramic radiographs than intraoral radiographs are the (choose all that apply):
   a. Mandibular foramen
   b. Palate
   c. Mandibular condyle
   d. Hyoid bone
   e. Mental foramen
5. Proper patient positioning for a panoramic exposure includes all of the following except:
   a. The Frankfort plane parallel to the floor
   b. The tongue relaxed in the floor of the mouth
   c. The midsagittal plane perpendicular to the floor
   d. The patient's chin in the chin rest
   e. The spinal column erect

Case-Based Critical Thinking Exercise

1. A patient presents for a routine dental examination. A panoramic radiograph is prescribed. The panoramic radiograph is exposed and exhibits a radiopacity inferior and distal to the angle of the mandible, as indicated by the *arrows* in the accompanying panoramic radiograph.

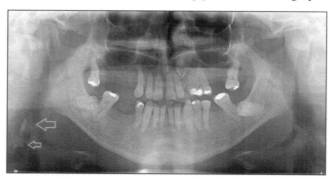

   a. Describe the finding, including the radiographic appearance and location.
   b. List the possibilities of what the finding could represent.
   c. Explain what the role of the dental professional is in identifying and managing this finding.
   d. Discuss the implications of this finding.

Identify the following panoramic exposure errors:

1. The artifact on the accompanying panoramic radiograph is as a result of:

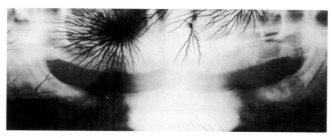

   a. Underexposure
   b. Static electricity
   c. Overexposure
   d. The operator removing the film from the box too slowly
   e. The operator placing the thyroid collar on the patient

2. The panoramic error showing a horizontal radiolucent band above the apices of the maxillary teeth is generally caused by:

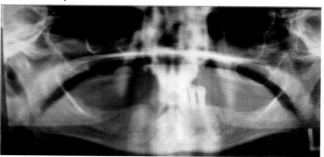

   a. A lead apron
   b. Static electricity
   c. The soft palate
   d. Cleft palate
   e. The patient's tongue not being placed on the palate

3. This panoramic image shows circular RO images on the film that are a result of:

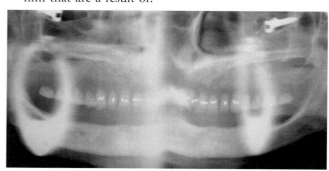

   a. Not removing bracelets
   b. Not removing facial jewelry
   c. Ghosting of facial jewelry
   d. Both a and c are correct
   e. Both b and c are correct

4. The anterior teeth in the accompanying panoramic radiograph appear blurred and narrowed. In addition, the spinal column is superimposed on the ramus. The cause of this error is most likely that:

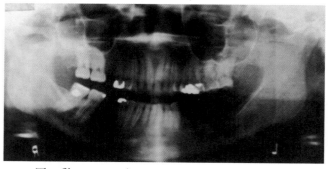

   a. The film cassette's movement was interrupted
   b. The patient's head was tilted up
   c. There was static created
   d. The patient was positioned too far forward
   e. The patient is positioned too far back

5. The dark vertical band on the accompanying radiograph is due to:

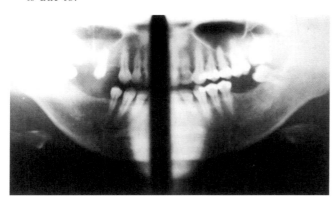

a. Underexposure
b. Fogged film
c. Interruption of the cassette movement
d. Inadequate closure
e. All of the above answers are incorrect

Bibliography

Carter LC, Haller AD, Nadarajah V, et al: Use of panoramic radiography among an ambulatory dental population to detect patients at risk of stroke, *J Am Dent Assoc* 28:977–984, 1997.

Friedlander AH, Garrett NR, Norman DC: The prevalence of calcified carotid artery atheromas on the panoramic radiographs of patients with type 2 diabetes mellitus, *J Am Dent Assoc* 133:1516–1523, 2002.

Frommer HIT, Stabulas-Savage JJ: A sign of the times: contemporary dental imaging artifacts, *N Y State Dent J* 74:37–39, 2008.

Iannucci JM, Howerton LJ: *Dental radiography: Principles and techniques*, ed 5, St Louis, MO, 2016, Elsevier Saunders.

Langland OE, Langlais RP: *Principles of dental imaging*, Baltimore, MD, 1997, Williams & Wilkins.

Thompson EM, Johnson ON: *Essentials of dental radiography for dental assistants and hygienists*, ed 9, Upper Saddle River, NJ, 2012, Pearson Education, Inc.

White SC, Pharoah MJ: *Oral radiology: Principles and interpretation*, ed 7, St Louis, MO, 2013, Mosby.

13

Extraoral Techniques

EDUCATIONAL OBJECTIVES

Upon completing this chapter, the student will be able to:

1. Define the key terms listed at the beginning of the chapter.
2. List and explain the two main categories of the indications for use of extraoral projections in dental radiography.
3. Know the equipment that is needed for extraoral projections, in addition to the function of each of them listed. Also, discuss the film-screen combination used in extraoral techniques.
4. Describe the film sensitivity of extraoral film, the handling of these films in the darkroom, and the processing requirements for these films.

5. Discuss extraoral radiographic technique, including:
   - List and describe the six steps to be taken when exposing an extraoral projection for dental radiographic purposes.
   - State the indications for use; the receptor, patient, and central ray positioning; and the exposure settings for each of the extraoral projections mentioned in this chapter.

KEY TERMS

anteroposterior projection
cassette
cephalometric radiography
cephalostat
extraoral films

extraoral projections
grid
lateral oblique projection
lateral skull projection
maxillofacial radiology

posteroanterior projection
submentovertex projection
Waters' view

Introduction

The scope of dental radiology is constantly expanding; it is not limited to panoramic radiography and the intraoral periapical, bitewing, and occlusal films that have been previously described. There is an ever-increasing use of the term **maxillofacial radiology**, which is that specialty of dentistry concerned with performance and interpretation of diagnostic imaging used for examining the craniofacial, dental, and adjacent structures. There are many accessory techniques, intraoral and extraoral, using different imaging systems and film-screen combinations, different projections, and digital systems. Operators responsible for the maxillofacial area must be able to expose the area of interest in any way possible to obtain a diagnostic image. The extraoral techniques that are described in this chapter can be performed with conventional or digital radiography. As is the case with intraoral radiographs, dental professionals should be knowledgeable and skilled in these accessory techniques. However, some states have statutes that prohibit or limit some dental professionals from performing certain extraoral techniques. Information about these restrictions is readily available from the appropriate agencies in individual states.

Newer imaging techniques—such as tomography, computed tomography, and magnetic resonance imaging—also are used by dentists to make complicated diagnoses and treatment plans. They are discussed in Chapter 16.

Indications

There are two main categories of indications for the use of **extraoral projections**. The first is when patients cannot or will not open their mouths to allow the receptor to be placed intraorally. Handicapped patients may be unable to open their mouths for receptor placement, and uncooperative patients may simply refuse (see Chapter 18). Patients with trismus or temporomandibular joint (TMJ) ankylosis cannot open their mouths. These indications are very similar to those listed for panoramic radiography.

The second indication is when the area being radiographed is larger than or cannot be seen on intraoral projections. Many areas of the mandible and maxilla cannot be seen on intraoral images. The scope of dental treatment, as mentioned previously, is not limited to the teeth and alveolar bone; it may be necessary to radiograph areas, such as the angle and ramus of the mandible, to visualize impactions or the skull for orthodontic cephalometric radiography analysis. Extraoral radiographs can be used to image the TMJ, maxillary sinus, or lesions that grow so large that they cannot be captured completely on periapical or bitewing projections. Through a combination of extraoral radiographs, it is also possible to locate objects in the buccolingual dimension, which is necessary for implant evaluation and with occlusal radiography (see Chapter 10).

> **NOTE**
>
> In summary, extraoral projections can be used:
> - When the patient cannot or will not accept intraoral receptors
> - To view areas that require a large field size, as in evaluating the angle of the mandible, the ramus, the skull, the maxillary sinus, or the temporomandibular joint (TMJ)
> - For evaluating growth and development
> - To observe and radiographically examine impacted teeth and their surrounding area
> - To examine large lesions and conditions that cannot be viewed on intraoral radiographs
> - To examine traumatic conditions of the jaws

Equipment

The radiographic equipment needed to perform standard extraoral projections is minimal, because extraoral radiographs can be taken with a standard intraoral dental x-ray unit and dental chair. Conventional extraoral techniques require a regular dental x-ray unit, 8 × 10-inch or 5 × 7-inch cassettes intensifying screens, and cassette holders or angling boards. When using film as the receptor, the darkroom must have the capacity to process the larger film size. The use of grids, although optional, results in better image definition, because they are placed between the patient and the x-ray film to reduce the scattered radiation and thus improve image contrast.

X-Ray Unit

For extraoral radiographs, the x-ray machine must be positioned in the operatory so that a target-receptor distance (or focal-film distance [FFD]) of 36 inches can be achieved. This distance is necessary to get a sufficiently large divergent beam size at the patient's face so that the complete area of interest can be radiographed and seen on the image.

Cassettes

When films are used, they are contained in a carrier called a cassette. Cassettes can be rigid or flexible and are available in varying sizes corresponding to the size of the film used (Fig. 13.1). A cassette must be light-tight but allow the passage of x-rays to affect the film and intensifying screen contained in the cassette.

Cassettes must be marked with lead letters on the front side of the cassette to identify the left or the right side of

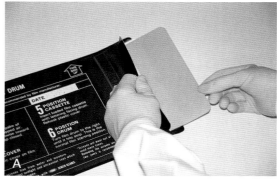
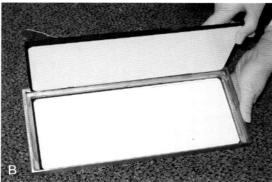

● **Figure 13.1** **A,** Front view of 8 × 10-inch cassette with marking letters. **B,** Rigid-type film cassette with intensifying screen. (From Bird DL, Robinson DS: *Modern Dental Assisting,* ed 12, St Louis, 2018, Elsevier.)

the processed film, or it will not be possible to orient the finished radiograph. Lead strips are available to imprint the patient's name and the date on the film as well. The cassettes have a front side that is usually composed of plastic and a back side that is made of metal to reduce scatter radiation. The front side of the cassette is the side that should face the patient and the source of radiation during an exposure.

Film-Screen Combination

The imaging system used in conventional, film-based extraoral radiography is a film-screen system (see Chapter 4). To reduce radiation exposure to the patient, the film is used in combination with intensifying screens. Previously in dentistry, to obtain better detail, some extraoral projections were taken with film alone in the so-called nonscreen technique. Today, with improved film quality and concern for radiation safety, all extraoral films should be taken using intensifying screens. The screen film used is more sensitive to the light emitted by the intensifying screens than it is to radiation. However, the film used must be sensitive to the type of light emitted by the particular screen (e.g., blue light or green light).

As mentioned in Chapter 4, extraoral film is available in 5 × 7-inch or 8 × 10-inch sizes. For panoramic radiography

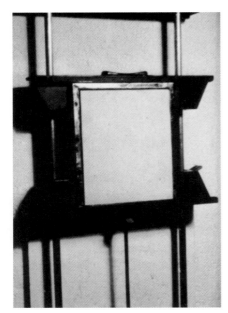

• **Figure 13.2** Cassette in a wall-mounted, film-holding device.

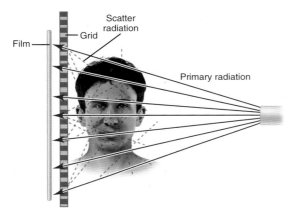

• **Figure 13.3** Grid. Note absorption of scatter radiation by radio-resistant strips of grid.

extraoral film is available in 5 × 12-inch and 6 × 12-inch sizes.

Holding Devices

Conventional extraoral cassette holders can be wall mounted or used on a tabletop if applicable. Holding devices have the advantage of standardizing techniques for comparison of films and preventing patient and film movement (Fig. 13.2).

Grids

The use of **grids** for extraoral radiography is not common in dental practice and is mostly confined to cephalometric and TMJ radiographs. The function of the grid is to decrease the amount of scatter radiation originating in the object (Fig. 13.3). This scatter degrades the image by decreasing the contrast. The grid is a thin plate composed of

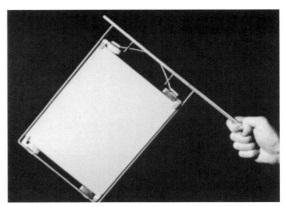

• **Figure 13.4** Piece of 8 × 10-inch film mounted on an extraoral processing film hanger.

radiotransparent and radio-absorptive strips that is placed in front of the cassette. The grid absorbs all radiation, leaving the object that is not at right angles to the film. In doing so, it decreases the effect of scatter on the diagnostic image. Grids are not used in intraoral radiography, because the secondary radiation does not greatly degrade the image as a result of the small field size. The panoramic units, with their narrow exposure field size, also do not need grids. Medical x-ray units use grids routinely. Extraoral radiographs taken with a medical x-ray machine have better-quality density and contrast than similar films taken with a dental x-ray unit because of the use of a grid.

Film Sensitivity and Processing

Extraoral screen films used with conventional extraoral radiography are more sensitive to light than are intraoral films. Therefore, what would be acceptable safelight conditions in the darkroom for processing intraoral films might fog the extraoral films. The films used in panoramic radiography are also especially sensitive to excessive safelighting and may not be merely fogged but ruined. Safelighting always should be checked by the coin test before processing extraoral films. It is also advised not to expose extraoral films to cell phone lighting while processing them in the darkroom. Consequently, it is advised to turn cell phones off before entering the darkroom or not to bring them in the darkroom at all.

Extraoral films are processed in the same manner as intraoral films, either manually or by automatic processors that can accommodate large-size film. For manual processing, the time-temperature method is used with the same fixation and washing time as with intraoral films. The only difference is that special sizes of film hangers are used (Fig. 13.4). Operators should take special care when processing the large films, because they are easier to scratch when more than one film is processed at a time.

Projections

As in intraoral radiography, certain factors must be known for every extraoral projection exposed, including (1) the

PROCEDURE 13.1 EXTRAORAL RADIOGRAPHIC TECHNIQUE

1. Proper infection control procedures should be performed for extraoral radiography, including covering or disinfecting the ear rods, chin positioner, headrest, bite block, or edentulous positioner.
2. Explain the procedure to the patient, place the double-sided lead apron (without a thyroid collar) properly on the patient (below the level of the clavicles), and remove all metallic objects in the head and neck region to be exposed.
3. Load the extraoral cassette in the darkroom under the proper safelight procedures for the film being used if using screen film. If you are using a digital system, follow the manufacturer's recommendations closely.
4. Set the exposure settings (kilovoltage, milliamperage, and exposure time) for the desired values according to the manufacturer's recommendations.
5. Place the receptor in the holding device.
6. Position the patient's head according to the projection, align the x-ray beam, and press the exposure button.

HELPFUL HINT

Remember that extraoral film is more sensitive to light than intraoral film. Be sure to double check that acceptable safelight conditions are being used before beginning to process the film, and do not expose the extraoral film to cell phone light.

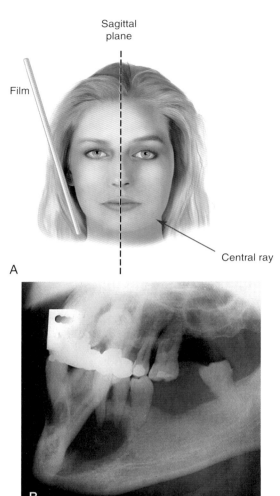

• **Figure 13.5** Lateral oblique projection. The central ray is directed at the receptor from beneath the opposite side of the mandible. **A,** Drawing. **B,** Radiograph.

clinical indication for use of the projection; (2) the relationship of the receptor to the patient; (3) the relationship of the central ray of the x-ray beam to the patient and the receptor; (4) the target-receptor distance (or FFD); (5) the point of entry of the x-ray beam; and (6) the exposure settings, including the exposure time, the kilovoltage and milliamperage unless it is preset, as it usually is in the newer dental x-ray units.

Lateral Oblique Projection of the Mandible

The lateral oblique projection of the mandible is used for surveying one side of the mandible entirely from the distal of the canine to the angle of the ramus, the ramus, condyle, and coronoid process. This projection is ideal for visualizing impactions, fractures, and large areas of pathologic conditions that would not be seen on periapical projections. It is not diagnostic anterior to the canine, because of the superimposition caused by the anterior curve of the mandible. Before the advent of panoramic radiography, it was the most commonly used extraoral technique for mandibular pathologic conditions and impactions.

Clinical Indication

To view mandibular third molar impactions, fractures, and pathologic conditions.

Receptor/Patient/Central Ray Position

An 8 × 10-inch or a 5 × 7-inch receptor may be used for this projection. The receptor is supported by the patient's shoulder or a holding device on the side of the mandible to be radiographed. The receptor is in contact with the cheekbone and mandible of the patient. The patient's head is inclined about 15 degrees away from the x-ray tube. The central ray is directed from under the opposite side of the mandible at right angles to the receptor.

Exposure Settings

The target-receptor distance (or FFD) is 14 inches. An average exposure time at 65 kV and 10 mA would be 5 to 10 impulses (Fig. 13.5).

Lateral Skull Projection

The lateral skull projection is used to survey the whole skull in the sagittal plane. The right and left sides of the

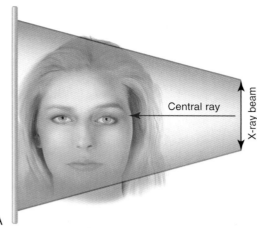

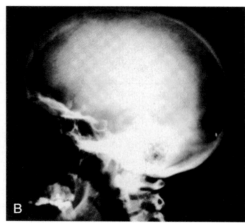

• **Figure 13.6** Lateral skull projection. The central ray is directed at the external auditory meatus at a minimum target-receptor distance of 36 inches. **A,** Drawing. **B,** Radiograph.

skull are superimposed on each other, with the side nearer the tube magnified slightly more than the side nearer the receptor.

Clinical Indication

Detection of pathologic conditions of the skull and cephalometrics. This projection is used in dentistry to detect fractures and systemic pathologic conditions that are also manifested in the jaws, such as Paget disease. It is the radiographic projection used by orthodontists to obtain lateral cephalometric radiographs.

Receptor/Patient/Central Ray Position

An 8 × 10-inch receptor is used. The receptor is held in position by the patient, supported on the patient's shoulder or by some supportive device. The receptor is positioned parallel to the sagittal plane of the patient's skull. The central ray is directed at the external auditory meatus at a target-receptor (or FFD) of 36 inches. The vertical angulation is zero degrees.

Exposure Settings

An average exposure time for an adult at 65 kVp and 10 mA would be 8 to 15 impulses (Fig. 13.6).

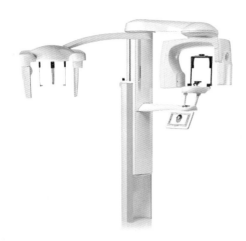

• **Figure 13.7** Orthoceph OC100 D direct digital cephalometric imaging unit. Note the cephalostat (head holder). The unit can also be used for panoramic digital imaging. (Courtesy GE Healthcare, Dental Imaging, Milwaukee, WI.)

If the lateral skull projection is to be used for cephalometric measurement, then a head-positioning device (cephalostat) must be used (Fig. 13.7). The cephalostat ensures that the patient's head is accurately aligned with the sagittal plane and allows reproducibility of the patient's position so that images taken during and after treatment are valid for comparison. As is shown in Fig. 13.7, there are digital radiographic units available that are used to take both panoramic and cephalometric radiographs particularly for orthodontic use.

Posteroanterior Projection

The **posteroanterior projection** is the companion projection to the lateral skull, used to survey the skull in the anteroposterior plane (coronal, frontal), and it provides a means of localizing changes in a mediolateral direction. Therefore, the left and right sides of the facial structures are not superimposed on each other, as in the lateral skull projection.

Clinical Indication

In dentistry, this projection is used to detect fractures and their displacements, tumors, and large areas of disease. It is not effective for studying the maxillary sinus because of the superimposition of other cranial structures on the sinuses. Although the anteroposterior projection shows the same area, the posteroanterior is preferred in dental radiography, because the structures that are of greatest interest are closer to the receptor in a posteroanterior than an **anteroposterior projection** and hence show less enlargement.

Receptor/Patient/Central Ray Position

An 8 × 10-inch receptor is used. The receptor can be held in position by the patient, but some type of receptor-holding device is preferable. The patient is positioned with the nose and forehead touching the receptor. The central ray

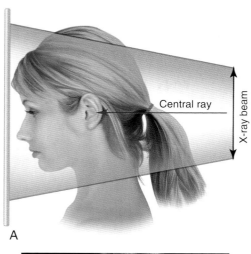

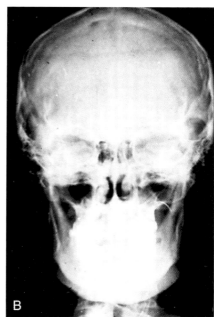

Figure 13.8 Posteroanterior projection. The central ray is directed at the occipital protuberance at a minimum target-receptor distance of 36 inches. **A,** Drawing. **B,** Radiograph.

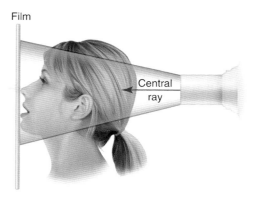

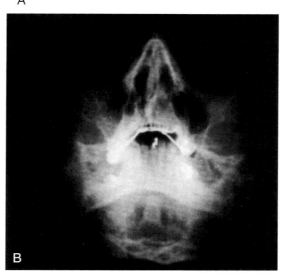

Figure 13.9 Posteroanterior projection of the sinuses (Waters' view). The central ray is directed perpendicular to the receptor at the occipital protuberance using a 36-inch target-receptor distance. **A,** Drawing. **B,** Radiograph.

is directed at a zero-degree vertical angulation, aimed at the external occipital protuberance (the prominent bump near the base of the skull). The target-receptor distance (or FFD) is 36 inches.

Exposure Settings

An average exposure time at 65 kV and 10 mA would be 8 to 15 impulses (Fig. 13.8).

Posteroanterior (Waters') View of the Sinuses

The Waters' view is a variation of the posteroanterior projection that enlarges the middle third of the face and is useful in the diagnosis of maxillary sinus and other pathologic conditions occurring in the middle third of the face.

Clinical Indication

To evaluate maxillary sinus pathologic conditions and facial fractures of the middle third of the face.

Receptor/Patient/Central Ray Position

It differs from the posteroanterior projection positioning in that the patient's mouth is kept open while the nose and chin are touching the cassette. The central ray is again directed at the external occipital protuberance, and a target-receptor distance (or FFD) of 36 inches is used.

Exposure Settings

An average exposure time at 65 kV and 10 mA would be 15 to 20 impulses (Fig. 13.9).

Submentovertex Projection

The submentovertex projection is used to detect fractures of the zygomatic arch and visualize the sphenoid and

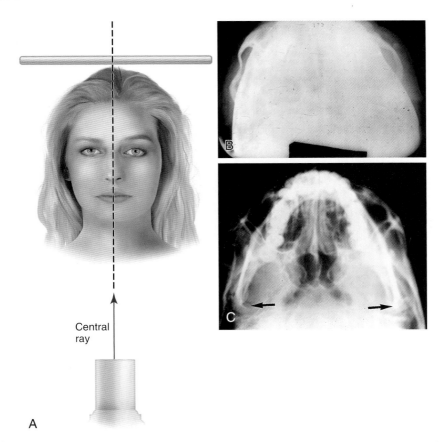

• **Figure 13.10** Submentovertex projection. **A,** Drawing shows that the central ray is directed from beneath the chin (menton) at 90 degrees to the receptor position at the vertex of the skull. **B,** Radiograph showing depressed fracture of zygomatic arch. **C,** Radiograph with *arrows* pointing to the condyles.

ethmoid sinuses, as well as the lateral wall of the maxillary sinus. It is also used in tomography as a scout image to determine the positions of the condyles.

Clinical Indication

To locate the position of the condyles, evaluate fractures of the zygomatic arch, and to view the sphenoid, ethmoid, and lateral border of the maxillary sinuses.

Receptor/Patient/Central Ray Position

The cassette is positioned on the vertex of the patient's skull, and the central ray is directed from underneath the patient's chin (menton) perpendicular to the cassette.

Exposure Settings

An average exposure time at 65 kV and 10 mA would be 8 to 10 impulses (Fig. 13.10).

Chapter Summary

- Extraoral radiography is performed with the receptor and source of x-radiation outside of the patient's oral cavity.
- Some of the general indications of use for the extraoral projections discussed in this chapter are when patients cannot or will not open their mouths to accept intraoral receptors, to obtain a larger field size, to evaluate growth and development in children, to view impacted teeth, and to examine large lesions and traumatic conditions in the head and neck region.
- Equipment that is needed for extraoral projections may include the conventional dental x-ray unit, film-screen systems, digital sensors, holding devices, grids, and a panoramic-cephalometric combination digital unit.

- When taking extraoral radiographs, the dental professional must follow the extraoral infection control procedures, explain the procedure to the patient, cover the patient with a lead apron, load the extraoral cassette if using screen film, follow the manufacturer's directions for digital extraoral procedures, set the desired exposure settings, have the patient remove metallic objects from the head/neck region, position the patient correctly, and then press the exposure button.
- This chapter discussed various extraoral imaging techniques. Ultimately, the choice of which projection is required depends on what information is needed for the diagnosis and treatment of the individual patient.

Chapter Review Questions

Matching

Match the extraoral projection in Column A with the indication for use listed in Column B.

Column A
1. Submentovertex projection
2. Lateral skull projection
3. Lateral oblique projection of the mandible
4. Posteroanterior projection
5. Waters' view

Column B
a. Survey one side of the mandible
b. Maxillary sinus pathology
c. Fractures, tumors, or large areas of disease
d. Orthodontic cephalometrics
e. Position of the condyles

Multiple Choice

1. Grids can be used in extraoral imaging to:
   a. Position the patient correctly
   b. Hold the receptor in place
   c. Prevent harmful effects of lead in the double-sided apron
   d. Absorb scatter radiation
   e. Manage the digital sensor
2. Intensifying screens are used in extraoral film-screen systems to:
   a. Decrease radiation exposure to the patient
   b. Reduce the radiation exposure time
   c. Secure the cassette
   d. Both a and b only
   e. Both b and c only
3. The projection that formerly was used primarily for third molar impactions prior to panoramic radiographs is the:
   a. Lateral skull projection
   b. Lateral oblique projection of the mandible
   c. Waters' view
   d. Submentovertex projection
   e. Posteroanterior projection
4. The projection primarily used for evaluation of the temporomandibular joint (TMJ) is the:
   a. Waters' view
   b. Posteroanterior projection
   c. Lateral oblique projection of the mandible
   d. Lateral skull projection
   e. Submentovertex projection
5. The Waters' view of the maxillary sinus projection enlarges the:
   a. Lower third of the face
   b. Middle third of the face
   c. Upper third of the face
   d. 3/4 of the head and neck region
   e. 2/3 of the head and neck region

Bibliography

Brooks SL, Brand JW, Gibbs SJ, et al: Imaging of the temporomandibular joint: a position paper of the American Academy of Oral and Maxillofacial Radiology, *Oral Surg Oral Med Oral Pathol Oral Radiol Endod* 83:609–618, 1997.

Iannucci JM, Howerton LJ: *Dental radiography: Principles and techniques*, ed 5, St Louis, MO, 2016, Elsevier Saunders.

Langland OE, Langlais RP: *Principles of dental imaging*, Baltimore, MD, 1997, Williams & Wilkins.

Thompson EM, Johnson ON: *Essentials of dental radiography for dental assistants and hygienists*, ed 9, Upper Saddle River, NJ, 2012, Pearson Education, Inc.

White SC, Pharoah MJ: *Oral radiology: Principles and interpretation*, ed 7, St Louis, MO, 2013, Mosby.

14

Radiography of the Temporomandibular Joint

Introduction

Patients with symptoms relating to the temporomandibular joint (TMJ) are not uncommon in dental practice. Patients may be referred for specialized treatment by other dentists or physicians when they are experiencing facial pain issues related to the TMJ. In these cases, they may bring previously exposed radiographs with them or may require new or additional radiographs to be taken. Some TMJ imaging can be done in the dental office, whereas some may have to be referred to advanced imaging centers for the appropriate radiographs. In either case, dental professionals should feel comfortable in dealing with these radiographic images focusing on the TMJ.

Anatomy of the Temporomandibular Joint

By understanding the hard tissue and soft tissue anatomy of the TMJ, a better understanding of the problems in imaging the TMJ can be appreciated. The joint is bounded laterally by the zygomatic arch and medially by the petrous ridge of the temporal bone. Structures that the dental professional should be able to identify on radiographs are the external meatus of the ear, the mastoid air cells, the mandibular

condyle, the mandibular fossa (glenoid fossa), the neck of the condyle, and the articular eminence. The internal and external pterygoid muscles and the articular disc (meniscus) are not seen with routine radiographic imaging (Figs. 14.1 and 14.2), because they have soft tissue components. Some of the structures associated with TMJ images are radiolucent, and some are radiopaque. The articular disc, which is a major source of TMJ disorders, is not seen on conventional radiographic images, because it is fibrocartilaginous and thus appears radiolucent on radiographic images.

The pathologic lesions associated with TMJ disorders that are seen on radiographs include fractures, benign and malignant tumors, arthritic changes, ankylosis, disc displacement, fibrous adhesions, and congenital absence of structures. Because the condyle is a mobile structure, it is beneficial to image it in various positions (e.g., open, rest, and closed).

Transcranial Temporomandibular Joint Projection

In addition to the panoramic view, the transcranial projection is also used in the dental office for TMJ radiography.

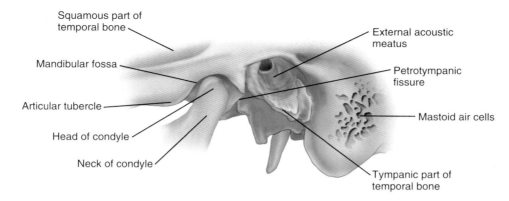

Squamous part of
temporal bone

External acoustic
meatus

Mandibular fossa

Petrotympanic
fissure

Articular tubercle

Mastoid air cells

Head of condyle

Neck of condyle

Tympanic part of
temporal bone

• **Figure 14.1** Sagittal view of the temporomandibular joint (TMJ).

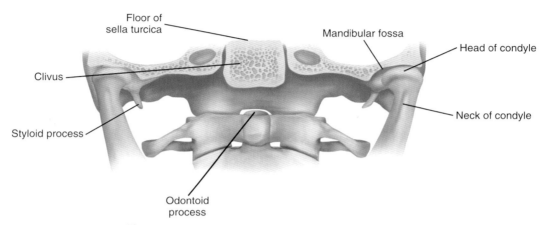

Floor of
sella turcica

Mandibular fossa

Clivus

Head of condyle

Neck of condyle

Styloid process

Odontoid
process

• **Figure 14.2** Coronal view of the temporomandibular joint (TMJ).

Clinical Indication

The clinical indication of the transcranial TMJ projection is to examine the articular eminence and the superior plane of the condyle, in addition to evaluating the condyle's mobility when the patient's mouth is opened. It can also be used to compare the joint spaces on the patient's right and left sides.

Receptor/Patient/Central Ray Position

A 5 × 7-inch receptor can be used if there is to be only one exposure. Usually, radiographs are taken of both the left and right condyles in both the open and closed position. Because the diagnostic area is relatively small, the four views can be placed on an 8 × 10-inch receptor when applicable. The patient's head is positioned parallel to the receptor with the side to be imaged closest to the receptor. The receptor can be supported on the patient's shoulder or on a positioning device in either the upright (vertical) or horizontal position. The point of entry for the central ray of the x-ray beam is on the opposite side of the head from the condyle being radiographed, approximately 2½ inches above and ½ inch in front of the external auditory meatus. The x-ray beam is directed at a vertical angulation of 20 to 25 degrees. The open surface of the position-indicating device approximates the skin.

Exposure Settings

An average exposure time at 65 kV and 10 mA would be 7 to 15 impulses (Fig. 14.3). Positioning boards (angling boards) are available to use with the transcranial technique. These boards also incorporate means to hold the patient in a fixed position while allowing movement of the receptor to give up to three exposures for each condyle (open, closed, and rest) on an 8 × 10-inch receptor.

Submentovertex (Basilar) Projection

Besides the clinical indications noted in Chapter 13, submental or basilar views can also be used to view the TMJ from the axial plane (Fig. 14.4), allowing visualization of the medial and lateral aspects of the condyle. The submentovertex projection is also used as a scout film for tomograms of the TMJ, because the projection will relates the position of the long axis of the condyles with the patient's midsagittal plane.

Panoramic Projection

A conventional panoramic projection shows both left and right joints in the lateral plane, as well as an overall view of the mandible and maxilla. These views can be used for screening

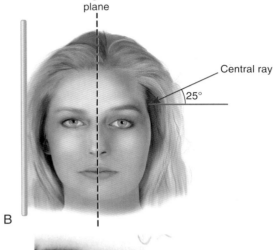

Sagittal plane

Central ray

25°

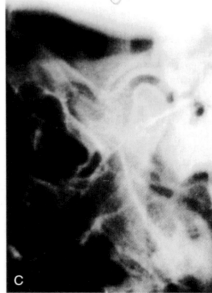

• **Figure 14.3** **A,** Transcranial temporomandibular joint projection. **B,** Drawing. **C,** Radiograph. (A, From Okeson JP: *Management of Temporomandibular Disorders and Occlusion,* ed 7, St Louis, 2014, Mosby.)

or as a scout film to detect any other existing condition that might be the cause of TMJ pathologic processes (Fig. 14.5). If the panoramic image shows a pathologic process, a more advanced projection can be used to formulate the diagnosis. Some panoramic units have specific programs for the TMJ that also allow the dental professional to take views in the

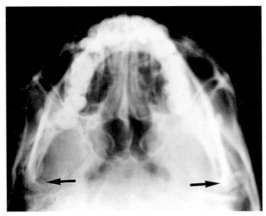

• **Figure 14.4** Submentovertex projection. Radiograph with *arrows* pointing to condyles.

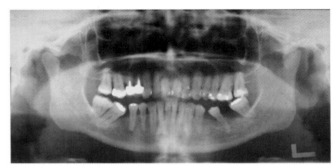

• **Figure 14.5** Conventional panoramic view of the temporomandibular joint (TMJ).

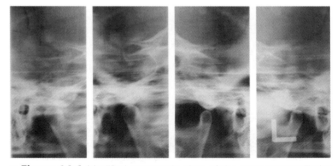

• **Figure 14.6** Modified panoramic view of the temporomandibular joint (TMJ).

open and closed positions. The glenoid fossa (mandibular fossa) and the condyle will be seen, but the articular disc will not (Fig. 14.6).

Conventional Tomography

Before the wide use of computed tomography (CT) scanning, conventional tomography was one of the better ways to examine the condyle radiographically. Dedicated dental tomographic units are available (Fig. 14.7) that produce tomographic images of the TMJ (Fig. 14.8). The images are better than panoramic projections, and in some ways equivalent to a CT scan for TMJ evaluation. Again, however, the articular disc is not seen, but the fossa, neck, and head of the condyle are seen.

Computed Tomography

As will be discussed in Chapter 16, CT and cone beam computed tomography (CBCT) imaging techniques facilitate viewing of an area in three planes and are excellent means for examining the bones of the TMJ. However, these scans do not include diagnostic images of the articular disc (Figs. 14.9 to 14.11).

Magnetic Resonance Imaging

Magnetic resonance imaging (MRI) is a very effective means for viewing soft tissue and thus for viewing the articular disc of the TMJ. Because the disc is an important factor in the TMJ pathologic processes, the use of an MRI should be considered. If one remembers the basic anatomy of the TMJ, the images are not difficult to read. What is radiolucent on a CT scan or radiograph will be opaque on an MRI, indicating high soft tissue density or a strong signal. What is radiopaque on a CT scan will appear lucent on a magnetic resonance image, indicating low soft tissue density or a weak signal (Fig. 14.12).

Arthrography

One of the means of radiographing soft tissue is to outline it with a radiographic opaque contrast medium (see Chapter 18). In the case of the articular disc, a contrast medium is injected into both the upper and lower joint space, thus outlining the disc (Fig. 14.13). Arthrography is an invasive procedure that may have complications if the contrast medium is not placed in the correct space. After considering the options, MRI is the system of choice when imaging the disc and other soft tissues of the TMJ.

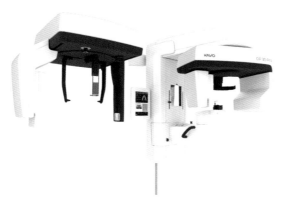

• **Figure 14.7** The Gendex GXDP 700 Series is a 3-in-1 system that provides digital panoramic, cephalometric, and 3D radiography. (Courtesy KaVo Kerr, Orange, CA.)

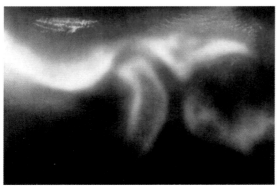

• **Figure 14.8** Tomographic view of the temporomandibular joint (TMJ).

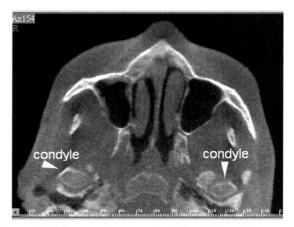

• **Figure 14.9** Computed tomography (CT) axial view of the temporomandibular joint (TMJ).

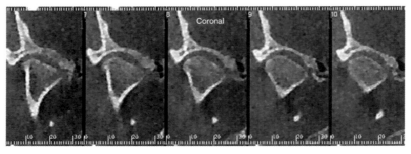

• **Figure 14.10** Computed tomography (CT) coronal view of the temporomandibular joint (TMJ).

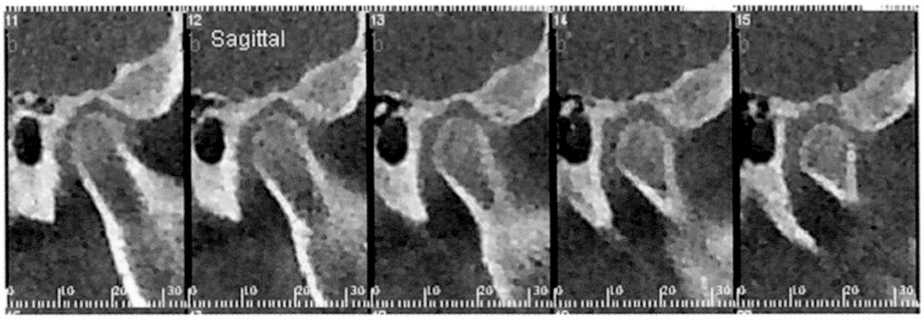

• **Figure 14.11** Computed tomography (CT) sagittal view of the temporomandibular joint (TMJ).

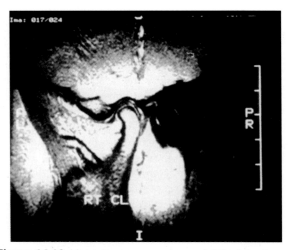

• **Figure 14.12** Magnetic resonance image (MRI) of the temporomandibular joint (TMJ) showing the articular disc.

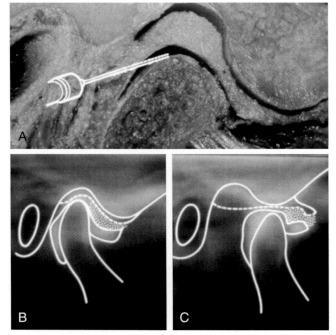

• **Figure 14.13 A,** Contrast medium is injected into the joint space. **B** and **C,** Arthrogram images of the temporomandibular joint (TMJ).

Chapter Summary

- Patients with TMJ issues are quite common in dental practice and may require appropriate radiographs to aid in the diagnosis and treatment of these issues.
- Various dental radiographic techniques can provide the images necessary for the clinical management of these patients.
- The choice of the imaging technique is determined by the origin of the signs and symptoms that the patient presents with.
- When the etiology of the patient's TMJ problems are related to the bony components of the area, x-ray images are recommended. These projections include the transcranial projection, submentovertex projection, panoramic projection, conventional tomography, CT and CBCT imaging.
- When the etiology of the patient's TMJ issue is related to the soft tissue structures of the TMJ area, it is recommended that the patient have an MRI taken, because this technique is more conducive to demonstrating the soft tissue components, especially the articular disc of the TMJ.

Chapter Review Questions

1. _____ is a very valuable means of viewing the articular disc of the TMJ.
   a. Tomography
   b. CT scanning
   c. CBCT scanning
   d. MRI
   e. Submentovertex projection

2. The TMJ is bounded laterally by the _____ and medially by the_____.
   a. Clivus, styloid process
   b. Odontoid process, head of the condyle
   c. Zygomatic arch, petrous ridge of the temporal bone
   d. Articular fossa, neck of the condyle
   e. External auditory meatus, mastoid air cells

3. Angling or positioning boards are used to hold the patient still and allow movement of the receptor while exposing the _____ projection.
   a. Submentovertex
   b. Tomographic
   c. Transcranial TMJ
   d. Panoramic
   e. Basilar

4. Some _____ units have specific programs allowing the TMJ to be viewed radiographically in an open and closed position on the right and left sides of the patient.
   a. Panoramic
   b. CT

   c. Conventional dental radiographic
   d. Transcranial
   e. CBCT

5. The _____ projection can be used to visualize the medial and lateral aspects of the mandibular condyle.
   a. Panoramic
   b. Transcranial
   c. MRI
   d. CT
   e. Submentovertex

6. An excellent means of examining the bones of the TMJ in three planes is produced by exposing a _____ on the patient.
   a. Submentovertex projection
   b. Periapical projection
   c. Panoramic projection
   d. CT image
   e. Transcranial projection

7. _____ is a means of radiographing the soft tissues associated with the TMJ with the use of an opaque contrast medium.
   a. Arthrography
   b. Conventional tomography
   c. CBCT scanning
   d. Panoramic radiography
   e. Cephalometric radiography

Bibliography

Iannucci JM, Howerton LJ: *Dental radiography: Principles and techniques*, ed 5, St Louis, MO, 2016, Elsevier Saunders.

Langland OE, Langlais RP: *Principles of dental imaging*, Baltimore, MD, 1997, Williams & Wilkins.

Thompson EM, Johnson ON: *Essentials of dental radiography for dental assistants and hygienists*, ed 9, Upper Saddle River, NJ, 2012, Pearson Education, Inc.

White SC, Pharoah MJ: *Oral radiology: Principles and interpretation*, ed 7, St Louis, MO, 2013, Mosby.

15
Digital Imaging

EDUCATIONAL OBJECTIVES

Upon completing this chapter, the student will be able to:

1. Define the key terms listed at the beginning of the chapter.
2. Discuss the following related to digital imaging:
   - Know the basic elements that are necessary to acquire a digital image.
   - List the three basic types of digital imaging systems and how they differ from each other.
3. State the three types of digital sensors that can be used in digital imaging.
4. Describe the following related to the nature of the image:
   - Define what a pixel is, and explain its role in the formation of a digital image.
   - List the advantages and disadvantages of digital imaging when compared to conventional film-based radiography.
5. State the components of the digital imaging technique and be able to apply them to clinical practice.
6. Discuss the types of digital systems, as well as the legal aspects of digital radiography in dentistry.

KEY TERMS

analogue
charge-coupled device (CCD)
complementary metal oxide
   semiconductor (CMOS)
detector
digital image
digitize
direct digital radiography

gray level
hard copies
image manipulation
imaging plate
indirect digital radiography
line pairs per millimeter
monitor
optically scanned digital radiography

paperless office
photostimulable phosphor (PSP)
pixels
RVG system
sensor
storage phosphor

Introduction

One of the most exciting technologies introduced in dentistry is digital imaging, along with the other computerized aspects of a dental practice. Instead of film or a film-screen combination, this digital imaging system uses electronic sensors to record the penetration of the x-ray photons and sends this information to a computer that digitizes (converts to numbers) these electronic impulses. This allows the computer to produce a diagnostic image on a monitor almost instantaneously. Digital imaging was introduced into dentistry in 1987 by Dr. Francois Mugnon with his RVG system (RadioVisioGraphy). Since that time, the market has exploded with numerous companies making competing products. This chapter does not focus on a particular digital unit, but it attempts to explain the basic principles of digital imaging, as well as the technique, advantages, and disadvantages of the system.

Digital Image

A digital image is an image formed by the use of an electronic sensor that is connected in some manner to a computer. Early in the development of digital imaging, it was often referred to as *filmless radiography*, but that term is no longer used to describe this imaging technique. The basic elements necessary to acquire a digital image are (1) an x-ray machine; (2) an electronic sensor or detector; (3) an analogue-to-digital converter; (4) a computer, which can be a laptop or desktop version; and (5) a monitor (Fig. 15.1).

Presently, there are three basic types of digital imaging systems (Fig. 15.2):

1. Direct digital radiography. This system uses a sensor wired directly (or through a WiFi system) to the computer with the sensor either a charge-coupled device (CCD) or a complementary metal oxide semiconductor (CMOS).
2. Indirect digital radiography (storage phosphor). This wireless system employs a photostimulable phosphor (PSP) plate and laser beam scanning to produce the image.
3. Optically scanned digital radiography. In this system, a finished processed radiograph is scanned and digitized in much the same way that a document is scanned. The new digitalized image can be manipulated in the same manner that direct and indirect images are.

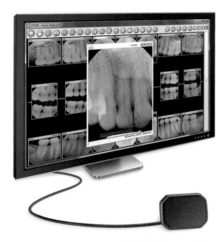

● **Figure 15.1** A full-mouth series of digital images. (Courtesy DEXIS LLC, Hatfield, PA.)

X-Ray Unit

The standard dental intraoral x-ray machine can be used for digital radiography, so it is not necessary to purchase a digital-specific unit. However, the unit must have a timer that can be adjusted to accommodate the digital receptors that require less time than conventional film. There are units available that have an icon picturing a computer that, when activated, automatically reduces the exposure time and provides the image quality and reduction in exposure times needed for digital radiography. These units can be utilized for both conventional and digital radiography. There are digital panoramic units available that combine the advantages of digital imaging with those of pantomography.

Sensors

The most critical part of a digital radiography system is the sensor that is placed in the patient's mouth. Presently, sensors are available that are equal in size to #0, #1, #2, #4, and panoramic films (Fig. 15.3). Direct sensors either have wires or are wireless devices that are linked to the image processor. The most common sensor in use is the CCD, which is a chip of pure silicon that is divided into a two-dimensional display called *pixels*. When either x-ray or light photons interact with a CCD (depending on the system used), an electric charge is created and stored. After the exposure is completed, the charges on the CCD are sequentially removed electrically, creating a continuous analogue output signal. An analogue signal represents data in a continuous mode, just like a wristwatch with hour, minute, and second hands. This information must be converted to digital units that can be assigned numbers.

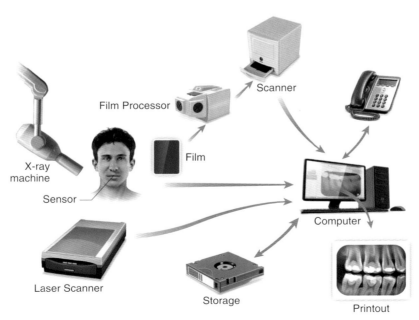

● **Figure 15.2** Different digital imaging systems.

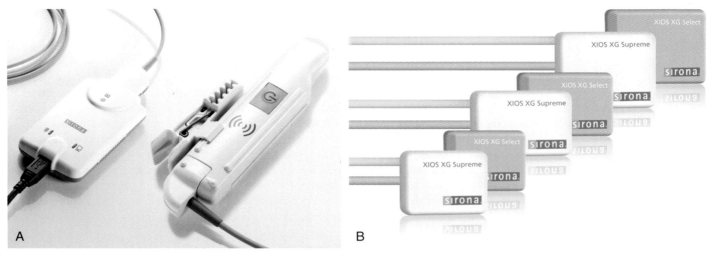

• **Figure 15.3 A,** Wired direct digital sensor. **B,** Various sizes of digital sensors. (A, Courtesy Dentsply Sirona, Charlotte, NC. B, Courtesy Dentsply Sirona, Charlotte, NC.)

An analogue-to-digital converter is used to convert the analogue output signal to a digital signal that is then sent to the computer. The CMOS sensors are also wired directly to the computer or are wireless devices that produce an instantaneous image. CMOS sensors have less power and are less expensive. CMOS sensors have more noise (lesser image definition) than the CCD and hold less diagnostic information. However, they are less fragile, and sensor replacement is less common.

A storage phosphor sensor (or PSP) produces images in a two-step process by using a reusable plastic imaging plate that is not wired to the computer and is thinner, less expensive, and less rigid than the CCD and CMOS sensors. PSPs can be manufactured for both intraoral and extraoral dental radiography. The phosphor material in the sensor stores the x-ray energy until it is scanned by a laser that digitizes the image and then transmits the image to the computer. Acquiring the image from the laser can take from 30 seconds to several minutes, depending on the number of images being scanned. The light released by the laser is captured as an electronic signal and is converted to a digital image that is seen on the computer monitor.

The sensors are reusable after the image has been erased and disinfected. The PSP is placed in a barrier envelope for infection control purposes before reusing it. It should be noted that a different PSP is used for each exposure, much like the use of film packets in conventional radiography. PSP sensors are also similar to conventional film in that they are flexible and are comparable in size, shape, and thickness. However, the laser scanning process and recharging of the PSP sensor do not necessitate that the room be completely dark like the use of standard film does.

Nature of the Image

A digital image is composed of structurally ordered areas called pixels. A pixel would be the digital equivalent of a silver halide crystal on conventional film, with the difference being that silver halide crystals are randomly positioned in the emulsion, whereas the pixel has a definite location that can be assigned a number (digit). The pixel is a single dot in a digital image; the image is made up of all the pixels or dots on the image. An analogy would be a photograph in a newspaper. In looking carefully at the newspaper image, you see that it is composed of multiple dots with varying degrees of black and white. When looking at the picture without looking at it so carefully, however, you do not see the dots but rather the entire picture.

Besides each pixel having a location, it also has a gray level that represents the photon penetration of the object (tooth) in that area. The pixel is represented in the computer by a number that indicates its location and photon penetration, and the total image is a table of numbers that can be manipulated (e.g., added or subtracted).

The pixels can be considered containers for numbers; the numbers vary from 0 to 256 (black to white). Hence there are usually 256 gray levels in an image. However, the human eye can only discern 32 gray levels. Diagnosis relies more on contrast discrimination (gray levels) than on spatial relations and definition. The fact that digital images have only 6 to 10 line pairs per millimeter discrimination as compared with 12 to 15 line pairs per millimeter for film is not that important as a disadvantage of digital imaging. Box 15.1 presents advantages and disadvantages of digital imaging.

Text continued on p. 182

• BOX 15.1   Advantages and Disadvantages of Digital Radiography

Before discussing the technique for digital radiography, we will consider its advantages and disadvantages. The following lists utilize conventional radiography as the means of comparison.

Advantages

- **Faster image acquisition.** The growing acceptance of digital radiography can be contributed to the dental professional's ability to view the digitized image on the monitor instantaneously or within minutes, depending on the digital method being utilized (i.e., direct or indirect digital radiography). This allows for immediate evaluation and interpretation of the digital image.
- **Overall procedure time is reduced.** Digital radiography is more time efficient in multiple ways than conventional film-based radiography. For example, in direct digital radiography, the same sensor and barrier sheath is used for all of the projections, the exposure time is reduced, and the processing and mounting steps are completely eliminated. Even though indirect digital radiography is not as time efficient as direct digital radiography, it does not take as long as conventional radiography.
- **Reduction in radiation dose.** A great deal of attention has been given to the fact that digital imaging requires much less radiation than film or film-screen combinations. The reduction is about 90% when compared with the exposure from D-speed film, about 60% when compared with E-speed film, and there is a 50% reduction when compared to F-speed film. This decrease in patient exposure is as a result of the increased sensitivity of the digital sensor to x-radiation.
- **Image adjustment and manipulation** (Fig. 15.4). Once the image is acquired, the computer can alter it in many ways. The image can be enlarged, darkened, or lightened (varying the density and contrast) or have selected areas magnified, colorized, or reversed.
- **Image storage.** Because the images are stored in digital form, the storage space required is minimal compared with mounted radiographs kept in a patient's chart. If the dental facility has electronic health records (EHRs), the images are accessible through the patient's EHR. In all available digital systems, stored images can be called up almost

instantaneously. In addition, images taken at different times can be placed on the monitor side-by-side for comparison.
- **Remote consultation.** The digital images can be transmitted to other dental offices or insurance companies if the intended receiver has the ability to receive the images. Instead of duplication of radiographs and reliance on the mail, the images are sent immediately to another practitioner, saving valuable time and labor.
- **Hard copies.** If teletransmission of the image is not possible, printouts, or hard copies, can be produced immediately, eliminating the need for duplication while preserving the integrity of the office records.
- **Patient education.** Patients seem to relate better to a digital image on a monitor than a radiograph or a series of mounted radiographs on a viewbox when the dentist is using them as a visual aid for case presentation. The reason may be that this is an electronic age; thus, patients may be used to the screen and close-up views. The ability to look at clinical images or radiographs on the same screen at the same time also helps in case presentation.
- **Environmentally friendly.** Because the silver salts found in film emulsion and processing chemicals are not used in digital imaging, there are no environmental and waste disposal issues. As discussed in Chapter 11, many states have laws governing the disposal of processing chemicals. This environmental issue is very important and appealing to both patients and dentists. In addition, no lead foil is used in digital radiography, which can also be hazardous to the environment, especially in large quantities.
- **Paperless office.** Most dental offices and clinics are now using computers for record keeping. Software that started out as a means of billing has been expanded to include treatment records, insurance forms, recall systems, and more. The final piece in the puzzle to make the use of the conventional dental chart obsolete is the digital image. With its addition, a paperless office makes every type of information about the patient available for immediate retrieval from the office electronic system. These records should be backed up by a duplicate disk that is stored at another location.

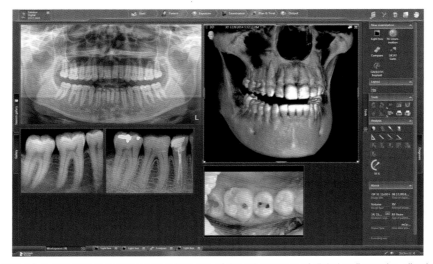

• **Figure 15.4** Magnification of images is just one of the advantages of digital radiography, allowing the dental professional to take closer look at areas of concern. (Courtesy Dentsply Sirona, Charlotte, NC.)

Continued

• **BOX 15.1** **Advantages and Disadvantages of Digital Radiography—cont'd**

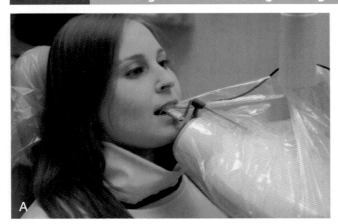

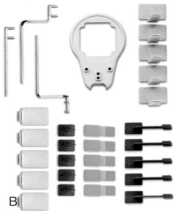

• **Figure 15.5** **A,** Charge-coupled device (CCD) sensor in patient's mouth. **B,** Beam alignment devices manufactured with adhesive backing to hold sensors in place. (Courtesy Dentsply Rinn, York, PA.)

• *Cross-contamination.* Computerized images are clean and sterile, because they are not touched by the operator's contaminated gloves when mounting or removing them from the chart or viewbox during an operative procedure.

Disadvantages

• *Sensor placement.* The main disadvantage or difficulty in digital radiography is sensor placement in the patient's mouth (Fig. 15.5A). The direct digital sensors are the same size as the standard #0, #1, and #2 dental film, but they are thicker and more rigid. Even though manufacturers have tried to make the sensors more user friendly, it may be difficult or impossible to obtain parallelism between the tooth and sensor in small or crowded mouths to follow the right angle/paralleling technique. However, paralleling instruments are available for use with direct digital sensors (see Fig. 15.5B). It should be noted that the storage phosphor systems use a thinner and slightly more adaptable sensor than the direct digital systems (Fig. 15.6); some practitioners feel that this gives the system a distinct advantage over the CCD-based (or CMOS-based) system.

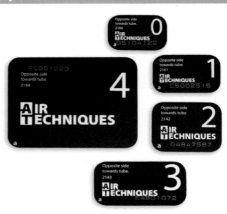

• **Figure 15.6** Intraoral phosphor sensors in various sizes. (Courtesy Air Techniques, Melville, NY.)

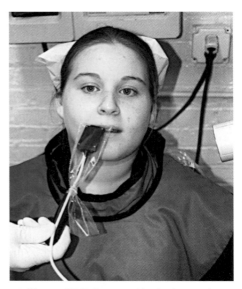

• **Figure 15.7** Sensor with plastic covering.

• *Definition.* As mentioned earlier, film provides better detail (12 to 15 line pairs per millimeter) than do digital images (6 to 10 line pairs per millimeter). Although this may be the case, the human eye cannot usually make this distinction in clinical situations. Also, the digital image can be altered to improve the visual image on the monitor.

• *Cost.* The initial cost of a digital system can be quite expensive. Although this may seem like a large expense at first, over time the savings in space, labor, storage, and more justify and amortize the start-up costs. Digital panoramic units can cost $25,000 or more. It is also important to consider maintenance and repairs when discussing continued costs of digital systems.

• *Fragility of sensors.* The intraoral sensors are really large silicon chips (Fig. 15.7); if dropped or abused, their replacement is costly. The cost of the sensor alone is considerably expensive. Therefore, careful handling of digital sensors should always be stressed in dental facilities.

PROCEDURE 15.1 THE DIGITAL IMAGING TECHNIQUE

The actual exposure technique for digital imaging at chairside is very similar to that of conventional radiography, with the exception of processing and the inclusion of computer knowledge and skills (Fig. 15.8).

The main difference between direct and indirect digital radiography is that the direct digital sensors are wireless or have wires that connect the system to a computer, are less similar to the film packet used in conventional radiography, and produce an instantaneous image on the monitor. The sensors used for both techniques are available in different sizes to accommodate varying patients. The operator should still maintain quality assurance in infection control, patient/operator protection, and chairside technique with digital exposures.

Operators are expected to protect themselves and the patient against unnecessary radiation exposure. Each patient should be draped with a lead apron and thyroid collar (Fig. 15.9). Operators are also expected to use sensor-holding devices and not use the patient's finger to stabilize the sensor when exposing images. Digital sensors should be covered with an infection control barrier and handled with extreme

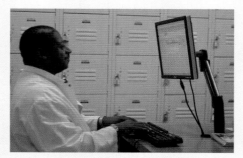

• **Figure 15.8** Operator accessing digital images.

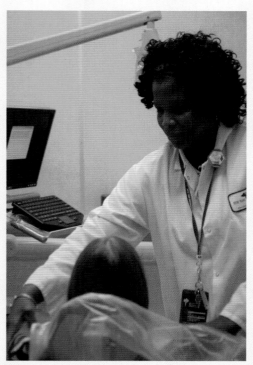

• **Figure 15.9** Operator placing lead apron/collar on patient.

caution and care, because they are very sensitive devices. The operator's position is maintained at least 6 feet from the source of radiation and behind an acceptable barrier.

Optimal chairside technique is extremely important in producing quality images and preventing overexposure to the patient. The operator must avoid retakes as much as possible. The spontaneous image of an error causes retakes to be less time-consuming than conventional radiography, but it still adds to the radiation burden of the patient. Some of the errors previously mentioned do not apply to digital radiography (reversed film, overbending of the film packet, double exposure, static electricity artifacts, processing errors), but most exposure errors (collimator cutoff, foreshortening, elongation, overlap, improper receptor placement) are still possible.

The Digital Full-Mouth Series

The digital full-mouth series is generally exposed using the paralleling technique with paralleling instruments. All principles of the paralleling technique are followed (refer to Chapter 9) with the digital sensor used as the receptor.

The following account includes the sensor, paralleling instrument, and position-indicating device (PID) position for each projection constituent of a full-mouth series. The combination of the digital sensor, paralleling instruments, and a collimated x-ray beam contribute to a decrease in radiation exposure to the patient.

> **NOTE**
>
> The operator may choose to place a cotton roll between the opposing arch and the bite piece to aid in patient comfort for any or all of the digital periapical projections. However, this technique is not recommended for bitewing projections.

Maxillary Central Incisors (Fig. 15.10)

The sensor is placed parallel to the teeth in both the vertical and horizontal planes and as close to the teeth as possible. The sensor is placed in the holder in the vertical position. The sensor placement in the patient's mouth may be difficult as a result of the rigidity of the digital sensors. However, the difficulty in placement may be remedied by increasing the distance of the sensor from the central incisors and resting the bite piece on the mandibular arch instead of on the incisal edges of the maxillary incisors prior to the patient gently biting on the bite piece. The center of the sensor is aligned with the junction between the central incisors. The central ray is aimed at the center of the sensor. The PID is placed perpendicular to both the sensor and the tooth in the vertical and horizontal planes. When a localizing device is being used, make sure that the ring is placed as close to the patient's face as possible and the PID is positioned as close to the ring as possible to decrease radiation exposure to the patient and to obtain proper contrast and density of the digital image.

Maxillary Canines (Fig. 15.11)

The sensor is placed parallel to the tooth in both the vertical and horizontal planes and as close to the tooth as possible. The sensor is placed in the holder in the vertical position for the canine projections. The placement of the sensor in the patient's canine region may be difficult as a result of the rigidity of the digital sensors. However, the difficulty in placement may be remedied by increasing the distance of the sensor from the canine and resting the bite piece on the mandibular arch away

Continued

PROCEDURE 15.1 THE DIGITAL IMAGING TECHNIQUE—cont'd

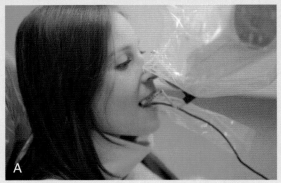

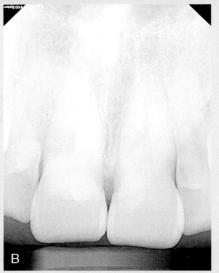

• **Figure 15.10** Maxillary central incisors. **A,** Sensor-holding device and position-indicating device (PID). **B,** Digital image.

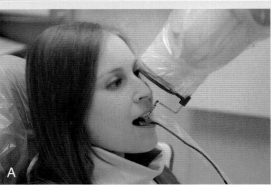

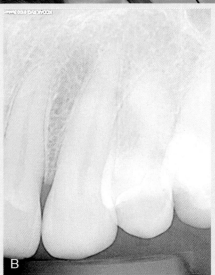

• **Figure 15.11** Maxillary canines. **A,** Sensor-holding device and position-indicating device (PID). **B,** Digital image.

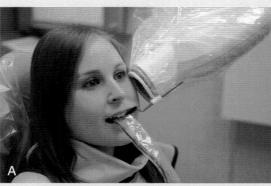

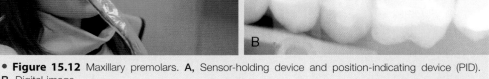

• **Figure 15.12** Maxillary premolars. **A,** Sensor-holding device and position-indicating device (PID). **B,** Digital image.

from the incisal edges of the canines prior to the patient gently biting on the bite piece. The center of the sensor is aligned with the center of the canine. The central ray is aimed at the center of the sensor. The PID is placed perpendicular to both the sensor and the tooth in the vertical and horizontal planes. When a localizing device is being used, make sure that the ring is placed as close to the patient's face as possible and the PID is positioned as close to the ring as possible to decrease

radiation exposure to the patient and to obtain proper contrast and density of the digital image.

Maxillary Premolars (Fig. 15.12)

The sensor is placed parallel to the teeth in both the vertical and horizontal planes and as close to the tooth as possible. The sensor is placed in the holder in the horizontal position for the posterior projections. The placement of the sensor in

PROCEDURE 15.1   THE DIGITAL IMAGING TECHNIQUE—cont'd

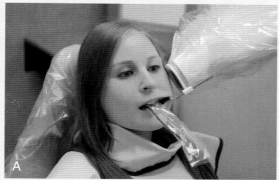

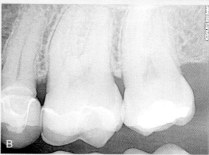

• **Figure 15.13** Maxillary molars. **A,** Sensor-holding device and position-indicating device (PID). **B,** Digital image.

the patient's mouth may be difficult as a result of the rigidity of the digital sensors. However, the difficulty in placement may be remedied by increasing the distance of the sensor from the premolars so that the sensor position may be in the middle of the palate. It is also helpful to rest the bite piece on the mandibular arch and guide the sensor into position as the patient closes their mouth. The center of the sensor is aligned with the center of the second premolar. The central ray is aimed at the center of the sensor. The PID is placed perpendicular to both the sensor and the tooth in the vertical and horizontal planes. Also, be sure that the sensor is parallel to the premolars in the horizontal plane to avoid overlapping of the premolar teeth on the digital image. When a localizing device is being used, make sure that the ring is placed as close to the patient's face as possible and the PID is positioned as close to the ring as possible to decrease radiation exposure to the patient and to obtain proper contrast and density of the digital image.

Maxillary Molars (Fig. 15.13)

The sensor is placed parallel to the teeth in both the vertical and horizontal planes and as close to the teeth as possible. The sensor is placed in the holder in the horizontal position for the posterior projections. The placement of the sensor in the patient's mouth may be difficult as a result of the rigidity of the digital sensors. However, the difficulty in placement may be remedied by increasing the distance of the sensor from the molars so that the sensor position may be in the middle of the palate. It is also helpful to rest the bite piece on the mandibular arch and guide the sensor into position as the patient closes the mouth. The center of the sensor is aligned with the center of the first molar, and the operator asks the patient to close down partially. Then, when the cheek is relaxed, the operator moves the sensor so that its center is aligned with the center

of the second molar and asks the patient to close fully on the bite piece of the sensor-holding device.

The central ray is aimed at the center of the sensor. The PID is placed perpendicular to both the film and the tooth in the vertical and horizontal planes. When a localizing device is being used, make sure that the ring is placed as close to the patient's face as possible and the PID is positioned as close to the ring as possible to decrease radiation exposure to the patient and to obtain proper contrast and density of the digital image.

Bitewing Projections (Fig. 15.14)

When the premolar bitewings are being radiographed, the center of the sensor is aligned with the center of the mandibular second premolar, and the biting surface of the sensor holder is held on the mandibular arch. While the operator holds the sensor in position, the patient is instructed to gently bite on the sensor-holding device. The operator should be sure that the patient is biting on the posterior teeth in centric occlusion and not holding the bite piece steady with the lips. The central ray is aimed at the center of the sensor. The PID is placed perpendicular to both the sensor and the tooth in the vertical and horizontal planes. Also, be sure that the sensor is parallel to the teeth being radiographed in the horizontal plane to avoid overlapping of the interproximal surfaces on the digital image. When a localizing device is being used, make sure that the ring is placed as close to the patient's face as possible and the PID is positioned as close to the ring as possible to decrease radiation exposure to the patient and to obtain proper contrast and density of the digital image. The procedure for radiographing the molars is the same as that mentioned earlier, except that the biting surface of the sensor holder is centered and held on the mandibular second molar. It should also be noted that there are sensor-holding devices available for use with digital vertical bitewing projections.

HELPFUL HINT

When exposing all bitewing and mandibular periapical projections, the operator must avoid placing the sensor on top of the tongue. The patient is asked to move their tongue away from the sensor. This tongue placement is requested to assure that the sensor is resting on the floor of the mouth and not on top of the tongue. If a receptor is placed on top of the tongue, the image will not show all of the radiographic information desired on the resultant image.

Mandibular Incisors (Fig. 15.15)

The sensor is placed parallel to the teeth in both the vertical and horizontal planes and as close to the teeth as possible. The sensor is placed in the holder in the vertical position. The sensor placement in the patient's mouth may be difficult as a result of the rigidity of the digital sensors. However, the difficulty in placement may be remedied by increasing the distance of the sensor from the central incisors. In some cases, it may be necessary to position the sensor further back in the floor of the mouth at the level of the molars. The operator may also start out with the sensor on an angle and then slowly bring the sensor into a parallel position with the closure of the mandible. The operator may also place an opened gauze pad under the sensor covering the floor of the mouth to prevent it from irritating the tissue in this area.

Continued

PROCEDURE 15.1   THE DIGITAL IMAGING TECHNIQUE—cont'd

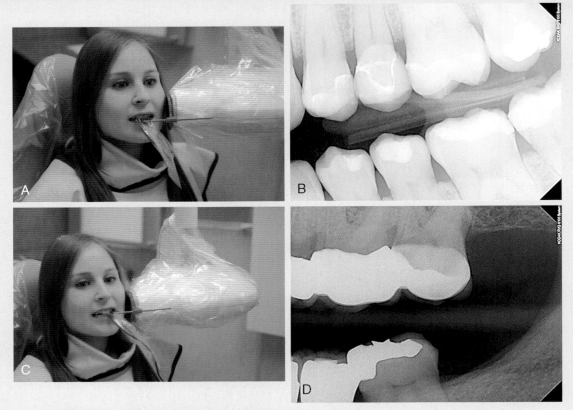

• **Figure 15.14** Bitewing projections. **A,** Sensor-holding device and position-indicating device (PID) for premolar bitewing. **B,** Digital image of premolar bitewing. **C,** Sensor-holding device and PID for molar bitewing. **D,** Digital image of molar bitewing.

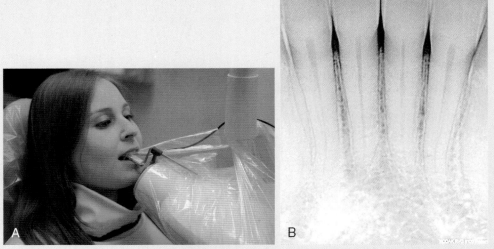

• **Figure 15.15** Mandibular incisors. **A,** Sensor-holding device and position-indicating device (PID). **B,** Digital image.

The center of the sensor is aligned with the junction between the central incisors. The central ray is aimed at the center of the sensor. The PID is placed perpendicular to both the sensor and the tooth in the vertical and horizontal planes. When a localizing device is being used, make sure that the ring is placed as close to the patient's face as possible and the PID is positioned as close to the ring as possible to decrease radiation exposure to the patient and to obtain proper contrast and density of the digital image.

Mandibular Canines (Fig. 15.16)

The sensor is placed parallel to the canines in both the vertical and horizontal planes and as close to the tooth as possible. The sensor is placed in the holder in the vertical position for

PROCEDURE 15.1 THE DIGITAL IMAGING TECHNIQUE—cont'd

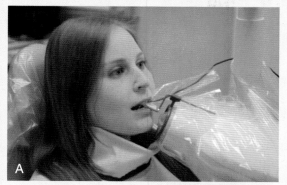

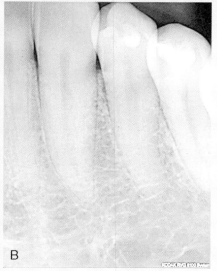

• **Figure 15.16** Mandibular canines. **A,** Sensor-holding device and position-indicating device (PID). **B,** Digital image.

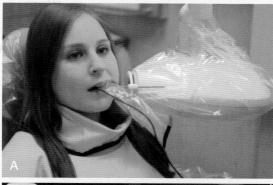

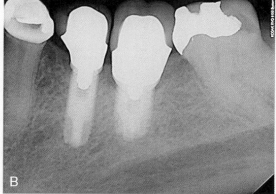

• **Figure 15.17** Mandibular premolars. **A,** Sensor-holding device and position-indicating device (PID). **B,** Digital image.

the anterior projections. The placement of the sensor in the patient's mouth may be difficult as a result of the rigidity of the digital sensors. However, the difficulty in placement may be remedied by increasing the distance of the sensor from the canine. In some cases, it may be necessary to position the sensor further back in the floor of the mouth. The operator may also start out with the sensor on an angle and then slowly bring the sensor into a parallel position with the closure of the mandible. The operator may also place an opened gauze pad under the sensor covering the floor of the mouth to prevent it from irritating the tissue in this area. Be sure that the sensor is placed below and not above the tongue. The center of the sensor is aligned with the center of the canine. The central ray is aimed at the center of the sensor. The PID is placed perpendicular to both the sensor and the tooth in the vertical and horizontal planes. When a localizing device is being used, make sure that the ring is placed as close to the patient's face as possible and the PID is positioned as close to the ring as possible to decrease radiation exposure to the patient and to obtain proper contrast and density of the digital image.

Mandibular Premolars (Fig. 15.17)

The sensor is placed parallel to the teeth in both the vertical and horizontal planes and as close to the tooth as possible.

The sensor is placed in the holder in the horizontal position for the posterior projections. The placement of the sensor in the patient's mouth may be difficult as a result of the rigidity of the digital sensors. However, the difficulty in placement may be remedied by increasing the distance of the sensor from the premolars so that the sensor position may be in the middle of the floor of the mouth. The operator may also place an opened gauze pad on the floor of the mouth, covering the entire mandibular arch, to prevent the sensor from irritating the tissue in this area. The anterior corner of the sensor will not curve to accommodate the arch; therefore, care must be taken to include the distal of the canine and the mesial of the first premolar on the image without causing unnecessary discomfort to the patient. Also, be sure that the sensor is parallel to the premolars in the horizontal plane avoid overlapping of the premolars on the digital image. The center of the sensor is aligned with the center of the second premolar. The central ray is aimed at the center of the sensor. The PID is placed perpendicular to both the sensor and the tooth in the vertical and horizontal planes. When a localizing device is being used, make sure that the ring is placed as close to the patient's face as possible and the PID is positioned as close to the ring as possible to decrease radiation exposure to the patient and to obtain proper contrast and density of the digital image.

Mandibular Molars (Fig. 15.18)

The sensor is placed parallel to the teeth in both the vertical and horizontal planes and as close to the teeth as possible.

Continued

PROCEDURE 15.1 THE DIGITAL IMAGING TECHNIQUE—cont'd

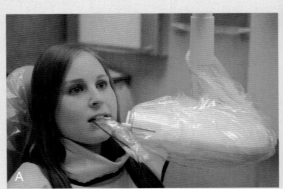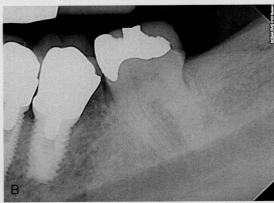

• **Figure 15.18** Mandibular molars. **A,** Sensor-holding device and position-indicating device (PID). **B,** Digital image.

The sensor is placed in the holder in the horizontal position for the posterior projections. The placement of the sensor in the patient's mouth may be difficult as a result of the rigidity of the digital sensors. However, the difficulty in placement may be remedied by increasing the distance of the sensor from the molars so that the sensor position may be in the middle of the floor of the mouth. The operator may also place an opened gauze pad on the floor of the mouth, covering the entire mandibular arch, to prevent the sensor from irritating the tissue in this area. The center of the sensor is aligned with the center of the first molar, and the operator asks the patient to close down partially. Then, when the cheek is relaxed, the operator moves the sensor so that its center is aligned with the center of the second molar and asks the patient to close fully on the bite piece of the sensor-holding device. The central ray is aimed at the center of the sensor. The PID is placed perpendicular to both the receptor and the tooth in the vertical and horizontal planes. When a localizing device is being used, make sure that the ring is placed as close to the patient's face as possible and the PID is positioned as close to the ring as possible to decrease radiation exposure to the patient and to obtain proper contrast and density of the digital image.

Types of Digital Systems

All of the systems mentioned differ in how they acquire the digital image and in availability of receptor plate size (e.g., panoramic). Once acquired, the systems do not vary greatly in how they display, adjust, store, or transmit the image.

Direct Digital Radiography

In direct digital radiography systems, the sensor, which is placed in the patient's mouth, is connected by a wire or a wireless device to the computer, and there is instantaneous image production on the monitor when the exposure is performed. Systems vary regarding the type of sensor used to capture the x-ray photons to affect the CCD or CMOS sensor. Some acquire the photons directly, whereas others use a fiberoptically coupled sensor that operates like a film-screen system, sending light photons to affect the CCD or CMOS sensor.

Indirect Digital Radiography (Storage Phosphor)

In indirect digital radiography (storage phosphor), a slightly flexible sensor, which is not connected by a wire or cable to the computer, is placed in the patient's mouth, and an exposure is made (Fig. 15.19). The sensor is then exposed, removed from the mouth, and processed by a laser beam with electronic data sent to the computer, which generates a digital image in 1½ to 5 minutes, depending on the number and types of sensor plates being processed. The plates can then be recharged and used again. Some types of digital scanners have a built-in heat sealer and bag cutter to maintain the sterility of the imaging plates.

Optically Scanned Digital Radiography

In optically scanned digital radiography systems, regular dental film is used to acquire the image with conventional film-based intraoral techniques. The film is then processed in the darkroom, the finished dry film is scanned, and the digital image is produced. This digitized image can be used in the same way as those that have been directly digitally acquired. With this method, it takes a great deal of time to acquire a digitized image, because complete film processing must be done before the image can be scanned and digitized. The most advantageous use of optically scanned digital imaging is in filing and storage of conventional images when EHRs are being utilized in the dental facility.

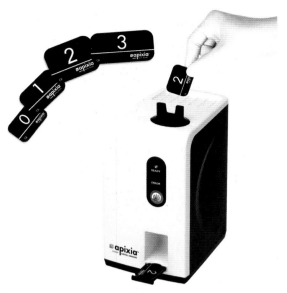

Figure 15.19 Storage phosphor imaging system. (Courtesy Apixia Digital Imaging, Industry, CA.)

Legal Aspects

One of the major concerns raised about all electronic information, including digital images, has been the reliability of the information and the possibility of image manipulation.

For example, conventional radiographs have been regularly admitted in court as evidence in cases for many years. With digital imaging, however, there is a possibility that if a jury learns that images can be altered, they may no longer look at the digital images as hard evidence. This concern has been largely overcome by the major manufacturers of digital radiographic systems by including "audit indicators" into their units that signal if and when an image has been altered.

Chapter Summary

- Digital radiography utilizes electronic sensors to record the penetration of x-radiation and transmits this information to a computer that digitizes these electronic impulses.
- There are three types of digital systems used in dental radiography: (1) direct digital radiography, (2) indirect digital radiography, and (3) optically scanned digital radiography.
- In intraoral digital imaging, an electronic sensor is placed inside the patient's mouth and is then exposed to x-radiation generated from a conventional dental x-ray unit. An electronic charge is produced on the sensor and is converted to a digital format. The image is then viewed on a computer monitor. Digital imaging and electronic sensors are also utilized in extraoral digital radiography. Infection control and radiation safety procedures are employed with both intraoral and extraoral digital radiography.
- The advantages of digital radiography when compared to conventional film-based radiography include faster image acquisition, an overall decrease in procedure time, reduced radiation exposure, image adjustment and manipulation, easier image storage, remote consultation, hard copy production, more convenient patient education, is environmentally friendly, creates a paperless office with EHRs, and more efficiency in avoiding cross-contamination.
- The disadvantages of digital radiography when compared to conventional film-based radiography include difficult sensor placement, less image definition, expensive initial costs, and fragility of the expensive sensors.

Chapter Review Questions

Multiple Choice

1. Direct digital and indirect digital radiography differ in:
   a. The type of sensors used
   b. The time it takes for an image to appear on the computer monitor
   c. The thickness of the sensor
   d. The radiographic unit used
   e. All of the above except d
2. When compared to D speed film, digital radiography reduces patient exposure by:
   a. 50%
   b. 60%
   c. 99%
   d. 90%
   e. 85%
3. All of the following statements regarding digital radiography are true except:
   a. The sensors are more sensitive to radiation than conventional film
   b. The image is best seen on the computer
   c. Direct digital sensors are difficult to place
   d. The conventional x-ray unit cannot be used
   e. The image can be altered

4. Pixels are considered containers for numbers, and the numbers vary from 0 to 256 (black to white), which means that there are usually 256 gray levels in an image. However, the human eye can only discern 52 gray levels. (Indicate all that apply.)
   a. Both statements are true.
   b. Both statements are false.
   c. The first statement is true, and the second statement is false.
   d. The first statement is false, and the second statement is true.
   e. The statements are related.

Critical Thinking Exercise

1. You are asked to give a presentation on the topic of digital radiography to a group of dental professionals. The following is a list of questions that was submitted by the audience members and compiled by the organization you are speaking on behalf of, be sure to include the answers to these questions in your presentation:
   a. What is the difference between direct and indirect digital radiography?
   b. Do I have to replace the radiographic unit in our dental facility if our facility is transitioning from conventional to digital radiography?
   c. Does digital radiography decrease radiation exposure to the patient? Please explain.
   d. Can I dispose of the lead apron and thyroid collar in my office when switching to digital radiography?
   e. What are photostimulable phosphor (PSP) plates, and how are they used in dental radiography?
   f. What is the difference between CCD and CMOS sensors?
   g. Can the digital image be altered?
   h. Can digital images be used as evidence in a court of law?
   i. What is the laser scanner used for in indirect digital radiography?
   j. Can I scan my conventional radiographic images and incorporate them in my electronic health records (EHRs)? Please explain.
   k. Are digital images more useful for patient education than conventional film images?
   l. How does the placement of CCD sensors differ from film placement in the patient's mouth?
   m. What are some helpful hints we can use when placing and exposing digital sensors?
   n. Is a digital system expensive to set up in a dental office? If so, how do you justify the initial costs?
   o. What is the advantage of using PSP rather than CCD sensors?
   p. What other facts could you provide in support of our switching from conventional to digital radiography?

Bibliography

Dunn SM, Kantor ML: Digital radiology, facts and fictions, *J Am Dent Assoc* 124:38–47, 1993.

Iannucci JM, Howerton LJ: *Dental radiography: Principles and techniques*, ed 5, St Louis, MO, 2016, Elsevier Saunders.

Jones GA, Behrents RG, Bailey GP: Legal considerations for digitized images, *Gen Dent* 44:242–244, 1996.

Mouyen F, Benz C, Sonnabend E, et al: Presentation and physical evaluation of radiovisiography, *Oral Surg Oral Med Oral Pathol* 68:238–242, 1989.

Tsang A, Sweet D, Wood RE: Potential for fraudulent use of digital radiography, *J Am Dent Assoc* 130:1325–1329, 1999.

White SC, Pharoah MJ: *Oral radiology: Principles and interpretation*, ed 7, St Louis, MO, 2013, Mosby.

16

Advanced Imaging Systems

EDUCATIONAL OBJECTIVES

Upon completing this chapter, the student will be able to:

1. Define the key terms listed at the beginning of the chapter.
2. Describe the following related to computed tomography (CT) scanning:
   - Explain the procedure for CT scanning.
   - Describe the functions of the axial, coronal, and sagittal planes of the human body.
   - List the advantages and disadvantages of CT scanning.
3. Discuss the following related to cone beam computed tomography (CBCT) imaging in dentistry:
   - Describe the role of CBCT imaging in dentistry.

- State the process for acquiring the image in the CBCT technique.
- Discuss the advantage of the CBCT procedure when compared with CT scanning in dental imaging.
- List the indications for use of CBCT imaging in dentistry.
4. Discuss the mechanism of image acquisition in magnetic resonance imaging (MRI) imaging, as well as the role that MRI imaging plays in dentistry.
5. Define nuclear medicine and discuss its role in medical imaging.

KEY TERMS

axial plane
bone window
computed tomography (CT) scanning
cone beam computed tomography
  (CBCT)
coronal plane
CT number
DICOM images
field of view (FOV)

gamma camera
Hounsfield unit
image acquisition
magnetic field
magnetic resonance imaging (MRI)
matrix
multiplanar reconstructed (MPR)
  images
radiofrequency

sagittal plane
scan
signal intensity
soft tissue window
software
target tissues

Introduction

With the introduction and now common use of advanced imaging techniques, such as computed tomography (CT) scanning, magnetic resonance imaging (MRI), cone beam computed tomography (CBCT), positron emission tomography (PET), and digital imaging (see Chapter 15), the field of dental radiology has greatly expanded. These new techniques can be used by dentists to image structures in ways that were previously unavailable. The use of CBCT scans for diagnosing lesions and planning implant cases and the use of MRI to visualize soft tissue components of the temporomandibular joint (TMJ) and assess pathologic conditions are now accepted as standard procedures in dental radiology. Although CT scanners and MRI units are not found in most general dental offices except in the ever-increasing dental radiology specialty practices, the dental professional should have some familiarity with these newer imaging systems, because patients may have to be referred

for such imaging, or copies of the images may be brought to the office by the patient for opinions and interpretation. Therefore, an overview of these imaging systems is included in this chapter.

Although different sources of energy are used (x-radiation in CT and radiofrequency energy in MRI), a common theme in these imaging systems is the use of tomography and the absence of film as the sensing device and the use of electronic detectors that send electrical impulses to a computer, which then stores or generates an image on a monitor.

As a result of the use of CBCT imaging in dentistry, dental imaging is not limited to two-dimensional imaging any longer. CBCT imaging provides a three-dimensional (3D) view of the structures in the oral cavity. This imaging technique furnishes more detailed information in formulating an enhanced and accurate interpretation of structures in the oral cavity.

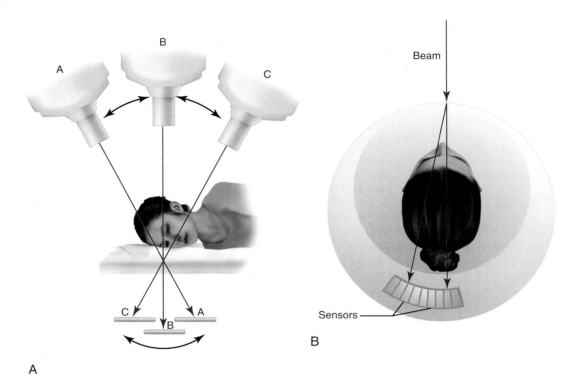

• **Figure 16.1 A,** Tomography. Note the film as the image receptor. **B,** CT scan. Note the sensors as the image receptor.

Computed Tomography Scanning

CT was introduced into the field of radiology in the early 1970s. In contrast to conventional radiographic techniques in which film or film-screen combinations are used to produce images, CT images are computer generated. However, CT still uses ionizing radiation as the energy source.

CT scanners produce digital data measuring the extent of the x-ray penetration through the patient. The **image acquisition** is done in a tomographic mode with the source of the radiation or the detectors traveling 360 degrees around the patient. Fig. 16.1 shows the comparison between tomography and CT scanning.

In CT, a finely collimated x-ray beam is directed through the patient to a series of electronic detectors or sensors. These detectors send electrical impulses that are digitized and stored by the computer. In medicine, this is called the **scan**, and it is usually done in the axial plane with the patient positioned in a large, doughnut-shaped unit that contains the x-ray tube and the sensors (Fig. 16.2). Originally, all scans were done in the axial plane, thus leading to the name *computerized axial tomography (CAT) scan*. The "A" has been dropped, because some initial scans are done in other planes than the **axial plane** (a plane that divides the body into inferior and superior regions). These images can be reformatted and viewed in the **coronal plane** (a vertical plane that divides the body into anterior and posterior regions), **sagittal plane** (a vertical plane that divides the body into right and left regions), and axial plane

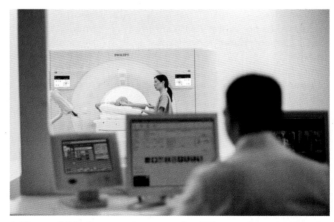

• **Figure 16.2** Computed tomography (CT) scanning unit. Note the patient in the scanner, the technician at the computer, and the image on the screen. (Courtesy Philips Medical, Andover, MA.)

(Figs. 16.3 and 16.4). Fig. 16.5 is a diagram illustrating all of the orientation planes.

The computer can generate an image based on the digitized data it has received. This image can be (1) displayed on a monitor, (2) reformatted into other planes in two or three dimensions (which cannot be done in digital dental radiography), (3) adjusted for optimum viewing of hard and soft tissue, (4) stored on a disk, (5) produced as a printout (hard copy), and (6) transmitted to other locations. Once the scan has been completed, the patient can be dismissed, because all subsequent image reconstruction manipulation can be done by the computer.

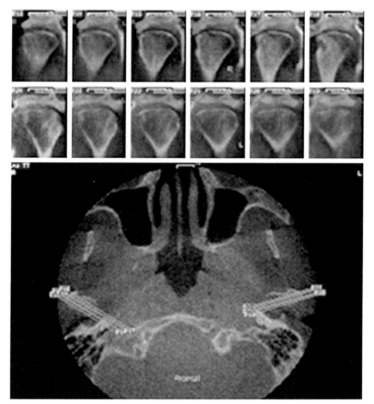

• **Figure 16.3** Computed tomography (CT) scan in the axial plane. Note the gray soft tissue imaging and the radiopaque bone.

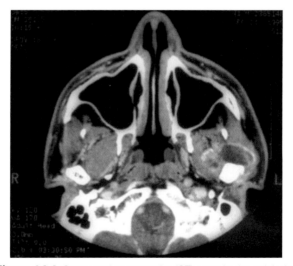

• **Figure 16.4** Computed tomography (CT) scan in the axial plane. Note the gray soft tissue imaging and the radiopaque bone.

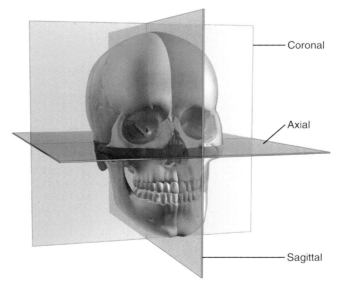

Coronal

Axial

Sagittal

• **Figure 16.5** All orientation planes.

The computer collects the x-ray beam penetration data in a grid pattern called a matrix, much like the digital imaging described in Chapter 15. Each square in the matrix is made up of pixels, which represent the density of a small volume of tissue. Because each pixel is digitized, it can be assigned a CT number, which represents the density of a particular area that has been penetrated by the x-ray beam. CT numbers are also called Hounsfield units, in honor of one of the developers of this radiographic imaging technique. CT numbers range from +1000 to −1000, with 0 being water, bone being +1000, and air being −1000. For example, fat tissue is about 100 Hounsfield units. Because the density of tissue has been assigned a number, one can narrow the densities that can be displayed. This is called *using a window*, and there can be either a bone window or a soft tissue window (Figs. 16.6 and 16.7). Box 16.1 presents the advantages and disadvantages of CT.

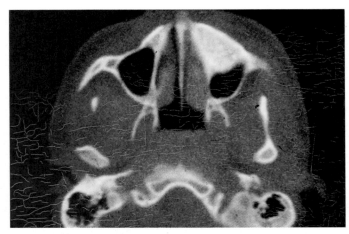

• **Figure 16.6** Computed tomography (CT) scan with a bone window. Decide which maxillary sinus is abnormal.

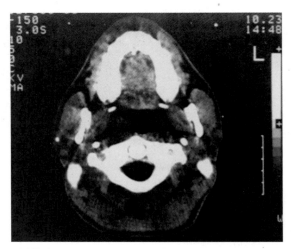

• **Figure 16.7** Computed tomography (CT) scan with a soft tissue window.

• BOX 16.1   Advantages and Disadvantages of Computed Tomography

Advantages

1. Eliminates the superimposition of images of structures superficial or deep to the area in question (tomography), which can be done in any plane. Images can be acquired in any plane, and the scan can reproduce images in any plane.
2. A computed tomography (CT) scan can enable one to distinguish between tissue density that differs from 1% to 2%, whereas at least 10% is needed for conventional radiography.
3. Images can be reformatted to another plane without the necessity of another scan. Some CT scanners can image the mandible and the maxilla on one scan.
4. Density and contrast can be adjusted using the CT numbers to create a bone or soft tissue window.
5. The enhanced image makes interpretation easier and more accurate.

Disadvantages

1. Increased radiation dose when compared with conventional film. Some of the newer cone beam units can reduce radiation by 90% when compared with older-design CT units. Many special software programs have been written for CT scanners that are specific for dental use in implant planning (Fig. 16.8). This software directs the computer in obtaining the desired images in three planes so that the site of the implant fixture can be determined. Not all CT units have implant software; thus, it is very important to ask whether the facility has the desired software program before referring a patient to a medical facility for an implant scan. However, cone beam computed tomography (CBCT) imaging is specifically designed for use in dentistry and is therefore recommended for three-dimensional (3D) imaging of the oral cavity. The use of CT scanning in the evaluation and planning of implant sites and evaluation of bone density has become a common application in dentistry and is rapidly becoming the standard of care for implant planning. The American Academy of Oral and Maxillofacial Radiology (AAOMR) has stated in their position paper on the use of x-rays in implants that "some form of cross-sectional imaging be used for implant cases," and CT is a form of cross-sectional imaging. Never before has it been possible to obtain multiple cross-sectional cuts with the speed and accuracy available now in implant evaluation.
2. The cost to the patient for a CT scan is quite considerable in comparison to, for example, a panoramic radiograph.
3. Significant artifacts are produced by metallic objects that are in the plane being scanned, such as metal dental restorations.

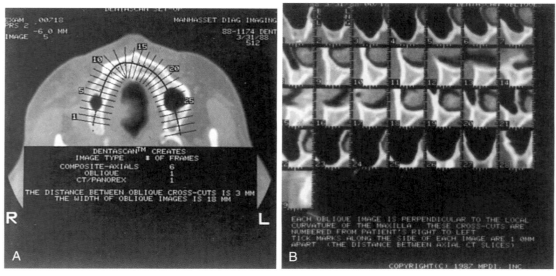

• **Figure 16.8** Computed tomography (CT) scan using software designed specifically for dental implant planning. **A,** Axial cut with numbered orientation planes that are seen in the corresponding vertical cuts in **B.**

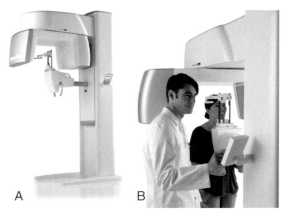

• **Figure 16.9** The NewTom VGi evo cone beam computed tomography (CBCT) unit, ideal for imaging the maxillofacial region. (Courtesy NewTom by Cefla s.c.)

Cone Beam Computed Tomography

A more recent means to acquire a CT image is by CBCT, also known as *cone beam volumetric tomography (CBVT).* Some of these CT scanners are dedicated to maxillofacial scans (NewTom 9000; Fig. 16.9A). The technique involves use of a round or rectangular cone-shaped x-ray beam on a two-dimensional x-ray sensor. This technique has the advantage of using less radiation, as well as less time acquiring the image as compared with medical CT scanning. The scanned series consists of 360 images, including transaxial, axial, and panoramic images. These CBCT units allow the patient to either be in the supine or upright position for exposure (see Fig. 16.9B). This option allows patients to have dental scans exposed without having to lie down in a confined space.

CBCT and CBVT represents a new generation of U.S. Food and Drug Administration–approved dental scanners that generate significantly less radiation than do traditional medical CT scanning devices. These CBCT (CBVT) scanners deliver comparable diagnostic images while adhering to the ALARA (as low as reasonably achievable) principle of using the least amount of radiation to obtain a diagnostic image. CBCT scanners are cost-effective and more accurate than conventional medical CT scanners. CBCT technology has many benefits, including reduced radiation exposure while creating 3D images of the anatomic structures of the mandible, maxilla, and related structures (Fig. 16.10). Given the fact that CBCT (CBVT) technology has greater accuracy than a dental periapical image, a panoramic projection, or even a medical CT scan, it is suggested that CBCT (CBVT) may be used in dentistry not only for dental implant planning, but also to evaluate impacted teeth, supernumeraries, oral pathologic conditions, and many more dental applications in multiple views (Fig. 16.11).

Acquiring the Image

To take a scan, the technician places the patient in position in the CT scanner and a preliminary scout image is exposed. This scout image helps the technician determine if the patient is positioned properly and calibrates the radiation dosage according to the hard and soft tissue densities. Once the head is in the correct position, the x-ray tube rotates 360 degrees once around the patient's head to take the desired images, which is similar to the technique used in panoramic imaging. The image produced is a 3D image as opposed to the former two-dimensional images that were produced in the past.

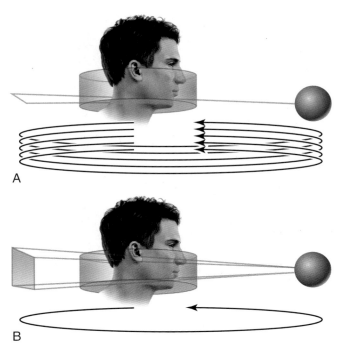

A

B

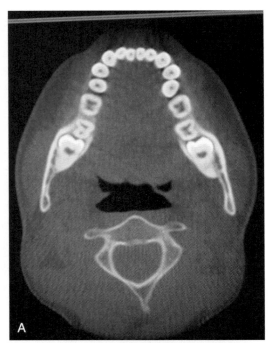

A

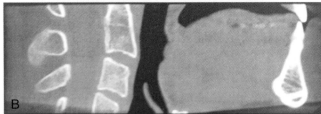

B

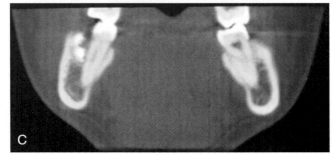

C

• **Figure 16.10 A,** Conventional computed tomography (CT) scan reformats a series of parallel helical slices, which incorporate small errors in final scan. **B,** Cone beam volumetric tomography (CBVT) captures volumes of data taken in one 360-degree rotation about a patient's head. Each volume "touches" adjacent volume to avoid distortion and error in reformatted studies.

• **Figure 16.11 A,** Cone beam computed tomography (CBCT) axial view. **B,** Cone beam volumetric tomography (CBVT; CBCT) sagittal view. **C,** CBVT (CBCT) coronal view.

Basic Information: Cone Beam Computed Tomography

The patient's maxillofacial area that is of interest when taking a CBCT image is known as the field of view (FOV). The CBCT unit takes multiple images of the FOV in a single scan. The digital receptor receives the information generated by the radiation exposure. This raw data is 3D, goes through reconstruction, and forms a pile of images known as DICOM images. These images are transferred to the software that allows the dental professional to view the area of interest (or FOV) in the axial, coronal, and sagittal planes. When these axial, coronal, and sagittal images are viewed simultaneously, they are referred to as multiplanar reconstructed (MPR) images.

Radiation Dosages

The average absorbed dose from a CBCT scanner is roughly 12.0 mSv (millisieverts), which is equivalent to or less than the radiation needed to take five periapical radiographs utilizing conventional film. This amount of radiation is similar to one-fourth of a typical panoramic machine. By comparison, medical CT scanners acquire images using effective doses 40 to 60 times these amounts; the radiation dose for medical CT scanners is based on the patient's weight, bone density, and whether one jaw or two jaws is being studied.

NOTE

The dental applications of cone beam computed tomography (CBCT) images include:
- Implant planning
- Endodontics
- Temporomandibular joint (TMJ) disorders
- Extractions
- Location of anatomic structures, such as the mental foramen and inferior alveolar nerve
- Orthodontics
- Trauma
- Assessment of abnormalities and lesions

Magnetic Resonance Imaging

MRI does not use ionizing radiation as the energy source but rather another type of energy wave from the electromagnetic spectrum, that is, radiofrequency energy (see Fig. 1.4). Because these wavelengths are long and cannot cause ionization, there is no radiation dose to the patient.

The patient is placed in a large magnet that is 10,000 times more powerful than the earth's magnetic field. The field is so powerful that all freestanding metal objects must be removed from the room, because they can become lethal objects if affected by the magnetic field. The magnetic field temporarily changes the alignment and orientation of the protons in the patient's body. Radiofrequency waves are applied to the realigned protons, and this radiofrequency energy is absorbed. When the radiofrequency signal ends, the protons release the absorbed energy, which is received by a sensor, and the information is transmitted to a computer that generates an image. Because MRI is actually based on measurement of proton density and 70% of the human body is water, of which protons are the major component, MRI is better for visualization of soft tissues and not as good for viewing bone, which has very little water. The images produced show strong signal intensity (white area) for soft tissue with many water molecules and show a weak signal (black area) where there are few water molecules. This is the exact opposite of radiation-generated images, in which bone is white (radiopaque) and soft tissue is black (radiolucent).

Presently, the main application of MRI in dentistry has been in imaging the articular fibrous disc of the TMJ and other soft tissue lesions (Fig. 16.12).

Nuclear Medicine

Nuclear medicine (radionuclide scanning, bone scanning) is a diagnostic radiation procedure using radioactive compounds that have an affinity for particular tissues (target

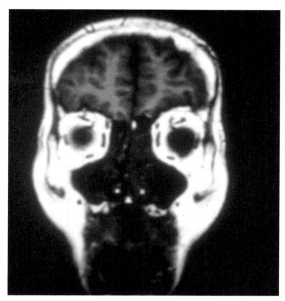

• **Figure 16.12** Magnetic resonance image (MRI) of the temporomandibular joint (TMJ). Locate and identify the condyle, articular disc, and the muscles.

tissues). These organ-specific compounds are injected into the patient, where they concentrate in the target tissue and are detected and imaged by a sensor called a gamma camera. In this manner, both the form and function of the target tissue can be studied. The injectable radiopharmaceutical material consists of an organic substance specific for a given tissue or structure and a nonspecific radionuclide (label). The image is recorded by a gamma camera, which detects the release of gamma rays in a given location and during a given period of time. The image is displayed on a cathode ray tube or stored in a computer. Radionuclide scanning is useful for examining bone and salivary gland tissue, as well as for investigating metabolic bone disorders, infection, and bone fractures.

Chapter Summary

- CT scanning is used in dentistry to produce enhanced images that makes interpretation easier and more accurate. The advantages of CT scanning include the elimination of superimposed images, the ability to reformat images on other planes, and the option of adjusting the density and contrast of the CT image. The disadvantages of CT scanning include an increase in radiation dose, a considerable cost to the patient, and significant artifacts caused by metallic objects in the patient's oral cavity.

- CBCT imaging is a type of CT scanning specifically used in dentistry to produce 3D images that provides the dental professional with a dimensionally accurate view of the desired area.
- MRI is used in dentistry to evaluate the fibrous articular disc of the TMJ. The images produced are more useful for soft tissue evaluation than for hard tissue evaluation.
- Nuclear medicine or radionuclide scanning is useful for examining salivary gland tissue and bony structures in dental imaging.

Chapter Review Questions

Multiple Choice

1. MRI is an effective means of visualizing:
   a. Bony structures
   b. Soft tissue
   c. Metallic objects
   d. Amalgam restorations
   e. The mandibular condyle
2. A diagnostic radiation procedure that uses radioactive compounds is known as:
   a. CBCT imaging
   b. MRI imaging
   c. CT scanning
   d. PET scanning
   e. Nuclear medicine
3. The plane that divides the body into superior and inferior regions is known as the:
   a. Coronal plane
   b. Cross-sectional plane
   c. Axial plane
   d. Sagittal plane
   e. Frontal plane
4. The 3D raw data produced when a CBCT image is taken and reconstructed is known as:
   a. The FOV
   b. Spatial resolution
   c. Contrast resolution
   d. A DICOM image
   e. A voxel
5. CBCT images can be used in dentistry:
   a. To evaluate lesions and abnormalities
   b. For implant planning
   c. To evaluate areas of trauma
   d. For endodontic assessment
   e. All of the above

Critical Thinking Exercise

1. A patient in your dental facility is referred for a CBCT to be utilized in the treatment plan for an implant procedure. Your task is to educate the patient about the CBCT particular to the patient's treatment plan. Be sure to include the following in your information session:
   a. What is CBCT imaging?
   b. What is the advantage of a CBCT procedure when compared to a medical CT scan?
   c. What is the procedure for acquiring a CBCT image?
   d. Other than implant planning, what other dental applications can CBCT images be used for?
   e. Is the radiation dose from a CBCT procedure harmful to the patient?
   f. What is meant by the term *3D imaging?*
2. A patient in your office is referred to a facial pain specialist for an MRI depicting the fibrous articular disc of the TMJ. You are presented with the task of educating the patient about an MRI and why it is prescribed for TMJ evaluation. Be sure to include the following in your informative session:
   a. Does an MRI use x-radiation as the source of energy for image production?
   b. Why is the MRI unit referred to as *a large magnet?*
   c. Why is it recommended that all metal objects be removed from the area when an MRI is being taken?
   d. What does the "magnet" do to the human body?
   e. What happens during an MRI procedure, and why is there a loud banging noise heard during the procedure?
   f. Why is an MRI used to view soft tissue rather than bony structures?
   g. Which structures are represented as "white" images on an MRI and which are "black?" How does this visualization differ from images produced by x-radiation?

Bibliography

Brooks SL: Computed tomography, *Dent Clin North Am* 37:575–590, 1993.

Iannucci JM, Howerton LJ: *Dental radiography: Principles and techniques,* ed 5, St Louis, MO, 2016, Elsevier Saunders.

White SC, Pharoah MJ: *Oral radiology: Principles and interpretation,* ed 7, St Louis, MO, 2013, Mosby.

Winter AA, Pollack AS, Frommer HH, et al: Cone beam volumetric tomography vs. medical CT scanners, *NY State Dent J* 71:28–33, 2005.

17

Quality Assurance

EDUCATIONAL OBJECTIVES

Upon completing this chapter, the student will be able to:

1. Define the key terms listed at the beginning of the chapter.
2. Discuss the following related to chairside technique:
   - State the significance of ensuring that all personnel are trained properly and monitored regularly in exhibiting high levels of chairside competence.
   - List the responsibilities that the supportive staff is responsible for in maintaining a sound dental radiographic quality-assurance (QA) program as recommended by the American Academy of Oral and Maxillofacial Radiology (AAOMR).
3. Discuss the following related to conventional radiography quality assurance, processing maintenance, and film maintenance:
   - Describe the QA constituents of monitoring and maintaining the x-ray units in a dental office.
   - Discuss the steps that the dental professional should take in assuring that the processing techniques,

   equipment, and darkroom are optimally monitored and maintained.
   - Explain the proper storage for dental radiographic film and the importance of checking the expiration date for a box of film.
4. Discuss the following related to extraoral radiography, lead contamination, and digital sensor maintenance:
   - Describe the steps in assuring the proper maintenance of the cassettes and intensifying screens that are used for extraoral radiography.
   - Know the main sources of lead used in dental radiography and the steps in preventing the harmful effects of this substance.
   - Discuss the steps in maintaining the integrity of the digital sensors used in dental imaging.

KEY TERMS

American Academy of Oral and
   Maxillofacial Radiology (AAOMR)
calibration procedure
Certified Radiation Equipment Safety
   Officer (CRESO)

darkroom maintenance
intra-office peer review
normalizing device
quality-assurance (QA) program
record keeping

reference film
step wedge

Introduction

One of the most important protocols in a dental office is a quality-assurance (QA) program. QA is a plan of action, concern, and responsibility to ensure that the x-ray images obtained in a dental office are of the highest quality, with minimal exposure to patients and dental personnel and resulting in the maximum diagnostic yield. An effective QA policy and administrative protocol that monitors the use of radiation in a dental office is the shared responsibility of all members of the dental team. QA programs fall into the following categories: chairside technique, monitoring of conventional and digital x-ray equipment, and darkroom equipment and procedures.

Chairside Technique

Maintaining high levels of chairside competence is the basis of any successful QA program. Using programs of self-evaluation, intra-office peer review, and continuing education, superior levels of chairside technique can be attained and retained, thus keeping retakes to a minimum. One should remember that every retake that is needed doubles the radiation to the patient for that image. The ultimate goal in dental radiography is to produce the most diagnostic radiographs with the least amount of radiation exposure to the patient. The criteria for radiographs given in Chapter 9 should be followed at all times. The task of reviewing radiographs can be assigned to any member of the office staff. The ability to accept criticism and perform self-criticism is an essential trait that must be developed. Each member of the dental team should ask for help and supervision instead of constantly repeating the same error. If a dental professional does not seek self-improvement, eventually a radiograph that is not diagnostic can become inappropriately acceptable. This type of imaging is useless and does the patient a disservice if committed repeatedly.

> **HELPFUL HINT**
>
> The remedy for an exposure error is usually the reverse of the cause. When an image is not diagnostically acceptable, the radiographer is responsible for troubleshooting the cause before retaking the image so that the error is not repeated. As Albert Einstein said, "The definition of insanity is doing the same thing over and over again and expecting different results." Although this behavior may not categorize the operator as actually being insane, it will add to the radiation burden of the patient unnecessarily.

In most dental practices, the supportive staff is most likely to be responsible for certain procedures, which the American Academy of Oral and Maxillofacial Radiology (AAOMR) groups into the following categories:

- Conducting proper chairside technique
- Making sure that all dental x-ray units are maintained properly and functioning optimally
- Properly storing and handling all films, digital sensors, cassettes, screens, grids, and processing chemicals
- Posting current technique charts, including a time-temperature chart for processing, x-ray exposure factors, x-ray equipment measurements, and darkroom maintenance schedules
- Accurate record keeping of films processed, mounted, and filed
- Maintaining proper conditions of processing tanks and automatic processors
- Maintaining optimal darkroom conditions by periodic checks for light-tightness and adequacy of safelighting, cleanliness procedures, and temperature control of solutions
- Maintaining the conditions of protective devices, such as lead aprons, thyroid collars, barriers, and receptor-holding devices

Also, it is the responsibility of the dental team to enforce the office infection control policy, because it concerns chairside technique and film processing.

Dental X-Ray Machine Maintenance

X-ray machines must be monitored and inspected on a regular basis. There are state and local agencies that provide inspection services as a component of their licensing and registration processes. Dental x-ray machines should be adjusted for accuracy at regular intervals. This action is referred to as a calibration procedure. X-ray machine calibration is performed by a competent technician to confirm that the radiographic equipment is functioning properly in producing consistently diagnostically acceptable radiographic images. The AAOMR has published an outline of preventive procedures for radiographic systems. In some areas, a health physicist or a Certified Radiation Equipment Safety Officer (CRESO) would perform the inspection. The type of inspection and calibration included in this group are checks on kilovoltage, milliamperage, output, timer accuracy, tube head stability, and x-ray beam alignment (Fig. 17.1).

The dental professional is responsible for maintaining the x-ray equipment and should report any equipment malfunctions, including tube head drift, head leakage, timing issues, and images that consistently do not meet diagnostically acceptable standards as a result of problems with the x-ray equipment.

Conventional Radiography Quality Assurance
Processing Technique

An effective QA policy for processing films and the dark-room is the shared responsibility of all dental professionals in the facility. Regardless of whether manual or automatic processing is used, a QA program in the darkroom is as important as and much easier to conduct than monitoring of the x-ray machine. First, for a darkroom QA program to be effective, the darkroom must be a darkroom and nothing else. The room should be a dedicated space rather than a place for general storage or for use as a dental laboratory.

At least monthly, and depending on the workload, the dental professional should check the safelighting, light-tightness, and accuracy of the timer and thermometer in the darkroom. If the processing tank lid is missing or the thermometer is broken, it should be noted and ordered. Charts showing when the various QA procedures were performed and by whom should be on the wall or in a dark-room logbook (Fig. 17.2). The dental professional should monitor the cleanliness of the countertops, the condition of the film hangers and clips, and the level and strength of the processing solutions.

As mentioned in Chapter 11, the test used to confirm the reliability of the safelight is known as the "coin test." This test is used to ensure that the safelight is acceptable for processing conventional film without exposing the film to unacceptable lightning, resulting in fogging or darkening of the radiographic image.

The chemical strength and level of solutions in both manual tanks and automatic processors must be monitored on a daily basis. This is the most critical part of a QA program. Processing solutions should be changed every 2 to 3 weeks depending on usage. Both manual tanks and automatic processors should be cleaned at least weekly depending on the workload of the office staff. There are better ways to determine when solutions should be changed than by just using the calendar or "eyeballing."

An easy way to obtain a rough estimate of solution strength in a dental office is to compare it with a standard or reference film (Fig. 17.3). A processed periapical film

NEW YORK UNIVERSITY COLLEGE OF DENTISTRY

RADIOLOGY QUALITY-ASSURANCE PROGRAM

Type of Unit: _____

Location: _____

kVp: _____

mA: _____

HVL: _____ mm of Al

FFD: _____ in

Average Exposure Time (F-speed film) _____ impulses

Output (Emission Rate) _____ mR/s

Calibration Date _____ Performed By: _____

EXPOSURES WITH EKTASPEED FILMS

Maxillary Anteriors   _____   Mandibular Anteriors   _____

Maxillary Premolars   _____   Mandibular Premolars   _____

Maxillary Molars   _____   Mandibular Molars   _____

Bitewings _____
Occlusals _____

Calculation of Facial Dose: Add up all exposure times
Divide by 60
Multiply by Emission Rate

DO NOT REMOVE THIS NOTICE

• **Figure 17.1** Form used to monitor dental x-ray machines.

of ideal density should be kept taped to the darkroom viewbox for comparison of densities of the films that are processed daily. A lessening of film density in the processed film indicates a weakened solution and signals the need for a solution change. Do not wait until the films lose their diagnostic usefulness to change the processing solutions. A better and more scientifically controlled way to make a test exposure is to use a step wedge at the beginning of each work day. This test exposure is done with a step wedge or a predetermined density (Fig. 17.4). The film is then processed and compared with standard film densities. With the normalizing device shown in Fig. 17.5, the processed film is placed in a slot, and the measured densities are moved until a visual match of densities is achieved. If the test densities are too light, the solutions are too weak or too cold. If the densities are too dark, the solutions are too concentrated or too warm. Either of these situations is unacceptable, and processing cannot begin until conditions are optimized. The strength of the fixer can also be gauged by noting the time needed to clear films. Fresh, full-strength fixer clears films in 2 to 3 minutes. If clearing requires more than 4 minutes, the fixing solution is weak and should be changed. It follows that usually developer and fixer solutions will require changing or replenishing at the same time.

Quality Control
Radiographic Processing Solution

Location _____   Month/Year _____

R = Replenished
CH = Changed Solution

Week Of	Monday	Tuesday	Wednesday	Thursday	Friday
	Maintenance	Maintenance	Maintenance	Maintenance	Maintenance
	Done by:	Done by:	Done by:	Done by:	Done by:
	Maintenance	Maintenance	Maintenance	Maintenance	Maintenance
	Done by:	Done by:	Done by:	Done by:	Done by:
	Maintenance	Maintenance	Maintenance	Maintenance	Maintenance
	Done by:	Done by:	Done by:	Done by:	Done by:
	Maintenance	Maintenance	Maintenance	Maintenance	Maintenance
	Done by:	Done by:	Done by:	Done by:	Done by:

• **Figure 17.2** Chart used to monitor processing solutions in the darkroom.

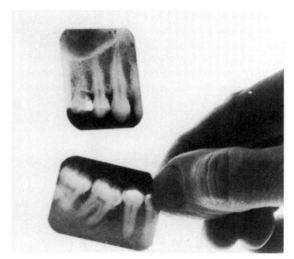

• **Figure 17.3** Reference film used to check solution strength by comparing densities.

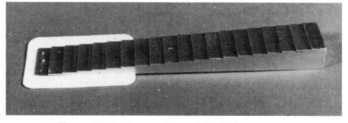

• **Figure 17.4** Step wedge and film before exposure.

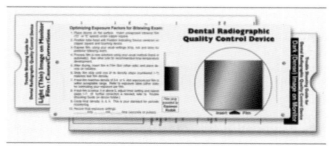

• **Figure 17.5** Dental radiographic quality control device. The radiograph is exposed under the copper and processed as usual. The resulting radiograph is inserted into the device and compared to the 7-density film strip. If it is too light or too dark, possible causes and corrections are indicated. (Courtesy Xray Quality Control, Vail, CO.)

Film Maintenance

Unexposed and unprocessed films, as well as solutions, should be stored in a cool, dry location. They never should be stored in an unventilated room near the heating system. Films should be stored at temperatures of 50° F to 70° F and between 40% and 60% relative humidity. Films should be used before their expiration date, and film boxes should be clearly marked. Older boxes should be placed on the front of the shelf in keeping with the "longest in, first out" rule.

Extraoral Radiography

The screens and cassettes that are used to produce diagnostic images in extraoral radiography should be checked and maintained on a regular schedule. The intensifying screens inside the extraoral cassettes should be cleaned with appropriate manufacturers' suggested solutions at least once a month. After cleaning the intensifying screens, the dental staff member responsible for maintaining them should apply an antistatic solution to the screens. If an intensifying screen is scratched, it must be replaced, because scratches and dirt on the screens cause unacceptable artifacts on the resultant radiographic images.

Lead Contamination

Lead contamination has been determined as being hazardous to humans and to the environment. One of the potential sources of lead exposure in the dental office that is not currently as common as it was in the past is the use of lead-lined boxes for film storage. Unexposed film was previously kept in the operatory in lead-lined boxes. Over time, the lead used to line the shielded boxes may oxidize and produce a white lead powder that may contaminate the stored intraoral film. This powder is about 80% lead and may be ingested by patients and operators. Fortunately, most dental offices currently store film out of the operatory or use stable metal dispensers. It is also important that all dental personnel appropriately dispose of the lead foil that is removed from the film packet in the dental office and that the proper agency confiscates it from the office.

Digital Radiography Quality Assurance

Digital Sensor Maintenance

The digital sensors used with direct and indirect digital radiography must be handled with proper care and maintained in optimum condition. These efforts ensure that they provide reliable service and adhere to infection control regulations.

The sensors used with direct digital radiography should be wiped with a disinfectant along with the sensor cable and then the sensor should also be covered with barrier sheaths before use to prevent sensor contamination. The sensor cable is carefully uncoiled, and the operator is expected to remove all tangles and sharp bends from the cable. The operator is encouraged not to soak the sensor in sterile solution or place it in an autoclave. The sensor or cable should not be clamped with a hemostat. The dental professional should avoid stepping on or rolling over the cable with the operator chair. The sensor cable is to be gently coiled and placed in a protective case after use. The phosphor plates used with indirect digital radiography should also be covered with an infection-control barrier before use. They are also not to be submerged in cold sterilizing solutions or autoclaved. All sensors are to be handled very carefully, and all effort should be made to maintain them in optimum condition to withstand years of successful daily use.

Chapter Summary

- A QA program is a plan of action, concern, and responsibility to ensure that the x-ray images obtained in a dental office are of the highest quality, with minimal exposure to the patients and dental personnel, which consequently results in the maximum diagnostic yield.
- A QA program is instituted in a dental facility to make certain that all equipment is functioning optimally, including the constituents of radiographic processing,
exposure, digital radiography, and that the elimination of hazardous material (lead) is addressed accordingly.
- The AAOMR suggests that a well-designed QA protocol in a dental office should include regular monitoring and testing of a dental facility's chairside techniques, x-ray units, films, digital sensors, cassettes, intensifying screens, grids, processing equipment, and processing chemicals.

Chapter Review Questions

Multiple Choice

1. A plan of action, concern, and responsibility to ensure that radiographic images used in dentistry for diagnosis and treatment are of the optimum quality is known as:
   a. A reference film
   b. A normalizing device
   c. A QA program
   d. Universal precautions
   e. The ALARA principle

2. Which of the following steps should be taken when ensuring the proper care and maintenance of digital sensors?
   a. The sensors should not be autoclaved.
   b. The sensors should be covered with a barrier sheath.
   c. The sensors cabled should not be stepped on.
   d. The sensor cable should be carefully uncoiled.
   e. All of the above.

3. _____ contamination has been determined as being hazardous to humans and to the environment.
   a. Phosphor
   b. Metallic
   c. Lead
   d. Processing solution
   e. Step wedge
4. After intensifying screens are thoroughly cleaned with the appropriate solution, they should be treated with:
   a. A solution containing alcohol
   b. An anti-contaminant
   c. An anti-radioactive solution
   d. An antistatic solution
   e. A soluble solution
5. A better and more scientifically controlled way to ensure the strength of the processing solutions is to:
   a. Use a step wedge at the beginning of each work day
   b. Add a replenishing solution
   c. Test the half-value layer (HVL)
   d. Empty the solutions every day
   e. Clean the processor roller daily

Critical Thinking Exercise

1. You have recently been designated as the QA manager in your dental facility. Your specific responsibilities are to make sure that the x-ray units and processing equipment are functioning properly. Discuss the steps you would take in accomplishing this assignment. Be sure to include the following in your discussion:
   a. A description of your plans to enlist a health physicist or a CRESO to perform the necessary calibration procedures and what they will specifically be checking for.
   b. A list of the equipment malfunctions that should be reported to the dental office manager.
   c. A schedule for checking the safelighting, light-tightness, and accuracy of the timer and thermometer in the darkroom.
   d. The test for confirming the reliability of the safelight in the darkroom.
   e. Three ways for checking the strength of the processing solutions.

Bibliography

American Dental Association Council on Scientific Affairs: An update on radiographic practices: information and recommendations, *J Am Dent Assoc* 132:234–238, 2001.

Eastman Kodak Co: *Quality assurance in dental radiography*, Rochester, NY, 1999, Health Science Division.

Iannucci JM, Howerton LJ: *Dental radiography: Principles and techniques*, ed 5, St Louis, MO, 2016, Elsevier Saunders.

Recommendations for quality assurance in dental radiography, *Oral Surg Oral Med Oral Pathol* 55:421–426, 1983.

18

Patient Management and Special Problems

EDUCATIONAL OBJECTIVES

Upon completing this chapter, the student will be able to:

1. Define the key terms listed at the beginning of the chapter.
2. Describe the general management techniques that a dental radiographer can employ while taking radiographs on patients.
3. Discuss the following related to treating patients with disabilities and special needs:
    • List the steps that the dental professional can take in treating a patient with mobility issues, including those who are wheelchair bound, in the hospital, homebound, bedridden, or in long-term care facilities.
    • Discuss some of the common developmental disabilities that dental professionals may encounter in the dental office and what technique adjustments are required in order to treat these patients.

• Discuss the modifications necessary when exposing radiographs on patients that are hearing or vision impaired.
4. Describe the techniques that are useful for managing pediatric patients in dental radiography.
5. List the areas in the oral cavity that can trigger the gag reflex and the various management techniques used to help the hypersensitive patient control this body defense mechanism.
6. List the localization techniques used in dental radiography and describe the clinical application for each technique.
7. Discuss the remedies that can be utilized when attempting to radiograph third molars; teeth undergoing endodontic treatment; and patients with anatomic constraints, such as tori, trismus, a narrow arch, or a shallow palate.

KEY TERMS

arthrography	hearing impaired	sialography
bedridden	localization	SLOB
buccal-object rule	marking grid	trismus
Clark's rule	physical disability	tube shift
developmental disability	radiopaque media	visually impaired
disability	radiopaque medium	wheelchair access
gag reflex	reverse bitewing	

Introduction

Patient management is important to all dental personnel involved with patient care in a dental facility. Patient understanding and consideration is a valuable tool in helping dental professionals perform their chairside duties. The dental team may be responsible for other patient management assignments, such as scheduling appointments, handling and screening telephone calls, and collecting fees. These duties also demand the use of understanding and empathy to manage patients successfully.

The dental professional encounters all types of personalities in the dental office. Some patients may be very apprehensive and tense about dental treatment, whereas others

are calm and cooperate easily. Some reveal their anxieties through behavioral and speech patterns; others may hide their anxieties.

Even with modern equipment, techniques, and attitudes, dentistry remains a stressful experience for some patients. As a profession, dentistry is still plagued by the image of the unpleasant experience. It is within this societal context that dental professionals must endeavor to serve patients. With the modern technologies available and an emphasis on behavior, this goal can be met.

Furthermore, dental radiographers must be able to alter their skills to fit the needs of the individual patient. This chapter introduces various ways of managing patients with a variety of specific needs including, but not limited to, patients with disabilities, pediatric patients, patients with a sensitive gag reflex, and patients with anatomic constraints that require an alternate method of receptor placement.

Management

One of the important roles of the dental professional is to try to relax the patient, which makes the work easier. The dental hygienist or assistant may be the first member of the office staff to greet the patient in the reception area. Patients like to be recognized and greeted by name. However, to conform to federal legislation (Health Insurance Portability and Accountability Act [HIPAA]) patients should not be addressed by their last names to ensure privacy (see Chapter 25). It is especially important to greet new or current patients with an appropriate phrase, such as, "We shall be with you shortly." "We" implies the team concept of treatment and stresses the importance of all of the constituents in the office, indicating that the whole dental team will take part in the active treatment.

In performing dental radiography, the dental professional also must develop an acceptable and respectful chairside manner. Patients must be made to feel comfortable and confident about the dental professional's ability to perform the radiographic examination.

In some dental offices, it is routine for any of the dental professionals to perform the radiographic procedures. As discussed in the preceding chapter, dental professionals should strive for a high level of clinical proficiency with efficient and confident work patterns. The dental professional can achieve these objectives through experience and honest self-evaluation and peer evaluation. The quality of the finished radiograph should be the same regardless of who performs the procedure. All members of the dental team should be held to the same standard of quality control.

When the dental professional is seating patients and draping them with the lead apron, some small talk may help to relax them. Patients want to know that the dental professional is interested in them and not just performing a mechanical procedure. This is not wasted time, because a relaxed, confident patient is much easier to work with.

Appearance is very important. All infection-control protocols must be followed. Hands should be washed; gloves, masks, protective eyewear, and protective clothing worn; and the prescribed infection-control procedures followed after the patient is seated in the dental chair so that the patient can take note of these procedures. If one sneezes, coughs, picks up something from the floor, or has to leave the treatment room, re-gloving is mandatory before resuming work.

The dental professional should always explain to the patient what procedures are to be performed and how many projections will be taken. Any questions that the patient has should be answered if the dental professional feels capable of doing so. If the question involves diagnostic judgments

or treatment planning that cannot be answered with confidence, it should be referred to the appropriate member of the dental team. Patients often ask about the need for radiographs and the potential radiation risk. Because these questions are usually asked before work begins, a well-answered question will give the patient confidence and lessen apprehension about having the radiographs taken. Answers to questions of this type are found in this text; the fears and concerns of the patient can be allayed by intelligent, meaningful answers.

Receptors must be placed in the patient's mouth, and directions must be given to the patient in a manner that indicates self-confidence. A patient likes to feel that the operator is in full control of the situation at all times. Instructions to the patient should be given in a firm but polite tone. In addition, dental professionals should encourage and praise patients for their cooperation in an effort to gain their confidence and mutual respect. Every patient is different, both in the anatomic configuration of the mouth and in physical and psychological makeup. This is the challenge of the profession—to perform one's duties and maintain standards of excellence even as the clinical situation changes. Through study, practice, and self-evaluation, these goals can be met.

Patients with Disabilities and Special Needs

A disability can be defined as a physical or mental condition that limits a person's movements, senses, or activities. These impairments often restrict the afflicted person's life activities. In the dental environment, it is imperative that all persons are treated equally and with the same level of respect. The dental professional should be able to modify radiographic techniques to meet the needs of each individual patient.

Physical Disability

The obstacles in treating patients with physical challenges in the dental office vary according to the degree of their disability. A physical disability may include problems with mobility, hearing, or vision. .

Mobility

With a patient confined to a wheelchair, it may be easier to radiograph in the wheelchair than to transfer the patient to the dental chair, as long as the procedure can be successfully accomplished with the patient's head positioned and supported properly. When transferring the patient, radiographers might ask patients how they would like to be transferred, and they may also assist the accompanying caregivers (if present) in transferring patients to the dental chair. Most local building codes require wheelchair access to the dental operatory so that the x-ray machine and patient can be maneuvered into the proper relationship.

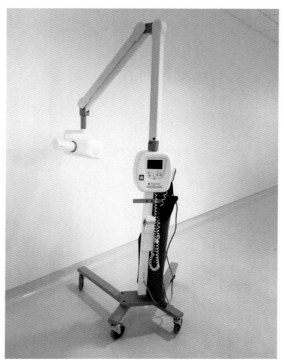

• **Figure 18.1** Portable dental x-ray unit. (From Bird DL, Robinson DS: *Modern Dental Assisting,* ed 12, St Louis, 2018, Elsevier.)

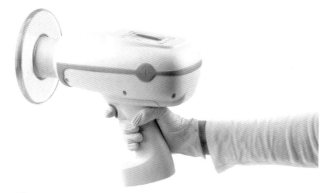

• **Figure 18.2** NOMAD Pro 2 handheld x-ray unit. (Courtesy Aribex, Charlotte, NC.)

Also, panoramic and other extraoral equipment have been manufactured to accommodate a patient in a wheelchair, allowing these projections to be useful with this type of patient.

Some homebound patients or those bedridden in hospitals and long-term care facilities may not be able to visit dental suites; their dental procedures and radiographs must be done at the bedside. In the past, mobile dental x-ray units could be brought to the bed and radiographs taken. For the patient in the supine position, it is easier to use a receptor-holding device with a localizing ring. In treating a patient at home or at a site that does not have a dental x-ray unit, portable x-ray units can be adapted for dental use and assembled on site (Fig. 18.1). If digital radiography is not available, then a small, portable, rapid-processing tank also should be brought along so that the radiographs can be processed and the patient treated during the same visit.

With the more recent introduction of the handheld portable dental x-ray machine, it is now possible to produce quality images and have the ability to utilize the unit outside of the dental facility in locations such as remote outreach sites, long-term care facilities, and hospitals. These units are lightweight and battery powered. The most popular of these systems are the Nomad models (Fig. 18.2). With this system, the receptor (film or sensor) is positioned in the patient's mouth while the exposure is made. The operator, while holding the device at chairside, directs it at the receptor in the patient's mouth and exposes it. The use of this device has raised the question of increased radiation exposure to both the patient and the operator in the past.

However, these Nomad units have recently been approved for dental use by the U.S. Food and Drug Administration. According to the manufacturers of the Nomad units, these handheld devices have a shield that potentially protects the patient and operator from unnecessary x-ray exposure.

Developmental Disability

Patients who are mentally disabled or have other physical conditions, such as cerebral palsy or autism, and are afflicted before the age of 22 (developmental disability) may present a management challenge in a dental facility. Unless there is complete cooperation while exposing dental images, the patient may move and render the radiographs useless. The degree of cooperation varies among patients. Problem situations should be recognized immediately. Repeated attempts may only excite the patient, subject the patient to unnecessary radiation, and prove fruitless. The dental professional should elicit the help of the patient's caregiver when applicable in obtaining diagnostic radiographs. The dental professional may also opt to take a panoramic or another extraoral projection as opposed to intraoral radiographs that require more tolerance and cooperation.

For a totally unmanageable patient or one with an extreme physical disability, radiographs may have to be taken with the patient under sedation or general anesthesia. These films are usually developed immediately or digital radiography is used, and the necessary dental procedures are performed while the patient is still anesthetized.

Hearing Impairment

The obvious challenge in treating hearing impaired or deaf patients is communication, as well as realization by the operator of the disability and how it may modify usual procedures. For example, the often-used command to the patient to "hold still" as the operator leaves the room to make an exposure is not applicable for patients with a hearing impairment. Depending on the patient's method of communication, instructions may have to be given through a translator, sign language, or in writing. Deaf patients can usually read lips, therefore, operators must be sure to remove their mask and always face the patients when speaking to them.

Vision Impairment

Visually impaired patients may have to be escorted into the operatory and directed or assisted into the dental chair. Because these patients cannot see what is going on, it is essential that the patient be kept informed of the treatment being rendered and why it is necessary. Patient education is extremely important. The dental professional must remember that the patient may have never seen a radiograph; thus, the explanation may require extra time and thought. An awareness of the disability is ultimately needed to treat visually impaired patients.

Pediatric Patients

The number and timing of radiographs for pediatric patients is discussed in Chapter 9 of this textbook. Dental radiography requires the complete cooperation of the patient. If the patient moves, the radiographic image is blurred and the image is rendered useless. In radiography, the patient must hold still while the exposure is made. The unknown is frightening to any child, and very few children know anything about x-rays. In fact, the dental radiograph may be their first introduction to radiography. The procedure must be explained to the child in terms that the child can easily understand. For example, the radiographer should talk of taking a "picture" of the tooth with a "camera" as opposed to using the terms "x-ray" and "radiography" to explain the procedure. Remind children that they must hold still when the picture is taken. Show children the film packet or digital sensor and possibly let them put it in their own mouths.

Children like to see pictures; it is sometimes helpful to show them what a radiograph of a tooth looks like. The dental professional should follow up with a promise to show them what their teeth look like on the finished radiograph. In certain instances, children have even been taken into the darkroom and allowed to help process the films. Children are fascinated by the darkroom with its tanks, automatic processing machines, and chemicals. Any effort expended to relax children and make them feel at ease will reap benefits at later appointments. If there is lack of cooperation and there is no emergency that requires immediate treatment, radiographs may be postponed to a second visit, in which the children may be more cooperative as they get to feel more at home in the dental office.

Children usually tolerate periapical receptors; the receptor can be held in place with a bite block or any receptor-holding device to perform either the paralleling or bisecting technique. It is advised to use a #0- or #1-sized receptor as opposed to the #2 adult-sized receptor with pediatric patients.

In children, it is acceptable to use the bisecting technique. If the child resists periapical receptor placement, have the patient close down on the receptor and increase

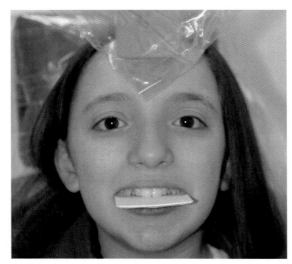

• **Figure 18.3** Technique for periapical projections that allows a child to bite on receptor. Note the increase in vertical angulation.

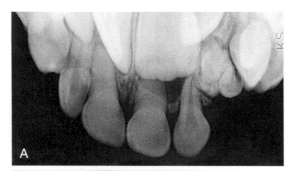

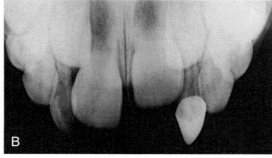

• **Figure 18.4** Radiographs taken by having the child bite the receptor. **A,** Adult-sized periapical receptor (note odontoma blocking tooth eruption). **B,** Occlusal image.

the vertical angulation to bisect the angle so that the procedure resembles an occlusal projection (Fig. 18.3). This type of projection is not as desirable as that obtained by the regular technique, but it is better than no image at all. This method will work for any area of the child's mouth, and a full-mouth series can be taken this way if necessary. Either an adult-sized or an occlusal receptor can be used for this technique (Fig. 18.4).

Reverse Bitewings

Some children have difficulty tolerating placement of the bitewing projection. When instructed to close on the tab,

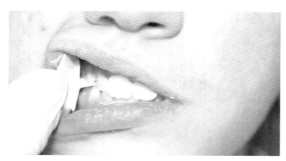

• **Figure 18.5** Receptor placement for a reverse bitewing radiograph.

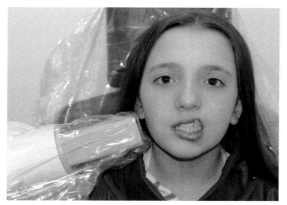

• **Figure 18.6** Tube position for reverse bitewing radiograph. Note that the central ray is directed from underneath the mandible of the opposite side while being aimed at the bitewing receptor.

NOTE

When the digital radiographic technique is used in a dental facility, it is advised to use the photostimulable phosphor (PSP) plate sensors rather than the direct digital sensors (charge-coupled device [CCD] or complementary metal oxide semiconductor [CMOS]) with pediatric patients. The PSP sensors are thinner and more flexible than the CCD or CMOS sensors and are easier placed and better tolerated in the small mouths of pediatric patients.

---

they push the lower part of the receptor out of the floor of the mouth with their tongue and then close their teeth on the receptor. If after repeated attempts proper placement meets with failure, a reverse bitewing technique can be substituted. In this method, the receptor is placed on the cheek side of the teeth in the buccal sulcus (Fig. 18.5). The child bites on the tab to hold the receptor in place, and the radiographer can position the receptor as the patient closes without the hazard of being bitten. The x-ray beam is directed extraorally from under the opposite side of the mandible as in a lateral oblique projection (Fig. 18.6). The resulting image will not have the detail of an intraoral bitewing radiograph but will be a useful substitute (Fig. 18.7).

If intraoral receptor placement is not possible for the child, an extraoral projection can be substituted. The view that is most diagnostic is also a slight variation of the lateral oblique technique. The cassette is positioned in the usual

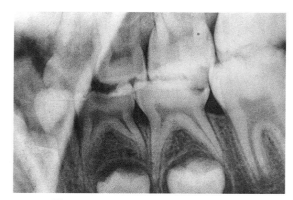

• **Figure 18.7** Reverse bitewing radiograph.

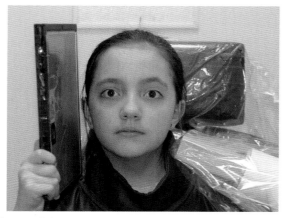

• **Figure 18.8** Lateral oblique technique for detecting caries and pathologic conditions in children. Note that the central ray is aimed from behind the angle of the mandible on the opposite side.

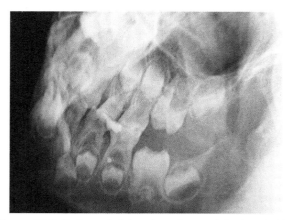

• **Figure 18.9** Radiograph taken through use of the lateral oblique technique.

way, but the central ray is directed from behind the angle of the mandible on the opposite side (Fig. 18.8). Again, the radiograph is not as diagnostic as an intraoral image but is better than none (Fig. 18.9).

If there is no extraoral cassette in the office, an occlusal receptor can be substituted but with the resulting increase of radiation exposure to the patient (Fig. 18.10). The radiograph produced will be of some diagnostic value

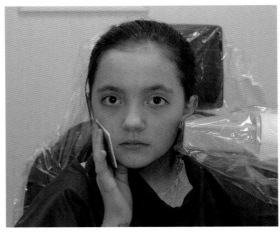

• **Figure 18.10** Occlusal receptor used as an extraoral receptor.

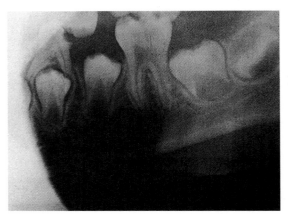

• **Figure 18.11** Radiograph produced by using an occlusal receptor extraorally.

(Fig. 18.11). Box 18.1 provides tips to help a dental professional take radiographs of a pediatric patient.

Special Problems

Gagging

Of all the problems one may encounter in intraoral radiography, gagging is probably the most troublesome. Gagging, more properly referred to as the **gag reflex**, is a body defense mechanism. The coughing and retching produced in the gag reflex are meant to expel any foreign body from the throat and thus protect the airway from obstruction. All patients have gag reflexes, with some more active and more hypersensitive than others.

The two types of stimuli for the gag reflex are psychogenic and tactile. Some patients start to feel the reflex coming on just by thinking about or anticipating the receptor placement. The areas that are most sensitive to tactile stimuli producing the gag reflex are the palate, base of the tongue, and posterior wall of the pharynx. Gagging occurs most often during exposure of the maxillary molar projection. The level of excitation of these reflexes varies from person to person. The patient with a low threshold

---

> • **BOX 18.1** **Helpful Hints for Radiographing the Pediatric Patient**
>
> 1. Be confident. Most children react favorably to the authority of a confident and capable operator. The dental professional must secure the child's confidence, trust, and cooperation. In addition, the dental professional must be patient and not rush through the radiographic procedures.
> 2. Show and tell. The typical pediatric patient is curious. The dental professional can use a "show and tell" approach to prepare the patient for radiographic procedures. Before beginning the procedure, the operator can show the child the equipment and materials that will be used and tell the child what will happen. The child should be encouraged to touch the tube head, receptor holder, and lead apron.
> 3. Reassure the patient. Children usually fear the unknown. The operator should reassure the patient and allay any fears about the procedures to prevent the uncooperative behavior of a frightened child.
> 4. Demonstrate behavior. The operator should demonstrate the desired behavior to show the child exactly what to do. For example, the radiographer can demonstrate "how to hold still" and then ask the child to do the same thing.
> 5. Request assistance. If a child cannot hold still or stabilize the receptor, the dental professional can ask the parent or accompanying adult to provide assistance. The adult can hold the receptor or the child during the exposure while wearing a lead glove, apron, and thyroid collar.
> 6. Postpone the examination. Only in emergencies and under general anesthesia should a child be forced to undergo a radiographic examination. It is much better to postpone the examination until the second or third visit rather than instill a fear of visiting the dental office.

for stimulation of the gag reflex presents more of a problem in intraoral radiography than those who are not quite as hypersensitive.

Very few patients, probably fewer than 0.1%, have a gag reflex so active that intraoral radiography is virtually impossible. The following are a set of generally accepted suggestions and techniques that can be used to prevent gagging and overcome it when it occurs. Not all techniques are applicable, nor will they prove successful with every patient. The dental radiographer must be able to determine which technique best suits the individual patient. It has been shown that the technique, authority, and self-confidence of the operator are major factors in preventing and suppressing gag reflexes during dental radiography.

Attitude

The operator should always maintain the appearance of being well trained and confident when dealing with patients. The patient wants to believe that the operator is so competent that it would be impossible for the receptor to slip and lodge in the throat. Firm positioning of the receptor-holding device with explicit instructions to the patient and proper body language are all necessary.

Think positively: Never mention the possibility of gagging. The worst thing the operator can say to a patient is, "This won't make you gag," or "Do you gag?" The patient may never have thought of gagging until reminded of the possibility.

Film Order and Technique

When taking a radiographic survey, the dental professional should start taking the anterior projections first and working posteriorly. The receptor placement in the maxillary molar area is the one most likely to excite the gag reflex. Once the reflex is excited, the patient may continue to gag even on anterior projections.

It is recommended to start the radiographic sequence as close to the midline as possible even when the radiographic prescription is for four bitewings only. It is advised to start with the premolar bitewings before exposing the molar bitewings.

When placing the receptor in the patient's mouth for maxillary molars and premolars, one should not slide the receptor along the palate. The receptor is placed in the desired position near the lingual surface of the teeth. Then, with one decisive motion, the receptor is brought into contact with the palate.

The exposure time for the desired exposure is always set before the receptor is placed in the patient's mouth. The tube head is positioned on the side of the patient's face that is to be radiographed, with the position-indicating device (PID) at the approximate vertical angulation. The object is to minimize the amount of time that the receptor has to remain in the patient's mouth. Preparations like these can save valuable seconds and lessen the likelihood of the patient gagging. Generally, the longer the receptor stays in the mouth, the greater the likelihood of gagging.

Deep Breathing

It is often helpful to instruct the patient to take deep breaths through the nose as the receptor is placed and remains in a gag-sensitive area, such as the palate. Why this works is debatable, but it may be that breathing through the nose prevents the rush of air across the sensitive tissues of the palate. Another explanation is that it gives the patient something to do and distracts the patient from thinking about gagging. The operator should use a firm tone of voice when instructing the patient to take these deep breaths and also may take some audible deep breaths to encourage the patient to do likewise. It is also advisable to instruct the patient to keep their eyes open during the procedure. This serves as a distraction as well, keeping the patient's mind off gagging.

HELPFUL HINT

It also helps to tell patients to keep their eyes open and not to close them when the receptor is placed and remains in their mouth. Patients who have a hypersensitive gag reflex have a tendency to immediately close their eyes during the radiographic procedure. This does not allow for any distraction and helps to keep the patient's thoughts focused on gagging.

Bite Blocks and Receptor-Holding Devices

Any receptor-holding device that requires the patient to bite and maintain pressure also may help to prevent gagging. Again, the patient is given something positive to do. Another tactile sensation, that of biting and the pressure of the bite block against the teeth, may distract the patient from thoughts of gagging.

Lozenges, Gargles, and Sprays

Lozenges, gargles, and sprays may be of some help in certain situations. The key is to make the patient believe that these over-the-counter antidotes will have an effect. This placebo effect has been seen in many other areas of dental practice.

Many viscous topical anesthetics (e.g., Cetacaine) are available for rinsing the mouth, gargling, or spraying the palate to produce a numbing sensation, intended to block the gag reflex. An undiluted mouthwash with high alcohol concentration may have some anesthetic effects on the palate. Many cough lozenges contain some local anesthetic; having the patient suck on a lozenge before radiography may be helpful. In all these cases, it may not be so much the anesthetic vehicle used as the manner of presentation to the patient that produces the desired results.

Hypnosis

Although the practice of hypnosis is out of the province of the dental professional, its use in dentistry should be mentioned. In intractable gaggers, hypnosis by trained, competent practitioners may be necessary to permit intraoral radiography.

Convincing a patient that something (such as, gagging) may not occur can be considered a form of hypnosis. An application of this principle is to tell gagging patients that the anti-gag nerve located in their neck or the temple is going to be pressed or tapped. There is no anti-gag nerve, and the temple does not control gagging either. However, the patient may not know this. If the area in the neck is pressed hard or the radiographer taps three times on the temple, some sensation will result, and the patient may become convinced that gagging will not occur. The power of suggestion often serves to foster the patient's mind control over the matter at hand. It also helps to tell patients that they could have control over the gag reflex themselves; often, this suggestion causes the patient to gain the control needed to suppress the gag reflex.

Salt

One of the more amusing techniques described in the literature to stop gagging is to place ordinary table salt on the tip of the tongue of the gagging patient. The salt is placed in the palm of the patient's hand; the patient is asked to touch the tip of the tongue to the salt and then raise the tongue to touch the palate. This method may be worth trying at least once in one's professional career.

For the intractable gagger, when all else fails, one must then resort to accessory techniques. Panoramic projections and other extraoral projections, previously discussed,

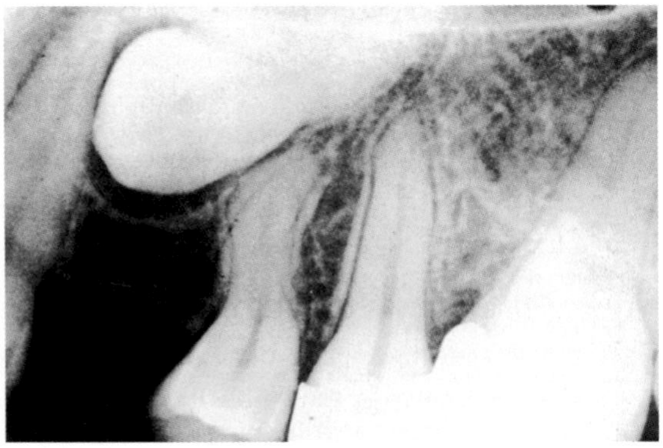

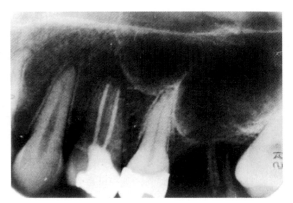

• **Figure 18.12** Impacted maxillary canine. Is the tooth positioned buccally or palatally to the alveolar ridge?

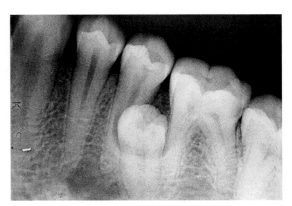

• **Figure 18.14** Localization by definition. Is the impacted supernumerary tooth more clearly defined than the rest of the teeth? If not, it is probably positioned buccally.

• **Figure 18.13** Maxillary first premolar with endodontic filling. Which canal is buccal and which is palatal?

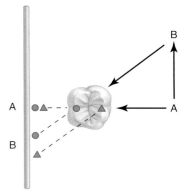

• **Figure 18.15** Buccal-object rule. As the tube position is shifted mesially (position *B*), the buccal object is seen to move relatively in the opposite direction, distally.

because of their extraoral receptor placement circumvent the gag reflex.

Localization Problems

Standard intraoral periapical and bitewing images show the teeth and bone in only two planes: superoinferior and anteroposterior. However, many clinical situations require a proper radiographic diagnosis to establish the position of structures in the buccolingual plane. Clinical examples include localization of impactions, foreign bodies, and areas of pathologic findings, as well as differentiating buccal and palatal roots in endodontic procedures (Figs. 18.12 and 18.13). This information is essential to the dentist before any treatment can be instituted.

The four techniques that can be used for localization are (1) definition evaluation, (2) tube shift, (3) right-angle technique, and (4) pantomography (panoramic radiography).

Definition Evaluation

Structures that lie closer to the receptor have better radiographic definition than those that are farther from the receptor. This is true for both intraoral and extraoral films. It is sometimes possible, depending on the quality of the radiograph, to determine the relative position of superimposed structures by determining which has better radiographic

definition. Because an intraoral receptor is positioned lingually in the patient's mouth, the superimposed structure that is more sharply defined is positioned lingually in relation to the other structures (Fig. 18.14). An advantage of this technique, when compared with the others that follow, is that it requires no further x-ray exposures of the patient. It is, however, the least reliable of the techniques mentioned and is not recommended.

Tube Shift

The **tube shift** method uses what is referred to as **Clark's rule**, or the **buccal-object rule** (Figs. 18.15 and 18.16). Its advantage to the practitioner is that it can be accomplished by using a standard periapical technique. To determine the relative buccolingual relationship between two structures that appear radiographically superimposed, a second radiograph is taken with a different horizontal angulation (or a horizontal tube shift). All factors remain the same for the second exposure, except that the tube is shifted about 20 degrees either mesially or distally. The point of entry, receptor position, and vertical angulation remain the same as in the previous projection. When the two radiographs are compared, the buccal object appears to have moved in the opposite direction from the direction of the tube shift when

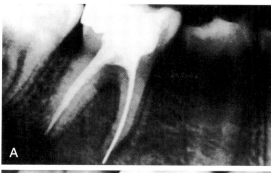

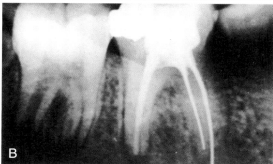

• **Figure 18.16** A and B, Radiographs illustrating the buccal-object rule. The tube in **B** was shifted mesially, indicating that the short endodontic point is in the mesiobuccal canal.

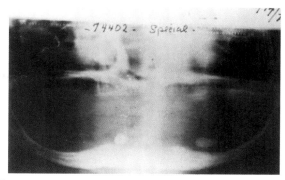

• **Figure 18.17** Localization of an object by a pantomographic redundant image.

compared with other structures on the radiograph (see Figs. 18.15 and 18.16). If the tube is shifted mesially by changing the horizontal angulation, the buccal object appears to have moved distally. Conversely, a distal shift results in the more buccal object moving mesially. Furthermore, if on the second radiograph the object does not appear to move after the tube is shifted horizontally, the object is said to be situated more lingually. This can be demonstrated on the fingers by holding the hand so that the second and third fingers are superimposed when sighting them from the side. Move the head either to the left or to the right (mesially or distally) and imagine the images of the fingers being recorded on the receptor. Two distinct fingers can now be seen and not the fingers superimposed. Now, apply the buccal-object rule. The key phrase is "same lingual, opposite buccal;" the acronym is SLOB. This procedure can also be applied to objects for use in the superior inferior plane.

Right-Angle Technique

The right-angle technique uses two projections taken at right angles to each other—first, a periapical projection and then an occlusal projection of the same area, for example. The planes radiographed are at right angles to each other. The occlusal techniques and examples are discussed in Chapter 10.

Pantomography

The redundant images produced in the anterior region by some older-model pantomographic units, such as the Panorex, can be used to localize objects in repeated areas. In viewing the image, the object in question will be seen

twice (once on each half of the image). A recommended technique is to compare the relative movement of the object with adjacent structures from one side of the image to the other with the direction that the clinician reads the image (e.g., left to right). The object seems to move in the same direction as the clinician's viewing movement if it is lingually positioned and in the opposite direction if it is on the buccal side (Fig. 18.17).

Third Molar Problems

The third molars are in an area of the mouth that is difficult to radiograph. In many cases, it may not be possible to position the receptor intraorally to visualize these areas adequately on radiographs. This is especially true if the teeth are impacted. In these cases, it may be necessary to use the extraoral and panoramic techniques described in Chapters 12 and 13. The entire third molar area must be seen to make a complete diagnosis. This means that the entire tooth and at least 3 mm of surrounding bone in every direction must be imaged. If it cannot be seen on periapical projections, other methods must be used.

Maxilla

As the receptor is placed increasingly more distally toward the patient's throat, the likelihood of exciting the gag reflex increases. It may be helpful to hold the receptor with a hemostat to maintain a minimum of contact with the palate. The receptor should be kept as parallel to the palatal vault as possible. To avoid distortion, the vertical angulation must be increased, with the resulting relationship of the central ray to the receptor looking very much like an occlusal projection.

Mandible

The most common difficulty in radiographing lower third molars is the inability to place the receptor distal enough to record the image of the whole tooth and root structure. This placement is prevented by the muscles of the floor of the mouth and tongue. To overcome this problem, the tongue can be deflected to the opposite side of the mouth by the operator's finger or a mouth mirror. The floor of the mouth is gently depressed, almost massaged, to relax the mylohyoid

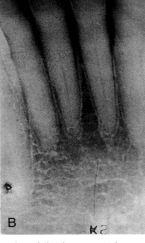

• **Figure 18.18** Periapical radiographs of the lower anterior region using a narrow anterior (#1) receptor seen in **A** and pediatric size (#0) receptor seen in **B**.

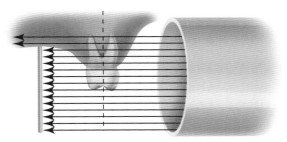

• **Figure 18.19** Problem of receptor placement in paralleling technique with patients who have low palatal vaults. Note that the receptor cannot be placed high enough to record the image of the root apices.

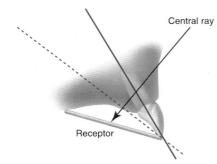

• **Figure 18.20** Vertical angulation overcomes the problem of a low palatal vault in the bisecting-angle technique.

muscle. While this is being done, the receptor is slid along the lingual surface of the mandible as far distally as possible. In certain horizontal impactions of the mandible, it may be necessary to distort the image in the horizontal plane to visualize the entire tooth with intraoral radiography. This is done by changing the horizontal angulation of the x-ray beam so that it is not at right angles to the receptor, which is the usual procedure. Instead, the beam comes from the distal side, and the central ray makes an acute angle with the receptor.

Receptor Placement Problems

Narrow Arch

In some mouths, it may be impossible to place anterior receptors properly without excessive bending, with resultant distortion of the radiographic image. This is a major problem when using direct digital radiography with its rigid sensor. The best way to overcome this problem is to vary the receptor size. The #1 narrow anterior receptor is recommended, although it may be necessary to use #0. There is no rule stating that one cannot use different-sized intraoral receptors in the same full-mouth series. Pediatric or narrow receptors may be used as the situation dictates (Fig. 18.18).

If radiographs show overlapping teeth, especially in the anterior region, it does not necessarily indicate that the images were taken improperly. If the teeth are overlapped in the mouth, they appear overlapped radiographically.

Shallow Palate

The shallow palatal vault presents a problem in the paralleling technique. Fortunately, this does not occur so often and severely that the bony structures make it impossible to place the receptor parallel to the long axis of the tooth and high enough to record the radiographic image (Fig. 18.19). In these rare cases, the bisecting-angle technique may be the better choice. Before changing techniques, one should always check to see that the receptor is in the midline, where

there is the greatest palatal height. The number of times that the paralleling technique cannot be used is quite small.

The bisecting-angle technique compensates for the shallow palate by increasing the vertical angulation. The receptor must be in the patient's mouth with a 3-mm border projecting beneath the incisal or occlusal edge of the teeth and the central ray bisecting the angle formed between the receptor and the long axis of the tooth (Fig. 18.20). As an alternative, the operator may choose to change the receptor size.

Lingual Frenulum

It is extremely difficult to radiograph patients who have a large, tight, lingual frenulum attached close to the tip of the tongue. These patients are sometimes referred to as "tongue-tied," because they cannot protrude their tongues very far out of their mouths.

The paralleling technique is not the method of choice for these patients, because the tight frenulum does not allow placement of the receptor deep in the floor of the mouth. One option is to use the bisecting technique. Because the receptor cannot be placed very deep in the mouth, negative vertical angulations in the range of −40 to −60 degrees can be expected. Another option is to hold the receptor at an angle and, as the patient starts to close and the mylohyoid muscle relaxes, to slowly place the receptor in a more upright, parallel position.

Tori

The maxillary torus (torus palatinus), if present, usually causes no problems in periapical radiography. It is located

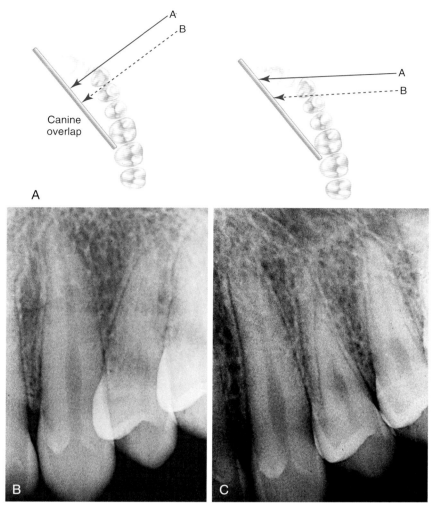

• **Figure 18.21** **A,** Changing horizontal angulation to prevent distal overlap of maxillary canine. **B,** Overlapped canine. **C,** Overlapping eliminated.

posteriorly in the midline of the palate and does not hinder periapical placement. The best way to radiograph a torus palatinus is by use of an occlusal projection.

The mandibular tori—or torus, as the case may be—are located on the lingual aspect of the mandible in the premolar area. Their presence prevents the placement of the receptor in its usual position. This difficulty is more accentuated in the bisecting-angle technique than in the paralleling technique. The receptor cannot be depressed into the floor of the mouth and still be kept close to the lingual surface of the teeth. The only possible solution is to place the receptor over the torus. This increases the angle between the receptor and the long axis of the tooth; increasing the vertical angulation to bisect the angle compensates for the change. In the paralleling method, with its increased object-film distances, the receptor is positioned behind the tori.

Canine Overlap

Overlapping the image of the mesial portion of the maxillary first premolar with the image of the distal surface of the canine is a common problem. The overlapping is caused by the large palatal cusp of the first premolar. The problem can be solved by changing the horizontal angulation so that the central ray comes more from the distal side, as in a premolar periapical projection (Fig. 18.21). Then, the palatal cusp is not superimposed. Overlapping does not occur in the mandible, because the first premolar has a very small lingual cusp.

Trismus

Trismus is the condition in which a patient is unable to open the mouth. It may be partial or complete and is usually caused by infection or trauma. To make an adequate diagnosis and identify the infected tooth or area, radiographs are necessary. If the patient's mouth cannot be opened at all, extraoral or panoramic projections are necessary. If there is partial opening, it may be possible to place an intraoral receptor by modifying the usual technique. A hemostat is used to hold the receptor, because it is much narrower than a receptor-holding device. The receptor is placed in the mouth by sliding it between the partially opened anterior teeth in the horizontal plane. Once beyond the teeth, the receptor can be turned to its proper vertical orientation. If possible, the patient then holds the hemostat with the receptor attached to it in position while the exposure is made.

Endodontic Problems

In patients undergoing endodontic treatment, it is necessary to take working and measurement images while the rubber dam is in place. The bisecting method can be used, with the patient supporting the receptor under the rubber dam with a bite block, but it is not recommended. Using the paralleling method with the dam in place is difficult because of the lack of working space in the mouth and the patient's inability to bite on any receptor-holding device, because of the presence of the rubber dam clamp and protruding endodontic files from the tooth. The best course is to disengage the rubber dam frame, keeping the saliva ejector in place, and position the receptor in a hemostat or "Snap-a-Ray" parallel to the tooth and held by the patient. This is especially true for digital radiography in which the sensor is thicker and more rigid than film. Care should be taken with the sensor-holding device not to damage the fragile sensor. There are also special receptor-holding devices with localizing rings that have an open bite piece to allow for the files and gutta percha to go through that are made specifically for endodontic radiography (Fig. 18.22).

Plastic rubber dam frames and saliva ejectors should be used to prevent superimposition of their images on the radiograph (Fig. 18.23). Punching a hole in a predetermined corner of the dam makes it easier to reorient the dam in the frame once the exposure has been made.

To save time and not have the patient sit in the chair with the rubber dam in place, rapid processing, as discussed in Chapter 11, can minimize working time and can be adequately diagnostic in endodontic working films.

Digital radiography with its instantaneous image formation is a very fast and effective approach to endodontic radiography. The working image is obtained quickly and is stored for archival life.

Grid Measurement

Some dentists use grid markings to quantify and evaluate bone levels or for endodontic measurements. Intraoral

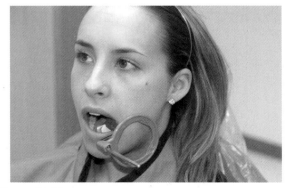

• **Figure 18.22** Endodontic receptor-holding device with localizing ring.

measurement grids are available that superimpose thin radiopaque or radiolucent lines in the vertical and horizontal planes in 1-mm gradations (Figs. 18.24 and 18.25). The marking grid is affixed to the front of the receptor when the exposure is made. No increase in exposure is necessary with the use of the marking grid. The measurement or

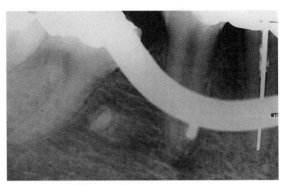

• **Figure 18.23** Radiograph with superimposition of rubber dam frame.

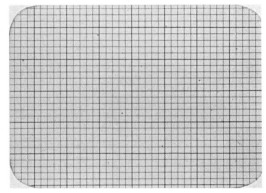

• **Figure 18.24** Intraoral grid placed on dental receptor.

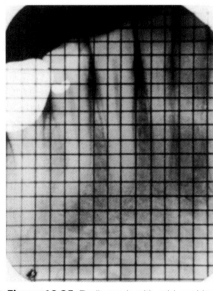

• **Figure 18.25** Radiograph with grid markings.

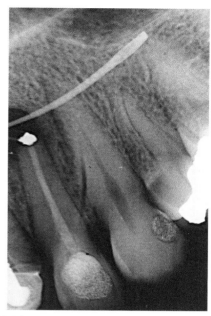

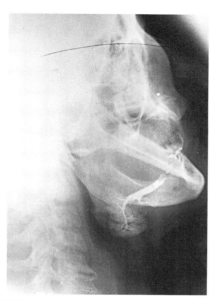

• **Figure 18.27** Sialograph outlining submandibular duct and gland.

• **Figure 18.26** Fistulous tract traced back from palatal opening to its origin by insertion of gutta-percha point.

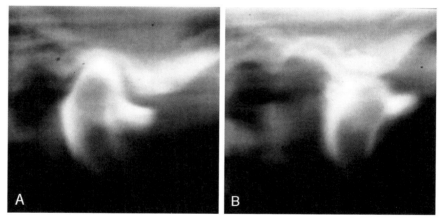

• **Figure 18.28** Arthrography of the temporomandibular joint (TMJ) in the closed **(A)** and open **(B)** positions. Note the radiolucent space between radiopaque areas that represents the articular disk.

marking grid should not be confused with the grid used in extraoral projections (see Chapter 13) to absorb object scatter. Furthermore, in digital radiography, endodontic measurement is easily accomplished directly through use of the corresponding computer program.

Radiopaque Media

The use of radiopaque media has many applications in dental practice. It is used routinely in endodontics, with the radiopaque file, to determine root length. Gutta-percha or silver points can be placed in periodontal soft tissue pockets to determine pocket depth and direction. Fistulous tracts can be traced to their origin using thin, flexible wire or gutta-percha points (Fig. 18.26).

The technique of sialography involves injecting radiopaque media into salivary ducts and glands and then visualizing these soft tissues radiographically. This method is used in diagnosing ductal and glandular obstructions, salivary stones, infections, and tumors of the major salivary glands. The contrast medium used is usually an iodine-containing formula in either an aqueous or oil suspension (Fig. 18.27). Contrast media are also used in radiographing the temporomandibular joint (TMJ) to visualize the articular disc with a procedure called arthrography (Fig. 18.28). Because the disc is fibrocartilage, it is not seen on radiographs; but if a radiopaque medium is injected into the upper and lower joint spaces, then the void between them represents the articular disc (see Chapter 14).

Chapter Summary

- Dental imaging techniques may be modified to accommodate patients with physical and developmental disabilities, including those patients with mobility, hearing, or vision impairment.
- Pediatric patients have special needs when managing them in the dental office, including technique modifications when exposing intraoral and extraoral radiographs on them. Care should be taken to gain pediatric patients' confidence when explaining procedures and helping them to feel comfortable in the dental office setting
- All patients have a "gag reflex;" however, this body defense mechanism is more sensitive in some patients than in others. There are various ways to manage patients with hypersensitive gag reflexes, including those that concern the operator's attitude, the exposure sequence and radiographic technique, deep breathing through the nasal cavity, and others.
- Other special-needs situations exist in dental radiography, including localization, third molar, and endodontic issues. It is necessary for the dental radiographer to know the appropriate remedies for these issues and to learn how to modify their patient management techniques accordingly.

Chapter Review Questions

Multiple Choice

1. The gag reflex is:
   a. Always more active with posterior projections
   b. Resolved with slow, deep breathing
   c. A body defense mechanism
   d. Both a and c only
   e. Answers a, b, and c are all correct
2. A reversed bitewing is usually used when:
   a. An adult patient gags
   b. A pediatric patient constantly cries
   c. A pediatric patient is not sitting in the chair properly
   d. An adult patient does not want radiographs
   e. A pediatric patient consistently moves the bitewing receptor out of the mouth with their tongue
3. The SLOB rule states that objects that move in the same direction when a second radiograph is taken for localization are usually positioned:
   a. Mesially in the mouth
   b. Lingually in the mouth
   c. Distally in the mouth
   d. Bucally in the mouth
   e. All of the above are incorrect answers
4. The best way to radiograph an impacted third molar is to:
   a. Ask the patient to hold the receptor with their finger to place it in the most posterior position possible
   b. Take a panoramic radiograph
   c. Use a bitewing projection
   d. Take an intraoral photograph
   e. Both a or c are acceptable techniques to capture impacted third molars on a radiographic image
5. When managing patients with a hearing impairment, the dental professional should:
   a. Face the patients when speaking to them
   b. Remove their mask when speaking to them
   c. Turn their backs on the patients when speaking to them
   d. Use sign language when communicating with them
   e. All of the above except c are acceptable answers

Critical Thinking Exercise

1. The office that you are employed in wants to publish a manual for the staff describing the technique modifications needed when exposing radiographs on patients with special needs. The office manager is asking for input from every member of the dental team. Your task is to list the suggested management techniques for each of the following special-needs situations:
   a. Endodontic radiographs
   b. Localization techniques
   c. Patients with anatomic constraints, such as a narrow arch, shallow palate, tight lingual frenum, tori, or trismus
   d. Hypersensitive gag reflex
   e. Pediatric patients
   f. Vision impairment
   g. Hearing impairment
   h. Mobility constraints

Bibliography

Iannucci JM, Howerton LJ: *Dental radiography: Principles and techniques*, ed 5, St Louis, MO, 2016, Elsevier Saunders.

Sewrine I: Gagging in dental radiography, *Oral Surg Oral Med Oral Pathol* 58:725–728, 1984.

White SC, Pharoah MJ: *Oral radiology: Principles and interpretation*, ed 7, St Louis, MO, 2013, Mosby.

19

Film Mounting and Radiographic Anatomy

EDUCATIONAL OBJECTIVES

Upon completing this chapter, the student will be able to:

1. Define the key terms listed at the beginning of the chapter.
2. Discuss the types of descriptive terminology used in radiography, including how the density of a structure determines its radiographic appearance.
3. Discuss the following related to mounting procedures:
   - State the advantage of mounting radiographs.
   - List the two techniques in mounting conventional films and state which is the preferred method.
   - List the two modes of mounting techniques that can be employed when utilizing a digital radiographic system.
   - List five helpful hints that can be used in mounting radiographs.

4. Describe the following related to radiographic tooth anatomy:
   - Know the radiographic appearance of the components of the tooth and surrounding bone and soft tissue structures.
   - Identify and describe the anatomic landmarks of the maxilla on radiographic images.
   - Identify and describe the anatomic landmarks of the mandible on radiographic images.
5. Identify common restorations on radiographic images.
6. Identify the anatomic landmarks on occlusal, panoramic, and other extraoral images.

KEY TERMS

alveolar bone
alveolar crest
anterior nasal spine
antral or inverted Y
buccinator shadow
cancellous bone
cementum
concavity
coronoid process of the mandible
cortical bone
dentin
enamel
external oblique ridge
floor of the maxillary sinus
floor of the nasal cavity
floor of the nasal fossa
foramen
fossa
genial tubercle
hamular notch
hamular process (hamulus)
incisive canal
inferior border of the mandible

inferior nasal concha (turbinate)
internal oblique ridge (mylohyoid ridge)
labial mounting
lamina dura
lateral fossa
lingual foramen
lingual mounting
mandibular canal (inferior alveolar canal)
mandibular foramen
mandibular tori (torus mandibularis)
maxillary sinus
maxillary torus (torus palatinus)
maxillary tuberosity
median palatine suture
medullary spaces
mental foramen
mental ridge
mounts
mylohyoid ridge
nasal fossa (nasal cavity)
nasal septum

nasolabial fold
nasopalatine (incisive) foramen
nutrient canals
periodontal ligament (membrane)
pneumatization
pterygomaxillary fissure
pulp
pulp canal
pulp chamber
pulp horns
radiolucent (RL)
radiopaque (RO)
ridge
septa
sinus
submandibular fossa
trabeculae
tuberosity pad
viewbox
x-ray
zygoma
zygomatic arch
zygomatic process of the maxilla

Introduction

The mounting of processed dental radiographs is another important function of the dental professional. It is much easier to view and interpret radiographs when the films are placed in mounts in their proper anatomic orientation. Properly mounted films make charting and examination a more orderly procedure. The mounted films are kept with or in the patient's chart. At each subsequent visit, the radiographs are placed on the viewbox for the dentist's referral. Care should be taken not to handle the mounted radiographs or the chart with contaminated gloves.

The finished radiographs are identified and oriented to the position in the mouth by the raised portion of the dot, teeth, and bony structures visible on each film. A thorough understanding of radiographic anatomy makes mounting an interesting and challenging procedure.

This chapter discusses the basic concepts of film mounting and the appearance and significance of radiographic anatomy on periapical, bitewing, occlusal, panoramic, and other extraoral projections.

Descriptive Terminology

Because this chapter deals with the processed radiograph in mounting and interpretation, certain terms are needed to describe the shades of black, white, and gray that appear. The appearance of any area (e.g., tooth, bone) on a radiograph is determined by the density of that area, the quality of the x-ray photons, and hence the penetration of the x-ray beam that reaches the film. With these terms, one can more accurately describe the radiographic findings. The black areas, where there is greater penetration of x-rays that reach the radiographs, are called **radiolucent (RL)**. The white areas, where there is little or no penetration, are called **radiopaque (RO)**. All structures are either RL or RO, but each category includes gradations. For instance, metallic fillings are more RO than enamel, but both are still RO. Caries appears RL, because the decay causes a lessening of density when compared with enamel and dentin.

> **HELPFUL HINT**
>
> A radiograph should never be referred to as an x-ray. One may say "x-ray film" or better still, "radiograph," but the term **x-ray** should only be used when referring to the beam of energy that is aimed at the receptor in the patient's mouth. The film is then processed to produce a radiograph.

Mounts

Various types of dental film mounts are available. **Mounts** are made for both pediatric and adult surveys and come with a full range of numbers of windows (Fig. 19.1). In addition to full-survey mounts, single-film, double-film, and bitewing survey mounts are also available (Fig. 19.2). Film mounts usually are made of cardboard or a celluloid-like material. The area around the film windows may be clear

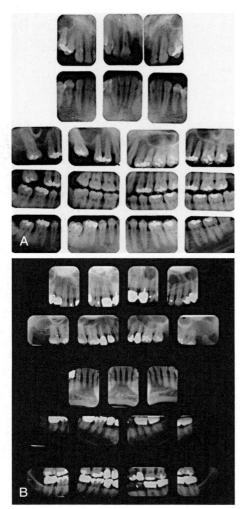

• **Figure 19.1** Full-mouth series mounted in clear celluloid **(A)** and opaque **(B)** mounts.

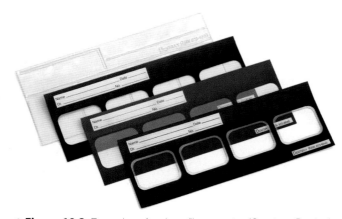

• **Figure 19.2** Examples of various film mounts. (Courtesy Dentsply Rinn, York, PA.)

or opaque. The opaque mounts are preferred, because the light is concentrated behind the radiographs and viewing is easier and more accurate. If the number of radiographs taken does not fill the mounts, the unused windows should be covered to prevent the light from distracting the viewer. The black opaque wrapper from the film packet is ideal for this, because it is the correct color and size and is easily placed in the mount.

The patient's name, chart number (if applicable), date, and the number of films taken should be recorded on each mount.

Mounting

Placement of the radiographs in their correct position in the mounts may seem challenging at first. However, if one develops a system based on understanding, this task can be mastered in a short time. The operators must always work on a clean, dry, light-colored tabletop so that they can see the radiographs easily when they are laid out. The radiographs are viewed on an illuminator, or viewbox, placed on or in front of the surface where the mounting is being done.

Every radiograph has an embossed or raised dot to help decipher the film orientation. The film packet is placed in the patient's mouth so that the side with the dot is always nearest the occlusal or incisal surfaces of the teeth. Manufacturers position the film in the packet so that the raised portion of the dot faces the x-ray machine when the exposure is made (Fig. 19.3). If the operator mounts the radiographs so that the raised portion of the dot is toward oneself, the operator is looking at the film as if facing the patient; the patient's left side is on the operator's right. This is called labial mounting (Fig. 19.4A). If the film is mounted so that the depressed side of the dot is toward the operator, the operator is looking at the films as if viewing them from a position on the patient's tongue looking out; the patient's left side is on the operator's left. This is called lingual mounting (see Fig. 19.4B). Both mounting systems have been used in dentistry, but the trend has been to adopt the labial mounting system as the technique of choice. The American Dental Association (ADA) recommends labial mounting for use in dental facilities. When receiving mounted radiographs

from another dental facility, the dental professional should always establish which mounting technique was used by the position of the orientation dot of the film or films in the mount.

Procedure

The proper size and number of film mounts is selected. The patient's name or identification number and the date the films were taken are entered on the mount. The patient's films are laid out on the clean, dry tabletop, and the empty mount is placed on the viewbox. The films are placed so that the dots are all one way, either facing toward or away from the operator. The films are then divided into three groups: bitewings, anterior periapical, and posterior periapical. The bitewing films are easily identified, because the crowns of both the upper and lower teeth are seen. The anterior and posterior periapical films are differentiated by the vertical orientation on the film for anterior teeth and the horizontal orientation for posterior teeth.

Dental professionals can differentiate the maxillary anterior films from the mandibular anterior films on the basis of root and crown shape and anatomic landmarks, which are discussed later in this chapter. To determine whether a film is from the patient's right or left side, the film is held up to the mount, and one imagines that the mount is the patient's face. Then, it is decided which is the mesial and which is the distal side of the radiograph, and the film is placed accordingly. When the anterior films have been placed in their proper position in the mount, the same routine is

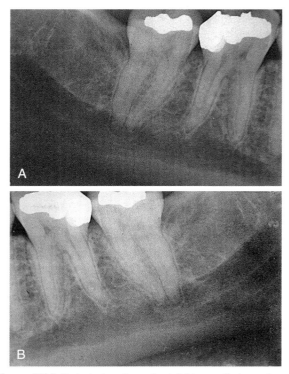

• **Figure 19.4** Periapical radiograph of right mandibular molar area. **A,** Labial mounting. **B,** Lingual mounting.

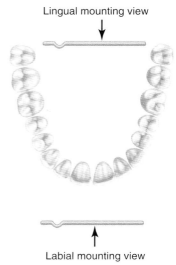

• **Figure 19.3** Raised dot on x-ray film and its orientation in film mounts for labial or lingual viewing.

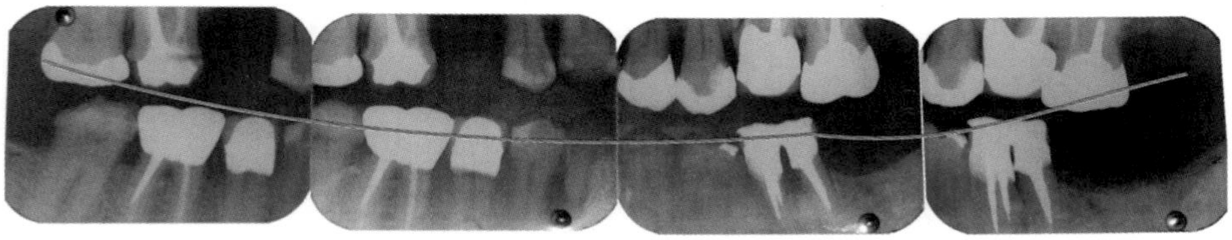

• **Figure 19.5** The "smile" appearance created by the curve of Spee.

repeated for the posterior films. Be sure that the maxillary radiographs are placed in the mount with the roots of the teeth pointing up and the mandibular radiographs are mounted with the roots of the teeth pointing down.

Bitewing radiographs show only the crowns of the teeth; there are no root shapes and few surrounding bony landmarks to aid in anatomic identification. However, the bitewing films can be mounted easily by orienting the curve of Spee (also called *von Spee's curve* or *Spee's curvature*), which is the curvature of the mandibular occlusal plane beginning at the tip of the lower incisors and following the buccal cusps of the posterior teeth, continuing to the terminal molar. Another method is to mount the bitewings first, then the posterior periapical radiographs, using the restorations on the bitewings to identify the posterior periapical projections. With this method, the anterior periapical radiographs are mounted last.

Some generalizations can be made about crown and root shapes seen on radiographs. The following hints will aid the dental professional in mounting films:

- The crowns of the upper anterior central and lateral incisors are wider and have longer roots than those of the lower central and lateral incisors. Because they are wider, the maxillary anteriors do not fit on one film like the mandibular incisors.
- Maxillary premolars usually have two roots; mandibular premolars have one root.
- Mandibular first and second molars usually have two divergent curved roots with bone clearly visible between them. This is particularly true of the first molar. Maxillary molars have three roots: two buccal and one palatal. The large palatal root obscures the interradicular bone.
- Most roots curve distally.
- The occlusal plane as it goes distally curves up in what is called the *curve of Spee*. When looking at the bitewing, one should imagine that the patient has a smile as the curve rises and an unhappy look if the curve incorrectly curves downward (Fig. 19.5).

HELPFUL HINT

Remember, even the unhappiest patient in the dental chair will appear happy in the radiographic mount if the orientation of the curve of Spee on the bitewing radiographs is correct. All patients are smiling when their bitewing radiographs are mounted properly. If they appear to be frowning, the bitewing radiographs are incorrectly mounted and should be corrected.

These aids, along with the anatomic landmarks that are described next in this chapter, enable the dental professional to properly orient radiographs in the x-ray film mount.

Mounting in Digital Imaging

In digital imaging, the arrangement of the images is either performed by the radiographer after the images are captured or set in the program's template during the radiographic procedure. There are some digital programs that enable the operator to "click and drag" the captured images to their appropriate window or frame on the template or mount on the screen of the computer's monitor after the images are captured. Other digital programs allow the operator to "click" on the appropriate frame on the monitor's template for the planned exposure before capturing the image. This "highlights" the corresponding window for the exposure so that when the exposure is taken, the image automatically appears in the respective window. For example, when dental professionals are taking a maxillary central incisor projection, they "click" on the frame for the maxillary central incisor before capturing the image. After the image is captured, it instantaneously appears in the respective window. Once the images are accepted and approved, the operator saves the images as a part of the patient's electronic health record (EHR).

Normal Radiographic Anatomy

To fully use and properly interpret radiographs, the dental staff must be thoroughly familiar with normal radiographic anatomy. This includes all of the structures seen on periapical, bitewing, occlusal, panoramic, and extraoral projections. The first consideration in interpreting a suspected lesion should be to differentiate it from a normal structure. This may often be challenging because of wide variations of normal gross anatomy in regard to size, shape, and location that may be further modified by age and use. Radiographically, these variations may be exaggerated by the projection and angulation used. Not all landmarks are always demonstrated on every full-mouth survey or individual image. When a dental professional is confronted with a suspicious lesion, the first things to consider are the anatomic landmarks normally seen in that particular area. Normal anatomy should be ruled out first when making a differential diagnosis.

In interpreting radiographic landmarks, dental professionals should keep in mind the gross configuration of the

NOTE

Knowing what structures are "within normal limits" on radiographic images is critical in being able to recognize when there is a radiographic sighting that is a cause for concern.

structure. A thick, bony structure such as a ridge or muscle attachment appears more RO because of increased object density. Any foramen, cavity, or concavity of bone produces an area represented on the image as RL because of decreased density. Radiographs, as two-dimensional representations of three-dimensional objects, produce superimpositions of many normal structures that can be misleading. Dental professionals should remember this when interpreting radiographic images.

Because radiographs are two-dimensional representations of a three-dimensional object, they do not portray depth; teeth may be superimposed on anatomic structures in the mandible, maxilla, or skull that may be millimeters in front of or in back of them. The best example is the roots of the maxillary molars and the maxillary sinus. Maxillary molar roots are rarely actually in the sinus, although they may appear that way on almost all molar radiographs (see Fig. 19.10).

Radiographic Tooth Anatomy

The component structures of the tooth and its supporting structures are defined on the dental radiograph because of their differences in density (Fig. 19.6).

Enamel is the densest and thus the most RO of the natural tooth structures. It is seen as a RO band that covers the crown of the tooth and ends in a fine edge at the cementoenamel junction.

Dentin is the next layer of tooth structure. It is not as highly calcified as enamel and thus not as RO. It composes the major part of the tooth structure and is seen in both the crown and the root portions. On a radiograph with poor contrast, it is difficult to see the border between the enamel and dentin (the dentinoenamel junction).

Cementum is the thin, calcified covering on the surface of the root of the tooth. It is difficult to distinguish cementum from dentin, because it is thin and its density is not very different from that of dentin. Cementum, however, is the outer covering of the root and dentin is the inner layer of tooth structure just outside of the RL core of the tooth known as the pulp. The pulp chamber and pulp canal are seen as a continuous RL space in the center of the crown and root of the tooth, respectively. The fingerlike projections in the coronal portion are called pulp horns. They are seen most often in young patients, because the pulp chambers of teeth become smaller with age and in some cases may become totally obliterated by secondary dentin.

The periodontal ligament (membrane) is seen as a RL line approximately 0.5 mm wide between the cementum of the root of the tooth and the lamina dura. There is always a periodontal ligament attaching the tooth to bone, but the periodontal membrane may not always be seen clearly on every root surface because of differences in horizontal angulation when the radiograph was taken.

The lamina dura is a RO line of cortical bone that surrounds the periodontal ligament. It represents the bony

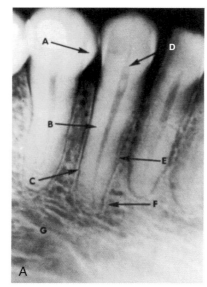

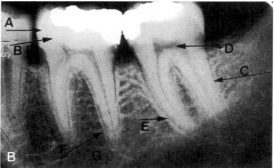

• **Figure 19.6** Normal radiographic tooth anatomy, anterior **(A)** and posterior **(B)** tooth: *A*, Enamel; *B*, dentin; *C*, periodontal membrane; *D*, pulp chamber; *E*, cementum; *F*, lamina dura; *G*, alveolar bone.

wall of the tooth socket. As with the periodontal ligament, it may not be seen on every surface because of angulation.

The alveolar bone is the bone that supports the tooth. It is composed of cancellous and cortical-compact bone. The cancellous bone is seen as a series of small RL compartments called medullary spaces. These spaces are separated by a RO honeycomb pattern called trabeculae. The superior part of the alveolar bone is referred to as the alveolar crest, which is composed of cortical bone. It should be noted that the mandible is a much denser bone than the maxilla; hence, the medullary spaces are smaller, and there is greater trabeculation in the mandible. The cortical bone is seen as a dense radiopaque structure that comprises the buccal and palatal plates of the maxilla, the buccal and lingual plates of the mandible, the inferior border of the mandible, the lamina dura, and the alveolar crest.

> ### NOTE
>
> The honeycomb pattern of the alveolar bone resembles the 3 × 3 grid used to play the game tic-tac-toe, with the horizontal and vertical lines representing the trabeculae and the spaces or boxes in between those lines representing the medullary spaces.

Text continued on p. 225

PROCEDURE 19.1 RECOGNIZING AND UNDERSTANDING RADIOGRAPHIC ANATOMY OF THE MAXILLA AND THE MANDIBLE

> **HELPFUL HINT**
>
> It is important to remember when visualizing the anatomic landmarks of the head and neck regions that radiographs of these structures are two-dimensional representations of three-dimensional objects. Therefore, these anatomic landmarks appear differently when comparing an actual skull view with the radiographic depiction of these structures.

Maxilla

Maxillary Incisor Area (Fig. 19.7)

The nasopalatine (incisive) foramen is seen as an oval radiolucency between the roots of the maxillary central incisors. In some radiographs, the incisive canal can be seen leading to the foramen. The foramen (an opening, hole, or passage in a bone) is actually in the anterior portion of the palate, but superimposition makes it appear to be located between the roots of the central incisors. The position of the nasopalatine (incisive) foramen on the radiograph may vary from just above the crest of the alveolar ridge to the level of the apices of the teeth because of anatomic variations and vertical angulation. In some cases, the shadow of the foramen may be superimposed on the apex of a central incisor and

must be differentiated from periapical disease. This is done by tracing the lamina dura and periodontal ligament space. These structures will be completely intact if it is a foramen and interrupted if an actual periapical pathologic condition is present.

The median palatine suture is seen as a thin radiolucent (RL) line running vertically between the roots of the maxillary central incisors. It must be differentiated from a fracture line, nutrient canal, and fistulous tract.

The nasal fossa (nasal cavity) is the paired RL structure superior to the apices of the maxillary incisor teeth. The fossa is also seen on the canine projection, where it may overlap or appear to adjoin the maxillary sinus. The radiopaque (RO) band that separates the left and right nasal fossa is called the median nasal septum. The septum ends inferiorly in the V-shaped RO anterior nasal spine.

The RO anterior nasal spine is near or superimposed on the nasopalatine (incisive) foramen. The radiopacity that sometimes projects into the nasal fossa from its lateral wall is the inferior nasal concha (turbinate). When the concha is very large, the thickness of the soft tissue may make it look RO.

The soft tissue and cartilaginous shadow of the tip of the nose and the soft tissue outline of the lip may be superimposed from the crest of the ridge to the crowns of the teeth. These soft tissue shadows are seen most clearly on

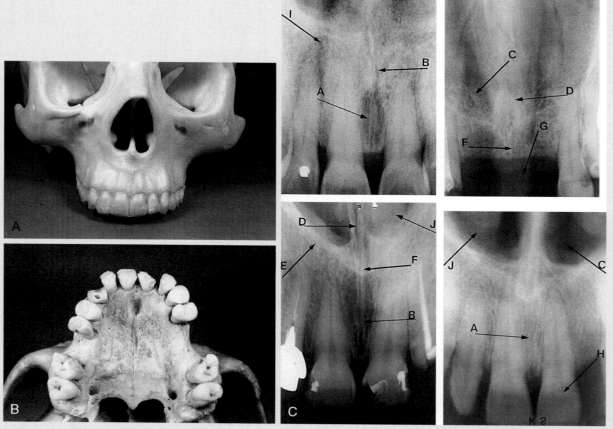

• **Figure 19.7** Maxillary central incisor area. **A** and **B**, Skull. **C**, Radiographs: *A*, Nasopalatine foramen; *B*, median palatine suture; *C*, nasal fossa; *D*, median nasal septum; *E*, floor of nasal cavity; *F*, anterior nasal spine; *G*, columella of nose; *H*, lip line; *I*, lateral fossa; *J*, inferior concha.

PROCEDURE 19.1   RECOGNIZING AND UNDERSTANDING RADIOGRAPHIC ANATOMY OF THE MAXILLA AND THE MANDIBLE—cont'd

edentulous images in which even the nares (openings) of the nose and the columella (separating column) are seen.

The lateral fossa is a depression in the labial plate in the lateral incisor region. It appears as a radiolucency between the lateral incisor and canine because it represents an area of thin bone.

Maxillary Canine Area (Fig. 19.8)

In the maxillary canine region, two large RL areas are seen. The more mesial area is the lateral aspect of the nasal fossa, and the more distal is the anterior extent of the maxillary sinus. In edentulous images, the RO Y, known as the antral or inverted Y, formed by the anterior and inferior border of the maxillary sinus as the arms and the floor of the nasal cavity as the stem, is useful in the mounting orientation of maxillary canine projections.

The RO soft tissue shadow of the nose may also show on canine area radiographs. In some projections, a RL area is seen distal to the canine and represents the nasolabial fold.

Maxillary Premolar Area (Fig. 19.9)

In the maxillary premolar area, the RL maxillary sinus may be seen either superimposed on, between, or above the apices of the teeth. It is not always visible because of vertical angulation of the x-ray beam and because the size and position of the maxillary sinus may vary from patient to patient. The floor of

the maxillary sinus appears as a RO line running horizontally along its lower border.

The floor of the nasal fossa may be seen as a RO line running horizontally at the superior portion of the maxillary sinus. Nutrient canals may be seen in the alveolar bone along with grooves for vessels in the walls of the maxillary sinus. Bony septum also may be seen in the maxillary sinus.

The edentulous premolar radiograph is identified by the presence of the maxillary sinus. It differs from the molar radiograph in the absence of the maxillary sinus in the mesial part of the image and the start of the RO zygomatic arch band at the distal portion of the image.

In some edentulous images, the shadow of the buccinator muscle is seen. The buccinator shadow makes part of the normally RL area below the ridge appear RO because of the increased density of the muscle.

Maxillary Molar Area (Fig. 19.10)

The maxillary sinus is a RL area that appears on periapical projections of the maxillary molar region. The sinus may be unilocular or compartmentalized by bony septa. RO spurs or ridges may project into the sinus; RL tracts or grooves, representing blood vessel positions, may be seen in the walls of the sinus. The size of the maxillary sinus varies greatly because of age, morphology, radiographic projection,

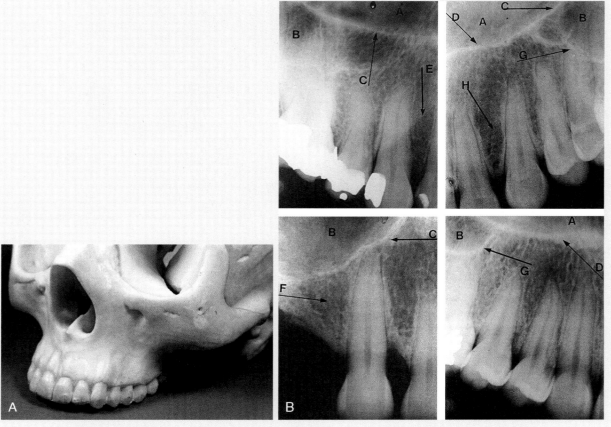

• **Figure 19.8** Maxillary canine area. **A,** Skull. **B,** Radiographs: *A,* Nasal fossa; *B,* maxillary sinus; *C,* septum of bone separating maxillary sinus and nasal septum; *D,* floor of nasal cavity; *E,* shadow of the nose; *F,* nasolabial fold; *G,* floor of maxillary sinus; *H,* lateral fossa.

Continued

PROCEDURE 19.1   RECOGNIZING AND UNDERSTANDING RADIOGRAPHIC ANATOMY OF THE MAXILLA AND THE MANDIBLE—cont'd

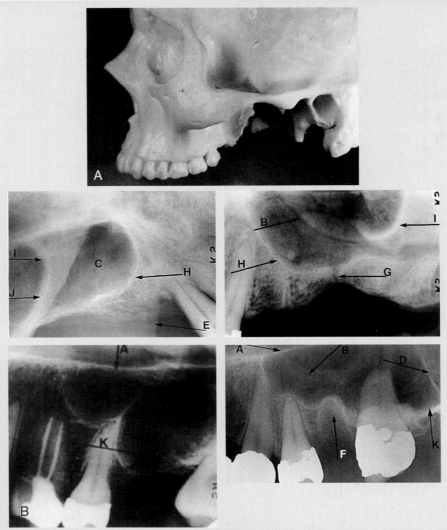

• **Figure 19.9** Maxillary premolar area. **A,** Skull. **B,** Radiographs: *A,* Floor of nasal fossa; *B,* nutrient canals in sinus wall; *C,* maxillary sinus; *D,* sinus septum; *E,* buccinator shadow; *F,* extraction socket; *G,* oral-antral communication; *H,* floor of maxillary sinus; *I,* zygomatic process of maxilla; *J,* zygomatic arch; *K,* pneumatization.

and vertical angulation used. A patient's sinuses may be asymmetric and may tend to enlarge or grow into areas of the alveolar ridge where teeth have been extracted. This process is called **pneumatization.** Just distal to the third molar ridge area is the **maxillary tuberosity.** This area of cancellous bone also may contain the posterior extension of the maxillary sinus. The large, fibrous buildup of soft tissue over the tuberosity may cause a slightly RO shadow on the radiograph and is called the **tuberosity pad.**

The **zygomatic process of the maxilla** is seen as a U-shaped radiopacity superimposed on the roots of the first and second molars and the maxillary sinus. The malar bone (**zygoma**), which is a continuation of the zygomatic process, appears as a broad, uniform RO band that extends posteriorly. Together with the zygomatic process of the temporal bone, they make up the **zygomatic arch.**

The **hamular process (hamulus)** is the RO projection that extends downward and distal to the posterior surface of the maxillary tuberosity. It is the inferior end of the medial pterygoid plate of the sphenoid bone. The RL area between the tuberosity and the hamular process is referred to as the **hamular notch** (Fig. 19.11).

In the distal inferior portion of maxillary molar radiographs, a large RO structure may be seen. This is the **coronoid process of the mandible.** When an edentulous series is mounted, this landmark is helpful in determining which is the most distal of the maxillary radiographs.

The **maxillary torus (torus palatinus)** is a lobulated bony growth in the midline of the palate. It is considered an anomaly and not anatomic landmark, because it does not exist in the anatomy of all patients. On a periapical radiograph, it appears as a dense, well-demarcated, RO area (Fig. 19.12).

PROCEDURE 19.1   RECOGNIZING AND UNDERSTANDING RADIOGRAPHIC ANATOMY OF THE MAXILLA AND THE MANDIBLE—cont'd

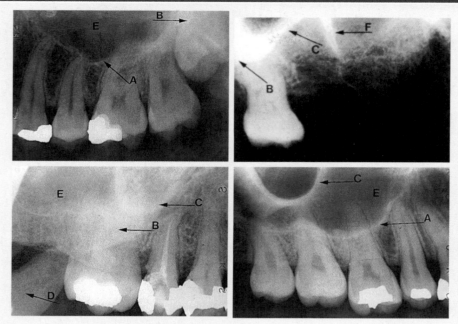

• **Figure 19.10** Maxillary molar area. *A*, Floor of sinus; *B*, zygomatic arch; *C*, zygomatic process of maxilla; *D*, coronoid process of mandible; *E*, maxillary sinus; *F*, septum in sinus.

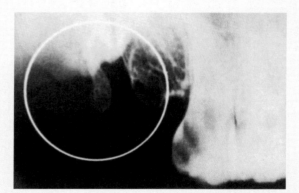

• **Figure 19.11** Posterior part of maxillary molar region. In the *circle* are maxillary tuberosity, hamular notch, and hamular process.

Mandible

Mandibular Incisor Area (Fig. 19.13)

In the mandibular central incisor area, just below the apices of the central incisors in the midline, there is often a somewhat circular radiopacity. This is the **genial tubercle**, which represents a bony growth on the lingual surface of the mandible to which the genioglossus and the geniohyoid muscles are attached. In the middle of the genial tubercle, a small circular radiolucency may be seen. This is the **lingual foramen**, which is the exit point from the mandible for the lingual branches of the incisive vessels. **Nutrient canals**, although found in all areas of the mandible and maxilla, are seen most easily in this area, because the mandibular bone is thin in this location and must be differentiated from fistulous tracts or fracture lines. They appear as RL lines that run vertically in the alveolar bone and terminate in small, circular,

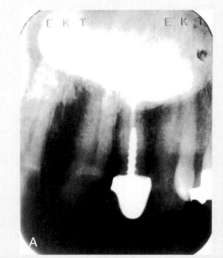

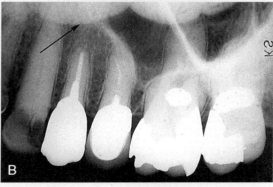

• **Figure 19.12** Maxillary torus. **A,** Anterior periapical. **B,** Posterior periapical.

Continued

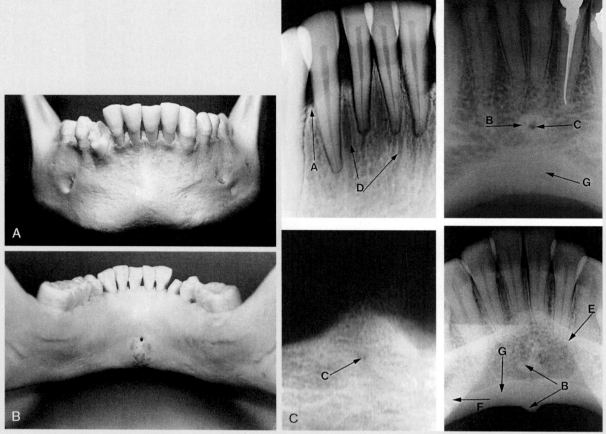

• **Figure 19.13** Mandibular incisor area. **A** and **B,** Skull. **C,** Radiographs: *A,* Alveolar ridge; *B,* genial tubercles; *C,* lingual foramen; *D,* nutrient canals; *E,* mental ridge; *F,* mylohyoid ridge; *G,* inferior border of mandible.

RL nutrient foramina. The nutrient canals are pathways for blood vessels and nerves.

The mental ridge is a broad V-shaped RO band that represents a ridge of bone on the labial aspect of the mandible. It arises bilaterally below the apical area of the canine and incisors and runs medially and upward toward the mandibular symphysis. The ridge, if superimposed on the apices of the teeth, may hinder diagnosis. The mental ridge should be differentiated from the internal oblique ridge (mylohyoid ridge).

The shadow of the lip is seen on anterior radiographs. That portion of the image not covered by the lip appears darker than the rest of the image, because there is no soft tissue attenuation in the area. The lip line, unless identified as such, can hinder radiographic interpretation.

The inferior border of the mandible is seen as a broad RO band that represents the thick cortical bone of this area. The inferior border of the mandible can be seen in all of the intraoral mandibular projections.

Mandibular Canine Area (Fig. 19.14)

The anterior extension of the internal oblique ridge and submandibular fossa can be seen in the canine area.

The edentulous mandibular canine may be difficult to orient in the mount. One should look for the genial tubercle on the mesial part of the image and possibly the mental foramen

in the distal part. The edentulous alveolar ridge crest slopes downward as it goes distally.

Mandibular Premolar Area (Fig. 19.15)

The mental foramen is seen as a round or oval radiolucency near the apices of the premolars. The mental foramen may be found between, below, or even superimposed on the apices of the premolars. The mental foramen may not be seen on all premolar periapicals because of horizontal angulation of either the central ray or the position of the foramen itself. It is through this foramen that the mental nerves and blood vessels emerge. In some cases, the RL mandibular canal may be seen leading directly to the foramen. The mental foramen, in many cases because of its superimposition on the apices of the premolar, must be differentiated from a periapical pathologic condition. Tracing the lamina dura and periodontal ligament space will again be helpful in distinguishing normal anatomy from a pathologic condition.

The termination of the external oblique ridge can be seen in this area, along with the internal oblique ridge, submandibular fossa, and inferior border of the mandible.

The mandibular tori (torus mandibularis), although not considered normal landmarks but rather considered anomalies, are included in this section because of their frequency in appearance. They are seen singularly or multiply, usually bilaterally on the lingual aspects of the mandible in or near the

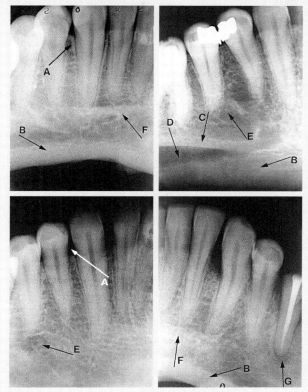

• **Figure 19.14** Mandibular canine area. *A,* Alveolar ridge; *B,* inferior border of mandible; *C,* internal oblique ridge; *D,* submandibular fossa; *E,* mental foramen; *F,* mental ridge; *G,* periapical pathologic condition.

premolar region. They appear as clearly outlined radiopacities (Fig. 19.16).

The edentulous premolar image is identified and oriented for mounting by the presence of the mental foramen and the ending of the external oblique ridge. The crest of the edentulous alveolar ridge tends to rise as it goes mesially.

Mandibular Molar Area (Fig. 19.17)

The mandibular canal (inferior alveolar canal) is seen as a RL band below the apices of the posterior teeth. It originates at the mandibular foramen and runs downward and forward to end at the mental foramen. It is bordered by thin RO lines.

The oblique ridges refer to the internal oblique ridge and the external oblique ridge. The external ridge, a continuation of the anterior border of the ramus, is seen as a RO line that passes diagonally down and forward across the molar region. The **internal oblique or** mylohyoid ridge is a RO line that runs from the medial and anterior aspect of the ramus downward and forward to end at the lower border of the symphysis. When these two ridges are seen together, the internal oblique ridge is the lower of the two RO lines.

> **NOTE**
>
> The external oblique ridge is higher and shorter, whereas the internal oblique ridge (mylohyoid ridge) is lower and longer.

The submandibular fossa is seen as a RL area below the internal oblique (mylohyoid) ridge. It represents an area of reduced thickness of bone caused by a depression on the medial surface of the mandible. This radiolucency may be accentuated by a prominent mylohyoid ridge and a thick, opaque, inferior border of the mandible.

Nutrient canals are seen commonly in the molar region, especially when it is edentulous.

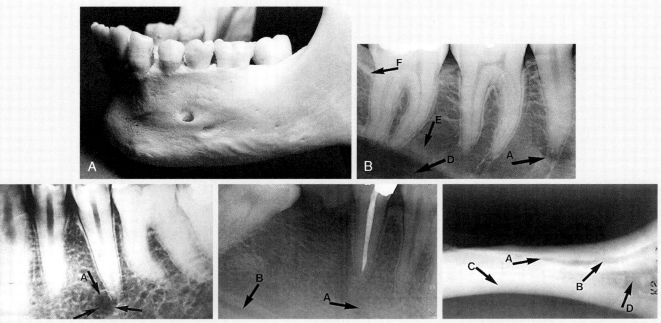

• **Figure 19.15** Mandibular premolar area. **A,** Skull. **B,** Radiographs: *A,* Mental foramen; *B,* mandibular canal; *C,* inferior border of the mandible; *D,* submandibular fossa; *E,* internal oblique ridge; *F,* external oblique ridge.

Continued

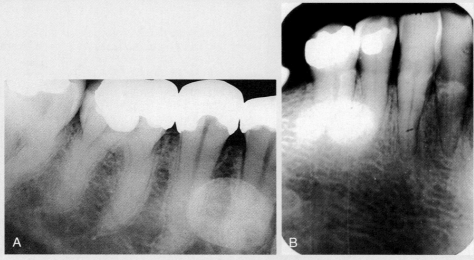

• **Figure 19.16** Mandibular tori. **A,** Premolar projection. **B,** Canine projection.

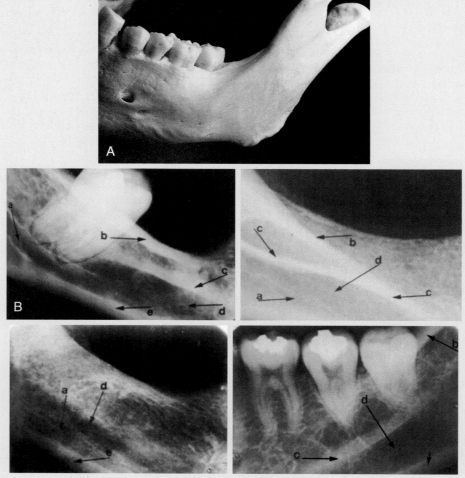

• **Figure 19.17** Mandibular molar area. **A,** Skull. **B,** Radiographs: *a,* Mandibular canal; *b,* external oblique ridge; *c,* internal oblique ridge; *d,* submandibular fossa; *e,* inferior border of mandible.

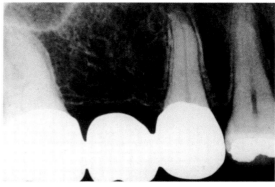

• **Figure 19.18** Fixed bridge and amalgam restoration. Note that the acrylic facing of the pontic does not appear on radiograph. Also note the difference in radiopacities between the amalgam and the cement base in the premolar.

Restorations

As with tooth and bone structure, the density of the restoration determines its appearance on radiographs. Metallic restorations (such as, gold inlays, crowns, foils, posts, pins, or silver amalgam) are the most RO areas seen on radiographs (Figs. 19.18 and 19.19). One can identify them only on the basis of size and shape, not on the degree of radiopacity. The synthetic restorations used in anterior teeth (e.g., glass ionomers, laminates, composites, and acrylics) appear RL and may be mistaken radiographically for caries (Fig. 19.20). Some manufacturers of synthetic restorations now incorporate RO particles in their preparations to distinguish the restorations from caries (Fig. 19.21). Temporary or sedative fillings and cavity liners (such as, zinc oxide, calcium hydroxide, and zinc oxyphosphate cement) appear RO, because they contain some metallic elements (see Figs. 19.20 and 19.21). Porcelain jackets appear slightly RO, because the silicate from which they are made is a metal, with the RO cement being more apparent (Fig. 19.22A). Porcelain-fused-to-metal (PFM) crowns appear with distinct outlines of the metal, with the porcelain seen poorly or not at all (see Fig. 19.22). Endodontic fillings appear as radiopacities in the pulp and root canal chambers. Of the two types of endodontic fillings most commonly used, the silver cones appear more RO than the gutta-percha points. However, silver cones are not commonly used in contemporary dentistry. Compare the endodontic filling in Fig. 19.19A with the filling in Fig. 19.23. Other materials that can be seen are fracture wires (Fig. 19.24) and orthodontic bands and wires (Fig. 19.25).

Radiographic Anatomy for Panoramic Films

The normal radiographic anatomy for panoramic images is shown in Fig. 19.26. Some of the anatomic landmarks listed were described in the preceding section on periapical radiographs. Those landmarks commonly seen on

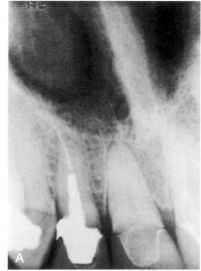

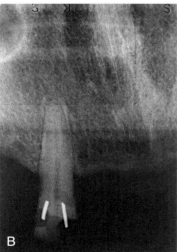

• **Figure 19.19** A, Gold post and core under porcelain jacket. B, Metallic pins under synthetic restoration.

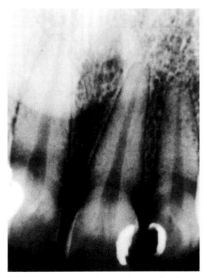

• **Figure 19.20** Radiolucent (RL) anterior synthetic restorations with cement bases.

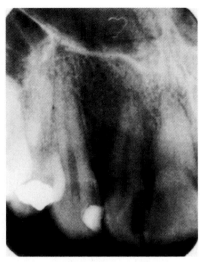

• **Figure 19.21** Radiopaque (RO) anterior synthetic restoration mesial to the canine. Mesial to the lateral incisor is a radiolucent (RL) synthetic restoration.

panoramic projections that are diagnostically important are also discussed here.

Mandibular Foramen

The mandibular foramen appears as an oval radiolucency at the origin of the mandibular canal at the midpoint of the ramus of the mandible.

Pharyngeal Airspace

The pharyngeal airspace appears as a bilateral, symmetric, RL band between the RO palatal line and the apices of the maxillary posterior teeth. It runs posteriorly and downward across the ramus and into the soft tissues of the neck. The appearance of the airspace on radiographs varies depending on the position of the tongue and thus the air above it and the state of contraction of the pharyngeal muscles. The diagnostic key for the airspace is the bilateral and symmetric appearance that can be followed running distally off the bone into the soft tissue.

Styloid Process

The styloid process is a RO projection that may be seen bilaterally projecting downward just posterior to the ramus of the mandible. The styloid ligaments attached to the process may calcify and give the appearance of an abnormally long styloid process. The calcification of the ligament may not be continuous or may start at the attachment of the ligament to the styloid process, giving the appearance of a fracture of the styloid process (Fig. 19.27).

Mandibular Condyle

The condyle, condylar neck, sigmoid notch, and coronoid process of the mandible are seen on panoramic films. Unless

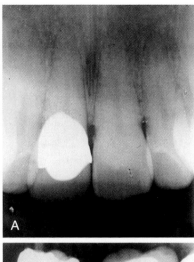

• **Figure 19.22** Porcelain-fused-to-metal (PFM) crown on an anterior tooth **(A)** and on a posterior tooth **(B)**. Note the different densities of the metal and porcelain components.

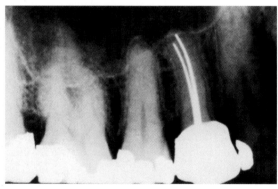

• **Figure 19.23** Silver cones used as endodontic filling material in the first premolar.

the unit has a variable focal plane, this is not the best way to view the condyle, because it does not lie within the usual focal trough. At best, the panoramic image can be considered a "scout film" to enable looking for gross changes in the maxilla or mandible.

Pterygomaxillary Fissure

The **pterygomaxillary fissure** is a fissure of the human skull. It is vertical and descends at right angles from the

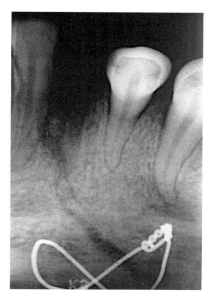

• **Figure 19.24** Healing mandibular fracture with intraosseous wires in place.

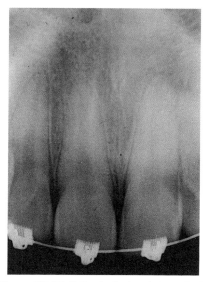

• **Figure 19.25** Orthodontic brackets and wires.

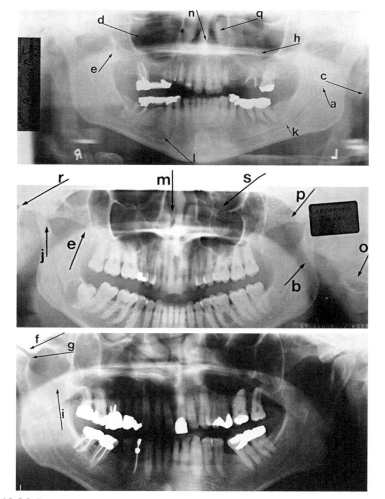

• **Figure 19.26** Panoramic film. *a,* Mandibular foramen; *b,* pharyngeal airspace; *c,* styloid process; *d,* maxillary sinus; *e,* coronoid process; *f,* articular eminence; *g,* glenoid fossa; *h,* hard palate; *i,* sigmoid notch; *j,* mandibular condyle; *k,* mandibular canal; *l,* mental foramen; *m,* nasal fossa; *n,* nasal septum; *o,* cervical vertebra; *p,* zygoma; *q,* inferior turbinate; *r,* external auditory meatus; *s,* Orbit.

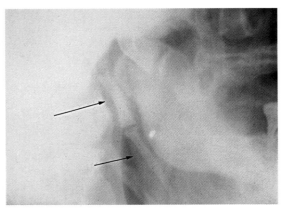

• **Figure 19.27** Calcified styloid ligament *(arrows)*.

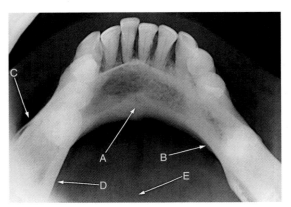

• **Figure 19.29** Mandibular occlusal film. *A,* Genial tubercles; *B,* interior border; *C,* buccal cortical plate; *D,* lingual cortical plate; *E,* shadow of tongue.

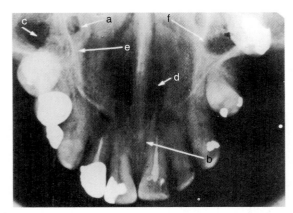

• **Figure 19.28** Maxillary occlusal film. *a,* Nasolacrimal duct; *b,* anterior palatine foramen; *c,* maxillary sinus; *d,* nasal fossa; *e,* lateral wall of nasal fossa; *f,* lateral wall of maxillary sinus.

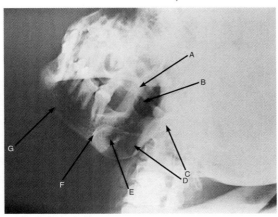

• **Figure 19.30** Lateral oblique projection of mandible. *A,* Coronoid process; *B,* sigmoid notch; *C,* condyle; *D,* pharyngeal airspace; *E,* mandibular foramen; *F,* mandibular canal; *G,* mental foramen.

medial end of the inferior orbital fissure; it is a triangular interval formed by the divergence of the maxilla from the pterygoid process of the sphenoid. It appears as an inverted teardrop on extraoral radiographs.

Occlusal Radiographs

When interpreting occlusal films, dental professionals must remember that the projection is in the superoinferior plane ("axial") and shows the third dimension not seen in periapical, bitewing, and panoramic films (Figs. 19.28 and 19.29). The type of occlusal projection used, right-angle or topographic (65 degrees), also should be considered, because the position of the landmarks varies depending on the angulation used.

Extraoral Projections

The most commonly seen and important landmarks for the extraoral techniques described in Chapter 13 are illustrated in Figs. 19.30 to 19.34.

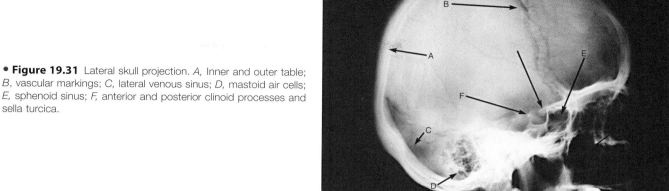

• **Figure 19.31** Lateral skull projection. *A,* Inner and outer table; *B,* vascular markings; *C,* lateral venous sinus; *D,* mastoid air cells; *E,* sphenoid sinus; *F,* anterior and posterior clinoid processes and sella turcica.

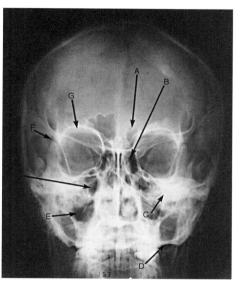

• **Figure 19.32** Posteroanterior view. *A,* Frontal sinus; *B,* ethmoid sinus; *C,* petrous ridge; *D,* base of skull; *E,* maxillary sinus; *F,* fronto-zygomatic suture; *G,* orbit.

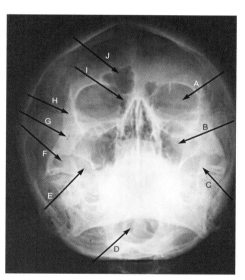

• **Figure 19.33** Posteroanterior view of sinuses (Waters view). *A,* Orbit; *B,* maxillary sinus; *C,* coronoid process; *D,* foramen magnum and vertebra; *E,* lateral wall of maxillary sinus; *F,* zygomatic arch; *G,* malar bone; *H,* frontozygomatic suture; *I,* ethmoid sinus; *J,* frontal sinus.

• **Figure 19.34** Normal temporomandibular joint (TMJ). *A,* External auditory meatus; *B,* condyle; *C,* articular fossae; *D,* articular eminence.

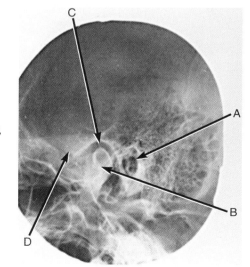

Chapter Summary

- It is easier to view and interpret radiographs when the films are placed in the mount in the same anatomic order as the teeth and anatomic structures appear in the patient's oral cavity. Properly mounted films make charting and examination a more orderly procedure. Digital radiographic techniques do not usually require a separate procedure for mounting the exposed images.
- The density of a structure directly affects its radiographic appearance. Structures that have considerable density appear RO, and areas with little or no density appear RL.

- The accurate mounting and interpretation of dental images is enhanced by the dental professional's knowledge regarding the radiographic appearance of the tooth structures and anatomic landmarks as they appear on periapical, bitewing, occlusal, panoramic, and other extraoral images.
- Knowledge of the normal anatomy on intraoral and extraoral radiographs is vital before the dental professional is capable of recognizing dental abnormalities.

Chapter Review Questions

Multiple Choice

1. Which of the following anatomic structures is better demonstrated on panoramic radiographs?
   a. Mandibular foramen
   b. Mental foramen
   c. Mylohyoid ridge
   d. Median palatine suture
   e. Coronoid process of the mandible
2. The radiolucent (RL) anatomic landmark represented by the letter C in the accompanying radiograph depicts the:

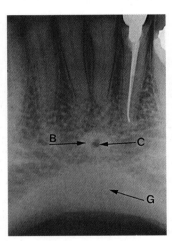

   a. Mental ridge
   b. Lingual foramen
   c. Genial tubercle
   d. Mental foramen
   e. External oblique ridge

3. The radiopaque (RO) structure distal to the hamular notch in this maxillary right posterior radiograph is known as the:

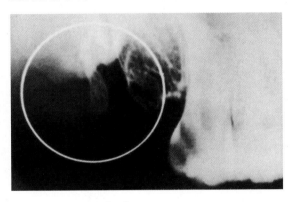

   a. Zygoma or malar bone
   b. Floor of the maxillary sinus
   c. Coronoid process of the mandible
   d. Hamular process
   e. Zygomatic arch
4. The RO structure seen superimposed over the roots of these maxillary posterior teeth represents:

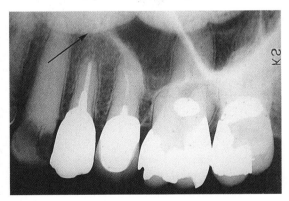

   a. Maxillary tori
   b. Bone trabeculation
   c. The internal oblique ridge
   d. Mandibular tori
   e. The inferior border of the mandible

5. The RL anatomic landmark represented by the letter C is the:

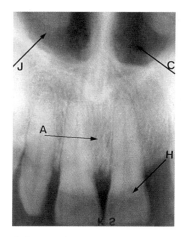

   a. Floor of the nasal cavity
   b. Median palatine suture
   c. Inferior nasal concha
   d. Nasal spine
   e. Nasal fossa
6. The most RO tooth structure is:
   a. Dentin
   b. Enamel
   c. Cementum
   d. Pulp chamber
   e. Pulp canal
7. The RL area lying below the internal oblique ridge in the mandible that represents an area of a reduced thickness of bone is called the:
   a. Mandibular canal
   b. Submandibular fossa
   c. External oblique ridge
   d. Mandibular tori
   e. Mental foramen
8. The U-shaped radiopacity superimposed over the roots of the first and second molars and the maxillary sinus is known as the:
   a. Hamular process
   b. Maxillary tuberosity
   c. Maxillary tori
   d. Zygomatic process of the maxilla
   e. Coronoid process of the mandible
9. The thin RO line of cortical bone that radiographically surrounds the periodontal ligament is known as the:
   a. Medullary space
   b. Nutrient canals
   c. Pulp canal

   d. Lamina dura
   e. Mental ridge
10. If the raised portion of the orientation dot is toward the operator when mounting radiographs, the mounting technique that is being employed is known as the:
    a. Curve of Spee mounting technique
    b. Lingual mounting technique
    c. Labial mounting technique
    d. Paralleling mounting technique
    e. Bisecting mounting technique

Radiographic Appearance of Common Anatomic Landmarks

Indicate whether the following anatomic landmarks appear RO or RL on radiographic images by circling the correct answer:

Maxillary Anterior Region
   Nasal septum: RO or RL
   Nasal fossa (nasal cavity): RO or RL
   Floor and walls of the nasal fossa (nasal cavity): RO or RL
   Median palatine suture: RO or RL
   Anterior nasal spine: RO or RL
   Incisive foramen (nasopalatine foramen): RO or RL
   Nasal concha: RO or RL

Maxillary Canine Region
   Inverted/antral Y: RO or RL

Maxillary Posterior Region
   Maxillary sinus: RO or RL
   Floor/walls/septa of the maxillary sinus: RO or RL
   Zygoma (of the maxilla): RO or RL
   Zygomatic arch (of the temporal bone): RO or RL
   Maxillary tuberosity: RO or RL
   Hamular notch: RO or RL
   Hamular process: RO or RL
   Coronoid process of the mandible: RO or RL

Mandibular Anterior (and Canine) Region
   Genial tubercles: RO or RL
   Lingual foramen: RO or RL
   Mental ridges: RO or RL
   Inferior border of the mandible: RO or RL
   Nutrient canals: RO or RL

Mandibular Premolar Region
   Mental foramen: RO or RL
   Inferior border of the mandible: RO or RL

Mandibular Molar Region
   Mandibular canal: RO or RL
   Submandibular (gland) fossa: RO or RL
   External oblique ridge: RO or RL
   Internal oblique ridge (mylohyoid ridge): RO or RL
   Inferior border of the mandible: RO or RL

Bibliography

Iannucci JM, Howerton LJ: *Dental radiography: Principles and techniques*, ed 5, St Louis, MO, 2016, Elsevier Saunders.
White SC, Pharoah MJ: *Oral radiology: Principles and interpretation*, ed 7, St Louis, MO, 2013, Mosby.

20

Principles of Radiographic Interpretation

Introduction

The inclusion of the following five chapters on interpretation in this text is not meant to imply that it is the dental professional's role to make the final radiographic diagnosis but rather to stress that interpretation is only one step in preparing a diagnosis on a patient. This step should be shared by all of the dental clinicians. At present, the final diagnostic role legally rests with the dentist, but certainly help and input from other members of the dental team should be encouraged. The purpose of Chapters 19 through 24 is to give dental professionals some basic understanding of radiographic interpretation, to stimulate interest, and to demonstrate the importance of producing an adequate diagnostic radiograph.

This chapter discusses the main differences between interpreting radiographs and ultimately formulating a definitive diagnosis. The diagnostic questions that the dental professional should ask in devising a differential diagnosis are included in this chapter as well.

Differential Diagnosis

The dictionary defines interpretation as "an explanation" and diagnosis as "the art or act of identifying a disease from its signs and symptoms." The interpretation of radiographs provides the signs or symptoms on which to build a diagnosis. Other signs or symptoms that may be part of a diagnosis are gathered by using the patient's chief complaint, dental and medical history, clinical examination, vitality testing, advanced imaging, biopsy, and laboratory tests. The steps that are to be taken in formulating a definitive diagnosis are: (1) identification of an area or structure that is questionable, (2) interpretation of what has been identified (differential diagnosis), and (3) diagnosis based on the interpretation (definitive diagnosis). Because the role of supportive dental professionals is included in steps 1 and 2, they need to develop interpretive skills to identify all normal anatomic structures, both tooth and bone, and artifacts that may be visible on intraoral, panoramic, and other extraoral radiographs. The dental professional also must be able to differentiate deviations in radiographic form and density from normal structures.

To produce adequate diagnostic films, the dental professional must know what relevant information is being sought from the radiograph. This base of knowledge makes exposing the radiographs a more challenging, interesting, and rewarding process. If dental professionals know how periapical pathologic conditions appear radiographically, they also will understand the necessity of seeing the entire periapical area of the tooth in question to make a proper diagnosis. For example, if dental professionals know how

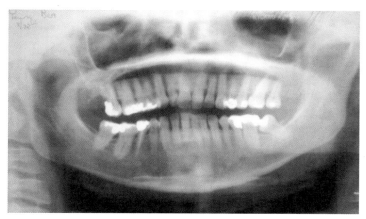

• **Figure 20.1** Panoramic radiograph with third molar impaction.

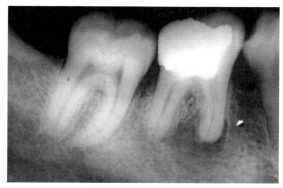

• **Figure 20.2** Pulp capping.

difficult—and, in some cases, how impossible—it is to interpret caries on radiographs with horizontal overlapping of the teeth, they will be motivated to prevent or correct this error in technique to produce adequate diagnostic images.

Diagnostic Questions

There are certain radiographic questions that diagnosticians should ask themselves and be able to answer to help make a proper differential diagnosis. Further analysis of the differential diagnosis will lead to the definitive diagnosis. The list that follows contains questions to gather recommended clinical and radiographic information with which diagnosticians should be familiar.

Preliminary Questions

- What is the patient's chief complaint? Often, this gives important information that helps focus the diagnosis.
- What were the clinical findings that prompted the dental professional to request the radiographs?
- What radiographic projections are available, and what additional images should be ordered? The dental professional should start with the basic intraoral images, and then progress if necessary to an occlusal projection, extraoral radiograph, panoramic view (Fig. 20.1), and finally a cone beam computed tomography (CBCT) scan or, in some cases, a magnetic resonance image (MRI).
- Have periapical and bitewing radiographs been taken recently? Previous images may give a history of treatment (e.g., signs of pulp capping bring periapical pathologic process to the forefront of the diagnostic possibilities; Fig. 20.2).

Questions That Follow the Preliminary Radiographic Examination

- Is a bone or soft tissue pathology suspected?
- What does the vitality test reveal? About 70% of all pathologic conditions seen in the jaws are the result of nonvital teeth and their sequela.

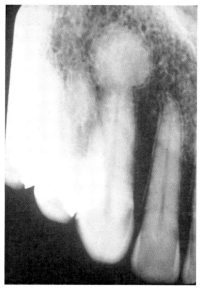

• **Figure 20.3** Radiopaque (RO) lesion.

- Is the lesion radiolucent (RL), radiopaque (RO), or mixed (both RL and RO components; Figs. 20.3 to 20.5)?
- Could the suspected "lesion" be an anatomic landmark (Fig. 20.6)? Landmarks are located in specific areas throughout the oral cavity and are well within normal limits.

HELPFUL HINT

When distinguishing between whether a radiographic finding is an anatomic landmark or a suspicious lesion, it is important to know the radiographic appearance (radiopaque [RO] or radiolucent [RL]) of the anatomic landmarks and their respective locations.

- Where is the lesion located? Is it in the mandible, the maxilla, or elsewhere? Certain lesions are seen more in one jaw than the other or can usually occur in one location (e.g., a nasopalatine cyst; Fig. 20.7).
- Is the lesion a unilateral or bilateral lesion (Fig. 20.8)? Most (but not all) bilateral findings are normal anatomic landmarks.

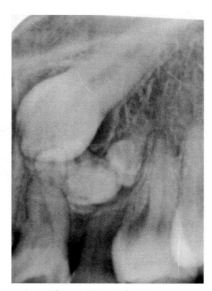

• **Figure 20.4** Mixed lesion.

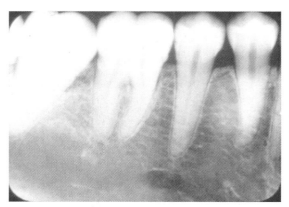

• **Figure 20.6** Normal anatomy.

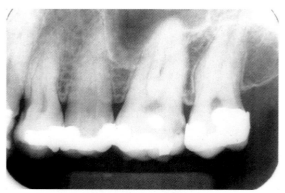

• **Figure 20.5** Radiolucent (RL) lesion.

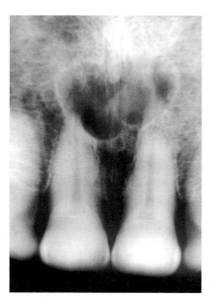

• **Figure 20.7** Nasopalatine cyst.

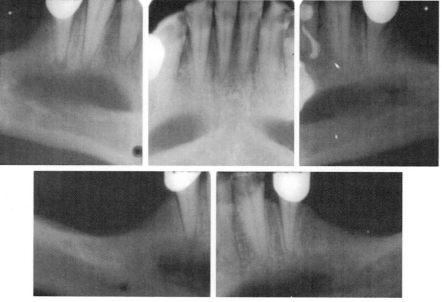

• **Figure 20.8** Bilateral lesion.

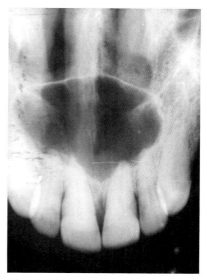

• **Figure 20.9** Lesion with distinct borders.

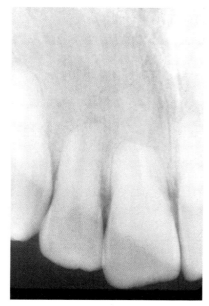

• **Figure 20.11** Root resorption.

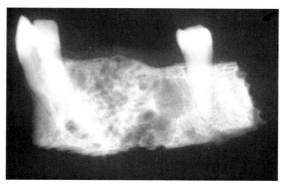

• **Figure 20.10** Multilocular lesion.

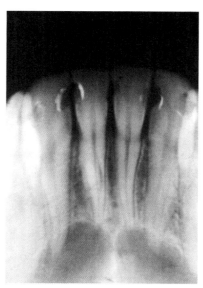

• **Figure 20.12** All the borders of the lesion are not seen.

- What is the size and shape of the lesion (expressed in millimeters)?
- Are the borders of the lesion well defined (Fig. 20.9)? Well-defined lesions are the signs of a benign lesion, whereas poorly defined borders suggest a malignant growth.
- Is the lesion unilocular or multilocular (Fig. 20.10)?
- How has the lesion affected the teeth in the area? Has there been root resorption or root displacement (Fig. 20.11)?
- Can the lesion be seen in the three planes? If not, then further imaging is needed.
- Can all the borders of the lesion be visualized (Fig. 20.12)? If not, then further imaging is necessary.
- If previous images of the lesion are available, what is the rate of growth of the lesion? Certain lesions (e.g.,

malignancies) have rapid growth, whereas cysts and benign lesions grow slowly.
- Have all impacted teeth and edentulous areas been visualized? Just because the area is edentulous does not mean that radiographs are unnecessary. An occult pathologic process may be present.

Chapter Summary

- The dental professional is responsible for exposing and interpreting radiographs. The interpretation will ultimately lead to the formulation of a definitive diagnosis and treatment plan for the patient.

- The three steps that are taken in forming a diagnosis are: (1) identification of an area or structure of concern, (2) radiographic interpretation of what has been identified (differential diagnosis), and (3) a diagnosis based on the radiographic interpretation (definitive diagnosis).

- The lesions that are observed on the radiographic images must be described and documented in terms of their appearance (RO, RL, or mixed), size, and location.

- Dental professionals should be capable of answering the proper diagnostic questions needed to formulate the appropriate diagnosis for their patients.

Chapter Review Questions

Matching

Match the term in Column A with the appropriate description in Column B.

Column A	Column B
1. Unilocular lesion	a. Appears "light" on a radiograph
2. Radiopaque lesion	b. A test used to decide if a tooth is vital or nonvital
3. Bilateral lesion	c. Occurs on one side of the oral cavity
4. Radiolucent lesion	d. Appears light and dark on a radiograph
5. Mixed lesion	e. Has one chamber
6. Multilocular lesion	f. Occurs on both sides of the oral cavity
7. Unilateral lesion	g. Has more than one chamber
8. Vitality test	h. Appears dark on a radiograph

Critical Thinking Exercise

A new patient presents with pain and swelling in the area of tooth #12. The dentist requests that a periapical radiograph of tooth #12 be taken. The image reveals part of a radiolucency at the apex of tooth #12. Upon clinical examination, the dental professional notices exudate coming from the swelling on the buccal surface of tooth #12. List the steps that should be taken in formulating a differential diagnosis of the area of concern. Be sure to include the answers to the following diagnostic questions in your description.

a. What is the patient's chief complaint?
b. What were the clinical findings that prompted the dental professional to request the radiographs?
c. What radiographic projections are available, and what additional images should be ordered?
d. Have periapical and bitewing radiographs been taken recently?
e. Is a bone or soft tissue pathology suspected?
f. What does the vitality test reveal?
g. Is the lesion RL, RO, or mixed?
h. Could the suspected lesion be an anatomic landmark?
i. Where is the lesion located?
j. Is the lesion a unilateral or bilateral lesion?
k. What is the size and shape of the lesion?
l. Are the borders of the lesion well defined?
m. Is the lesion unilocular or multilocular?
n. How has the lesion affected the teeth in the area?
o. Can the lesion be seen in three planes?
p. Can all the borders of the lesion be visualized?

Bibliography

Iannucci JM, Howerton LJ: *Dental radiography: Principles and techniques*, ed 5, St Louis, MO, 2016, Elsevier Saunders.

White SC, Pharoah MJ: *Oral radiology: Principles and interpretation*, ed 7, St Louis, MO, 2013, Mosby.

21
Caries and Periodontal Disease

EDUCATIONAL OBJECTIVES

Upon completing this chapter, the student will be able to:

1. Define the key terms listed at the beginning of the chapter.
2. Discuss the following related to caries:
   - Understand the effect of caries and periodontal disease on the radiographic appearance of teeth and alveolar bone.
   - Recognize caries on radiographs, correlate clinical findings with radiographic findings, differentiate caries from anatomic features and restorative materials, as well as evaluate the extent of the carious lesion.

- Discuss the limitations of radiographs in caries detection.
- List and discuss the conditions that resemble caries on dental radiographs.
3. Discuss the following related to periodontal disease:
   - Identify the signs of periodontal disease on radiographs.
   - Recognize the extent of bone loss and identify the associated predisposing factors.
   - Discuss and list the classifications of periodontal disease.

KEY TERMS

abrasion
advanced caries
attrition
buccal caries
calculus
caries
cementoenamel junction (CEJ)
cervical burnout
composite

crown–root ratio
enamel hypoplasia
erosion
furcation
horizontal bone loss
incipient caries
infrabony pocket
interproximal caries
lingual caries

occlusal caries
open contact
periodontal abscess
periodontal disease
periodontal ligament space
triangulation
vertical bone loss

Introduction

One of the most significant reasons for attaining dental images of a patient's oral cavity is for caries detection. The dental professional should be skilled in identifying caries radiographically. The intention of this chapter is to describe the evidence of caries on radiographs and to discuss dental conditions that can resemble caries on radiographs. This chapter also discusses the importance of dental radiographs in the assessment of periodontal disease, the associated predisposing factors, and the stages of periodontal disease as seen radiographically.

Caries

Before beginning this discussion of caries interpretation, it is imperative to stress that all areas interpreted as caries must be confirmed by clinical examination. Many conditions can resemble caries; simple errors in diagnostic judgment can be prevented by clinical confirmation.

Detection of caries is probably the most common reason for taking dental radiographs. Caries are seen on radiographs as a radiolucency in the crowns and roots of teeth. The caries process is one of demineralization of the hard tooth structure with subsequent destruction. This decrease in density allows greater penetration of the x-rays in the carious area and resultant radiolucency on the dental image. The degree of radiolucency on a given image is determined by the extent of the caries in the buccolingual plane in relation to the density of the overlying tooth structure. Radiographic interpretation of caries can be misleading in regard to relative depth and position in the tooth, as well as differentiation from other radiolucencies. For this reason, technique factors (such as, proper vertical and horizontal angulation) and all of the other factors discussed in Chapter 9 are very important. Caries always are advanced further clinically than the radiographs indicate, because the bacterial penetration of the dentinal tubules and early demineralization do not produce significant changes in density to affect the penetration pattern. As a result, radiographs

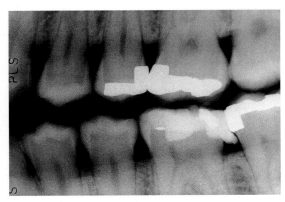

• **Figure 21.1** Bitewing radiograph showing incipient caries on the distal of the maxillary first premolar and the mesial of the maxillary second premolar. Note the temporary filling and excess on the distal of the mandibular first molar.

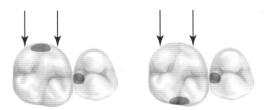

• **Figure 21.2** Buccal and lingual caries and relative effects on object thickness and the penetration of the x-rays when compared with interproximal caries.

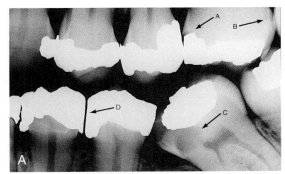

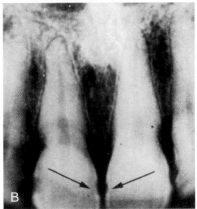

• **Figure 21.3** **A,** Interproximal caries on bitewing radiograph. *A,* Recurrent; *B,* incipient; *C,* advanced; *D,* open contact. **B,** Caries seen on periapical projection of maxillary incisors *(arrows).*

tend to minimize the actual extent of the carious lesions observed. The depth of the caries in relation to the pulp also can be misleading. Because the radiograph portrays a three-dimensional object in two planes, what may seem to be an obvious pulpal exposure radiographically may be the result of superimposition of images or improper horizontal angulation.

Incipient Caries

Caries that have only penetrated halfway through the enamel are called **incipient caries** (Fig. 21.1). This type of caries may be difficult to detect radiographically, because the size and density of the tooth structure have not undergone enough of a change to be radiographically evident. In fact, some clinicians, because of the possibility of remineralization, may elect not to restore these areas and just observe them for further changes.

Most **advanced caries** involving dentin in either the crown or the root of the tooth appear on properly exposed radiographs. However, small, deep occlusal, buccal, or lingual carious lesions may not be seen, because the decrease in density caused by the caries is small compared with the total buccolingual density of the tooth (Fig. 21.2).

Interproximal Caries

It is in the diagnosis of interproximal decay that radiographs are most important. **Interproximal caries** are best seen on

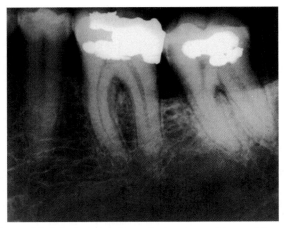

• **Figure 21.4** Periapical radiograph showing caries, mesial second molar.

bitewing radiographs (Fig. 21.3). If the paralleling technique is used, caries also appear clearly and undistorted on well-taken periapical projections (Fig. 21.4). In the bisecting-angle technique, the vertical angulation may distort or even mask interproximal caries. This is especially true of recurrent decay under old restorations. Bitewing radiographs are also useful in detecting poor contact, fit, contour, overhangs, and broken restorations (Fig. 21.5; see Fig. 21.3). To repeat, all of these findings may be obscured because of incorrect horizontal angulation, which results in an overlapped image that does not show the interproximal

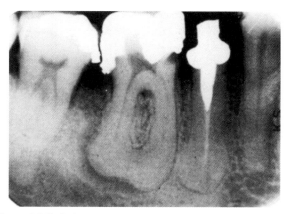

• **Figure 21.5** Caries seen on a periapical radiograph. Note the faulty contour on restorations and periapical radiolucency.

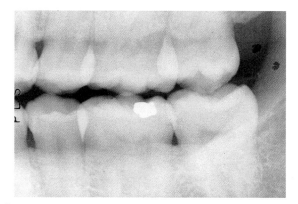

• **Figure 21.6** Bitewing radiographs showing horizontal overlapping.

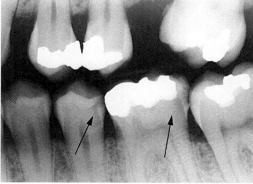

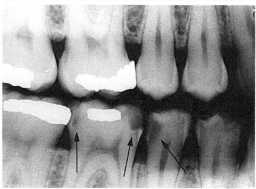

• **Figure 21.7** Interproximal caries *(arrows).*

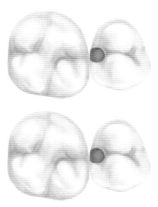

• **Figure 21.8** The effect of contact point on caries interpretation.

surfaces clearly and therefore does not have diagnostic value (Fig. 21.6).

The first radiographic sign of interproximal caries is a notching of the enamel, usually just below the contact point. As the caries progress inward, they assume a shape that resembles a triangle lying on its side with the apex of the triangle toward the dentoenamel junction. As it invades the dentin, the caries spread along the dentoenamel junction and proceed toward the pulp in a roughly triangular pattern (Fig. 21.7).

The radiographic appearance of interproximal caries is affected by the size and shape of the contact of the tooth involved. A tooth with a broad contact point does not show the caries as well as one with a narrow contact point, because of the greater density of the tooth structure surrounding the caries (Fig. 21.8).

Occlusal Caries

A careful clinical examination will detect occlusal caries earlier than radiographic interpretation. The absence of radiographic findings is a result of the superimposition of the dense buccal and lingual cusps on the relatively small carious area in the occlusal pits and fissures. Occlusal caries are not seen radiographically until they have reached the dentoenamel junction, at which point it appears as a

horizontal radiolucent line. As the decay progresses into the dentin, it appears as a diffuse radiolucent area with poorly defined borders. This appearance differentiates it from advanced buccal or lingual decay, which has more defined borders. This radiographic differentiation is always confirmed clinically (Fig. 21.9).

Very often, radiographs of teeth with deep or broad occlusal pits and fissures show radiolucencies that resemble caries. These normal variants can be differentiated by clinical examination.

Buccal and Lingual Caries

Early lesions on buccal and lingual surfaces may be very difficult, if not impossible, to detect radiographically

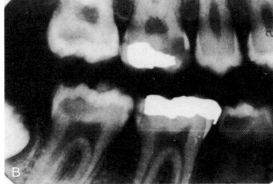

• **Figure 21.9 A,** Occlusal caries in mandibular first molar. **B,** Advanced occlusal caries in maxillary second molar and pulpal exposure in mandibular second molar. List the other carious lesions shown on this image.

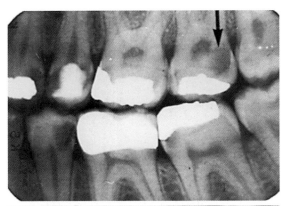

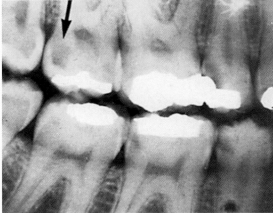

• **Figure 21.10** Buccal caries, as indicated by *arrows*. List the other carious lesions on these images.

because of the superimposition of the densities of normal tooth structures. As the caries progresses, the radiolucency is characterized by its well-defined borders. The differentiation is identified more easily with a thorough clinical examination. It is impossible to judge the relationship of buccal or lingual caries to the pulp on radiographs, because the depth of the caries lies in a geometric plane that is not recorded radiographically (Fig. 21.10).

Conditions Resembling Caries

There are various radiolucencies seen on dental radiographs that may be mistaken for caries. The final diagnosis of caries is always made by corroborating the clinical examination with the radiographic findings.

Cervical Burnout

Cervical burnout appears as a radiolucent band or notches at the neck of the tooth in the area of the cementoenamel junction (CEJ). It is contrasted because the part of the tooth apical to it is covered by bone and hence is more radiopaque, whereas the area of the tooth occlusal to it is covered by enamel and is also radiopaque. In addition to these differences in densities caused by enamel and bone, the concave root contours below the CEJ appear as radiolucencies. Cervical burnout is what some might consider to be an "optical illusion" and is most often observed when there has been no loss of the alveolar bone that provides

the radiographic contrast. It is seen most often in the mandibular incisor and molar areas (Fig. 21.11).

Abrasion, Attrition, Erosion, and Enamel Hypoplasia

Radiographically, cervical abrasion may resemble caries, because it causes a wearing away of root structure and results in a decrease in density in the affected area. The radiolucency produced by the abrasion is usually a well-defined horizontal defect seen at the CEJ. Evidence of secondary dentin formation and pulp recession in response to the irritant also may be seen radiographically.

Attrition, which is defined as occlusal wear on teeth, is easily visualized clinically and radiographically by the absence or thinning of the occlusal enamel and dentin. This loss of tooth material is seen as a radiolucent area (Fig. 21.12).

Erosion of the teeth results from a chemical action not involving bacteria on the tooth surface. Areas of erosion appear as radiolucent defects on the tooth, particularly on the crown of the tooth. The erosive margins may be either well defined or diffuse. A clinical examination usually resolves any questionable lesions when distinguishing them from carious lesions. Enamel hypoplasia can also be confused with a carious lesion on radiographs. Enamel hypoplasia is a defect associated with a reduced thickness of enamel that

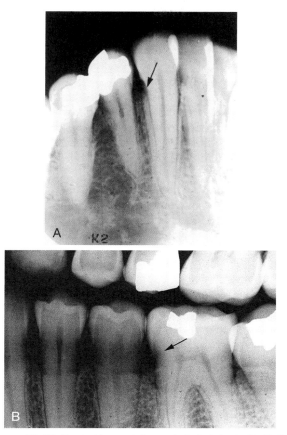

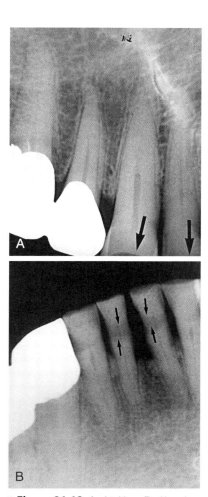

• **Figure 21.11** Cervical burnout *(arrows).* **A,** Anterior teeth. **B,** Posterior teeth.

• **Figure 21.12 A,** Attrition. **B,** Abrasion.

is formed during the developing stages of the enamel. Clinical examination can aid in distinguishing between this enamel defect and caries.

Indirect Pulp Capping

A radiolucent shadow under a metallic restoration may not always indicate recurrent decay but may indicate a previous indirect pulp capping. To avoid a carious pulp exposure in this technique, the last remaining portion of decayed tooth is not excavated. A sedative base and permanent restoration are placed with the hope that secondary dentin will be laid down to protect the pulp and, because of the seal and anaerobic conditions, caries will not progress any further. Radiographically, the indirect pulp-capping procedure shows the radiolucent band of the unexcavated decay near the pulp chamber with a sedative base and permanent restoration (Fig. 21.13).

Restorative Materials

Restorative materials (such as, silicates, acrylics, and some composites) may resemble caries radiographically (Fig. 21.14). Contemporary brands of composite filling material have had radiopaque materials added to their formulation. One can differentiate between caries and the radiolucent filling on the basis of the regular geometric outline of a cavity preparation and the presence of a radiopaque cement

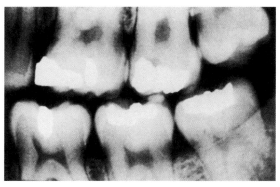

• **Figure 21.13** Indirect pulp capping. Note radiolucent area under restoration in maxillary second molar.

base (Fig. 21.15). However, all base and pulp-capping formulations that have a metallic component (e.g., zinc oxyphosphate, zinc oxide, calcium hydroxide) appear radiopaque (Fig. 21.16).

Periodontal Disease

The proper diagnosis and evaluation of periodontal diseases can be made only with a combination of radiographic

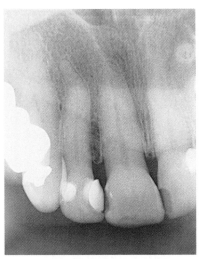

• **Figure 21.14** Radiolucent restorations in central incisors. The mesial and distal surfaces of the lateral incisor have synthetic restorations with radiopaque material added.

and clinical examinations. Periodontal disease has both soft tissue and bony components. There are radiographic limitations in both aspects of the disease process. Soft tissue (gingival) changes (such as, inflammation, hypertrophy, and recession) do not appear on radiographs, because all soft tissue is radiolucent. Bone loss in some areas may not be seen because of superimpositions of buccal and lingual alveolar bone. Dental professionals should remember that the radiograph portrays a three-dimensional disease process in two planes. Radiographic images of bone changes almost always show less bone loss than there is.

Despite these limitations, a proper periodontal diagnosis cannot be made without the appropriate radiographic prescription. Radiographs serve to (1) identify the risk factors, (2) detect early to moderate bone changes for which treatment can preserve the dentition, (3) approximate the amount of bone loss and its location, (4) help in evaluating the prognosis of affected teeth and the restorative needs of these teeth, and (5) serve as baseline data and as a means of evaluating posttreatment results.

Normal Periodontal Structures

To recognize disease, one must know the radiographic appearance of the "normal" anatomy. Periodontal anatomic structures identifiable on radiographs include supporting structures, such as the lamina dura, alveolar bone, periodontal ligament space, and cementum (see Fig. 19.6).

The normal crest of interproximal bone runs parallel to a line drawn between the CEJs on adjoining teeth at a level 1 to 1.5 mm apical to the CEJ (Fig. 21.17). The shape of the alveolar crest is primarily determined by the contact area of adjacent teeth and the shape of the CEJ. The alveolar crest is flatter in the posterior areas and more convex and pointed in the anterior regions. The interdental bone septum can be narrow in cases of close root proximity. In some patients, the roots of adjacent teeth are so close that there may be little to no cancellous bone present.

The lamina dura is seen radiographically as a thin radiopaque line surrounding the entire root and is continuous with the alveolar crest. The lamina dura represents the

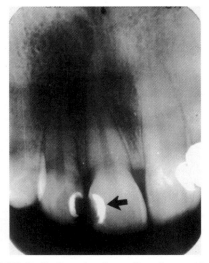

• **Figure 21.15** Synthetic restorations with radiopaque bases *(arrow)*.

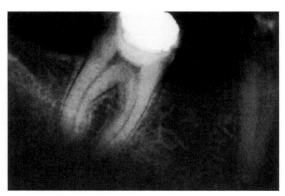

• **Figure 21.16** Radiopaque base and pulpotomy under metallic restoration.

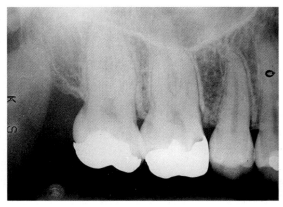

• **Figure 21.17** Ideal level of interseptal bone.

alveolar bone that lines the tooth socket. It may not be visible in all radiographs.

The periodontal ligament fibers traverse from the cementum to the alveolar bone. Because these fibers are soft tissue, they are not seen on radiographs, but the space that the fibers occupy is seen and referred to as the periodontal ligament space. Evaluating the width of the periodontal ligament space is an important part of a periodontal radiographic examination. The normal ligament space is about 0.5 mm. For example, in situations of occlusal trauma, an increase in the size of the periodontal ligament space is often seen.

Techniques

The paralleling technique with an appropriate target-receptor (focal-film) distance is the best method for evaluating periodontal disease. A full periapical survey taken in this manner and augmented by posterior, anterior, or vertical bitewings is the technique of choice. Vertical bitewings are especially useful for detecting bone loss of 5 mm or more radiographically.

The use of the bisecting technique with its inherent dimensional distortion provides a distorted representation of the level of bone present (see Fig. 10.11) and is not recommended for periodontal radiographic examinations.

Panoramic images are of some value in the diagnosis of periodontal disease, especially in the most advanced cases. However, panoramic projections should only be used if intraoral projections cannot be taken, because panoramic images do not have the detail and definition to evaluate periodontal disease, especially in the early stages of the disease.

Risk Factors in Periodontal Disease

The detection of local risk factors is one of the most important roles of radiography in periodontal disease. The management or prevention of early periodontal disease is much easier and has a higher success rate than efforts made once the disease has progressed. The detection and elimination of local irritants are essential steps in prevention or actual periodontal therapy. Reducing local risk factors increases the host response to disease.

Calculus

Both subgingival and supragingival calculi are the most common of all local irritants. Early deposits, small and not fully calcified, are not seen radiographically. Even when calcified, supragingival calculus, which is seen most often on the lingual surface of lower anterior teeth and the buccal surface of upper molars, is not seen clearly in its early stage because of superimposition of tooth structure (Fig. 21.18). Subgingival calculus on the proximal surfaces is detected more easily than supragingival calculus, although both are not easily observed in the early calcified stages. The calculus appears as an irregularly pointed radiopaque projection from the proximal tooth surfaces (Fig. 21.19). Horizontal

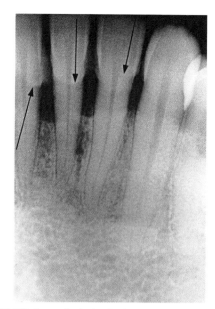

• **Figure 21.18** Supragingival calculus on lingual surfaces of lower incisors.

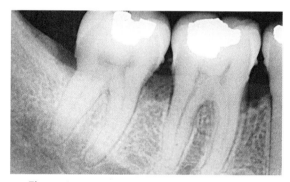

• **Figure 21.19** Subgingival calculus. Note bone loss.

bitewing radiographs are most helpful in discerning interproximal calculus in the posterior areas or vertical bitewings in the anterior or posterior areas.

> **NOTE**
>
> The dental professional should be aware of the radiographic limitations of characterizing subgingival and/or supragingival calculus by radiographs alone, because the gingival components are not visible on radiographs. For example, if a patient has advanced gingival recession clinically, calculus on the proximal root surface may appear to be subgingival on radiographic images but upon clinical examination can be found to actually be supragingival calculus deposits.

Restorations

Radiographic examination reveals restorations with open contacts, poor contours, overhanging and deficient margins, and caries, all of which are significant risk factors in periodontal disease (Figs. 21.20 to 21.22).

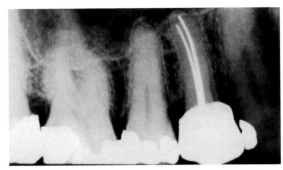

• **Figure 21.20** Overcontoured crown on premolar and bone response.

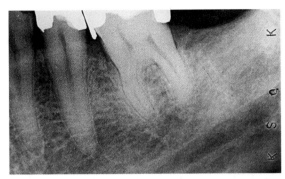

• **Figure 21.21** Restoration with open contact and overhang. Note the bony response.

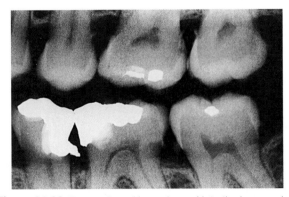

• **Figure 21.22** Restoration with overhang. Note the heavy calculus formation in other areas.

Anatomic Configurations

Only through radiographic examination can information about the size, shape, and position of the roots and the bone level of periodontally involved teeth be obtained. These factors are important in evaluating the present condition and planning periodontal and restorative therapy.

The crown–root ratio refers to the length of root surface embedded in bone compared with the length of the rest of the tooth. The greater the length of the tooth embedded in bone, the better the prognosis (Fig. 21.23). This becomes a critical factor when designing both fixed and removable prostheses.

Teeth that have an anatomically short root have a poorer prognosis periodontally than teeth with long roots. Teeth

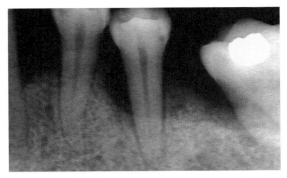

• **Figure 21.23** Unfavorable crown–root ratio.

with bulbous roots have more area for attachment than those with fine, tapered roots. In multirooted teeth, the space between the roots is important; teeth with widely spaced roots have a better periodontal prognosis. Adjacent teeth whose roots are close together have a poorer prognosis than those with adequate areas of interseptal bone.

Stages of Periodontal Disease

The classification system for periodontal disease was last revised in 1999. This framework classifies periodontal disease based on the amount of bone loss that can be identified radiographically as initially devised by the joint efforts of the American Dental Association (ADA) and the American Academy of Periodontology (AAP). The classifications are as follows: gingivitis (type I), mild or slight periodontitis (type II), moderate periodontitis (type III), and advanced or severe periodontitis (type IV).

Gingivitis (Type I)

Because gingivitis is a soft tissue change, there are no radiographic findings other than the presence of predisposing factors. Existing periodontal pockets, if there is no bone loss, will not be seen. Postoperative radiographs of extended surgery only show the new bone level and do not indicate healthy tissue and lack of pocket depth. Among the risk factors for gingivitis are medications that may cause gingival hyperplasia and inflammation (e.g., phenytoin [Dilantin], antiepileptic or anticonvulsant drug).

Mild or Slight Periodontitis (Type II)

The early stage of periodontal change is characterized radiographically by changes in the crest of the interproximal bone septum and triangulation of the periodontal membrane. Triangulation is the widening of the periodontal membrane space at the crest of the interproximal septum that gives the appearance of a radiolucent triangle to what is normally a radiolucent band. As mentioned earlier, the normal crest of the interseptal bone runs parallel to a line drawn between CEJs on adjoining teeth at a level 1 to 1.5 mm below the CEJ. The crest of the septa normally has a distinct radiopaque border. Fading of the density of the crest with cup-shaped defects appears in the early

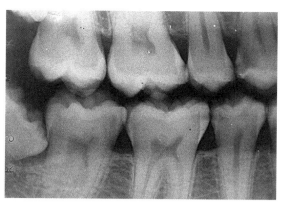

• **Figure 21.24** Early periodontal bone loss. Note the fading of density of the alveolar crest, slight cupping, and triangulation.

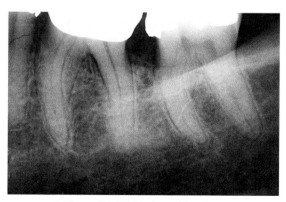

• **Figure 21.25** Moderate to advanced bone loss showing bifurcation involvement.

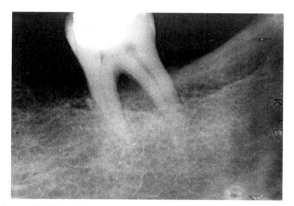

• **Figure 21.26** Horizontal bone loss.

stages of periodontal disease (Fig. 21.24) and is known as cupping.

Moderate Periodontitis (Type III)

In the moderate stages, bone loss shows up in both the horizontal and vertical planes. Radiolucencies appear in the furcations of multirooted teeth, indicating bone loss in these critical areas (Fig. 21.25). Horizontal bone loss is resorption that occurs in a plane parallel to a line drawn between the CEJs on adjoining teeth (Fig. 21.26). In vertical bone

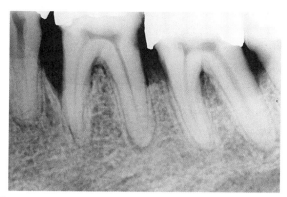

• **Figure 21.27** Vertical and horizontal bone loss. Note the early bifurcation involvement on the second molar.

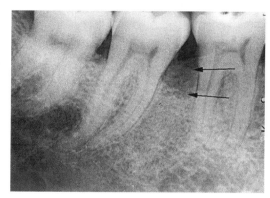

• **Figure 21.28** Different levels of buccal and lingual bone, as indicated by *arrows*.

loss, the resorption on one tooth root sharing the septum is greater than on the other tooth, the so-called infrabony pocket (Fig. 21.27). In this stage, the horizontal bone loss on the buccal or lingual surfaces may go undetected because of superimposition. Careful examination of the radiograph may reveal a difference in density, indicating different levels of bone on the buccal and lingual surfaces (Fig. 21.28).

Advanced or Severe Periodontitis (Type IV)

The advanced stage of periodontal disease is easily identified radiographically by the advanced vertical and horizontal bone loss, furcation involvement, thickened periodontal membranes, and indications of changes in tooth position (Figs. 21.29 and 21.30).

Periodontal Abscess

The radiographic signs of a periodontal abscess vary greatly. This diagnosis is dictated by an acute clinical manifestation. A periodontal abscess is caused by the blockage of an existing pocket; therefore, the radiograph of the acute episode may not differ greatly from previous images of the existing condition that produced the pocket. In other instances, there may be signs of rapid and extensive bone destruction (Fig. 21.31).

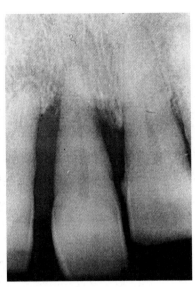

• **Figure 21.29** Advanced periodontal bone loss.

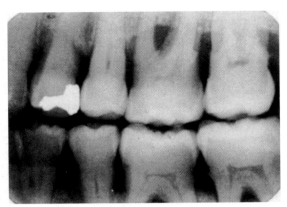

• **Figure 21.30** Trifurcation bone loss, upper first molar; bifurcation bone loss, lower first and second molars.

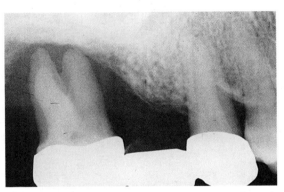

• **Figure 21.31** Periodontal abscess. Patient had acute buccal swelling and facial edema.

Chapter Summary

- Dental radiographs have significant diagnostic value in the identification of dental caries and periodontal disease.
- Radiographic evidence of caries should be confirmed by clinical examination. Both of these diagnostic processes are integral components of a definitive diagnosis and treatment plan.
- Radiographic examinations have both limitations and value in the identification of different types of carious lesions, including incipient caries, interproximal caries, occlusal caries, and buccal/lingual caries.
- Conditions that can resemble caries radiographically include cervical burnout, abrasion, attrition, erosion, enamel hypoplasia, synthetic restorations, and pulp capping.
- The identification of periodontal disease is reliant on both an equally effective radiographic and clinical examination.

- The limitations of a radiographic examination in the diagnosis of periodontal disease include a failure to view soft tissue structures involved in periodontal disease, the representation of only two dimensions of a three-dimensional structure or lesion, and the superimposition of the buccal and lingual alveolar bone.
- The risk factors for periodontal disease that can be identified radiographically include the presence of calculus, ill-fitting restorations, and various anatomic configurations of the roots of the periodontally involved areas in a patient's oral cavity.
- The classification of periodontal disease consists of four case types that include gingivitis, early bone loss, moderate bone loss, and advanced or severe bone loss.

Chapter Review Questions

Multiple Choice

1. The interproximal radiolucent lesions that the *arrows* are pointing to on the accompanying bitewing radiograph are identified as:

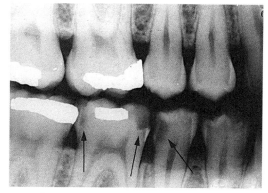

   a. Buccal caries
   b. Interproximal caries
   c. Horizontal bone loss
   d. Interproximal calculus
   e. Lingual caries

2. The bone loss between the roots of tooth #19 is specifically known as:

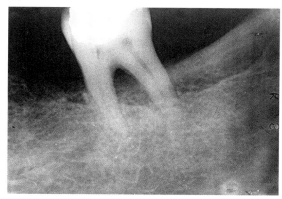

   a. Trifurcation involvement
   b. Horizontal bone loss
   c. Vertical bone loss
   d. Periapical bone loss
   e. Bifurcation involvement

3. The radiopaque calcified deposit on the mesial of tooth #30 and tooth #31 is identified as:

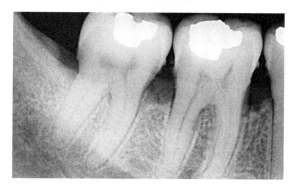

   a. An enamel pearl
   b. A denticle
   c. An overhang
   d. Interproximal calculus
   e. Gutta percha

4. The bone loss on the mesial of tooth #19 is classified as:

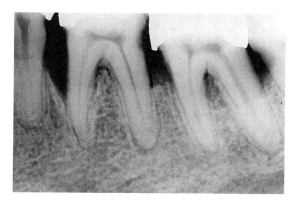

   a. Vertical bone loss
   b. Horizontal bone loss
   c. Medullary bone loss
   d. Trifurcation bone loss
   e. Cervical burnout

5. The radiolucencies on the distal of tooth #8 and mesial of tooth #9 are:

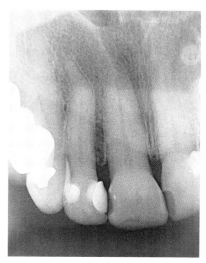

   a. Base materials
   b. Synthetic restorations
   c. Interproximal caries
   d. Gold restorations
   e. Amalgam restorations

6. As for periodontal prognosis, teeth that have tapered roots will:
   a. Be more resistant to caries
   b. Have a better prognosis
   c. Have a poorer prognosis
   d. Be less resistant to caries
   e. None of the above

Critical Thinking Exercise

1. A patient presents to the periodontal office where you are currently employed. The patient was referred by her general dentist's practice to receive a periodontal examination and consultation. The patient did not bring previously exposed radiographs with her. The patient has not had radiographs taken in more than 5 years. The patient presents with 6- to 8-mm pockets and appears to exhibit mobility on three of the posterior teeth. You are responsible for providing the sequence of care that is outlined for this patient. Be sure to include the following procedures and reasons for the procedures in your presentation:

   a. Clinical examination
   b. Radiographic prescription
   c. Radiographic evaluation
   d. Evaluation of the risk factors for periodontal disease that are present in the patient's mouth
   e. The apparent stage of the patient's periodontal disease

Bibliography

Armitage GC: Development of a classification system for periodontal diseases and conditions, *Ann Periodontol* 4(1):1–6, 1999.

Iannucci JM, Howerton LJ: *Dental radiography: Principles and techniques*, ed 5, St Louis, MO, 2016, Elsevier Saunders.

White SC, Pharoah MJ: *Oral radiology: Principles and interpretation*, ed 7, St Louis, MO, 2013, Mosby.

22

Pulpal and Periapical Lesions

EDUCATIONAL OBJECTIVES

Upon completing this chapter, the student will be able to:

1. Define the key terms listed at the beginning of the chapter.
2. Discuss the following related to pulpal lesions:
   - Discuss the role of dental radiographic images in the identification of pulpal lesions.
   - Describe the normal radiographic anatomic features of the pulp chamber and pulp canals, and state the significance of knowing how these normal structures appear radiographically.
   - State the appearance and identifiable characteristics of pulp denticles (or "pulp stones") and pulpitis.
3. Discuss the following related to periapical lesions:
   - Discuss the role of dental radiographic images in the identification of periapical lesions.

- State the appearance and identifiable characteristics of periapical cysts, periapical granulomas, periapical abscesses, periapical condensing osteitis, residual cysts, residual granulomas, internal resorption, and external resorption.
4. Discuss the three types of cemento-osseous dysplasias (CODs), including how they appear on radiographic images and where they generally appear in the oral cavity in addition to what demographic group is usually affected by these conditions.

KEY TERMS

calcification
cemento-osseous dysplasia (COD)
dentoalveolar abscess (dental abscess)
external resorption
florid cemento-osseous dysplasia
   (FLCOD)
focal cemento-osseous dysplasia
   (FCOD)

internal resorption
periapical cemento-osseous dysplasia
   (PCOD)
periapical condensing osteitis
periapical cyst
periapical granuloma
periapical lesions
pulp calcification

pulp denticle (pulp stone)
residual cyst
residual granuloma
residual periapical lesions
root resorption
secondary dentin

Introduction

Dental images are integral in the identification and evaluation of pulpal and periapical lesions. This chapter discusses various pulpal and periapical lesions, focusing on their radiographic appearance and discussing additional information about their other significant characteristics for the dental professional.

Pulpal Lesions

The most commonly seen pathologic condition after caries and periodontal disease is pulpal necrosis and subsequent periapical bone lesions. In fact, most pulpal and periapical lesions are the sequelae of caries, trauma, infrabony lesions, and advanced periodontal disease.

Anatomy

As shown in Chapter 19, the pulp chambers and pulp canals of teeth are seen radiographically as radiolucent areas, because they contain noncalcified material and are hence less dense than the tooth structure that surrounds them (Fig. 22.1). High-pulp horns and large-pulp chambers can occur in all age groups, not just in young patients in whom these findings are characteristic. The normal size and shape of the pulp chamber and canals change with age, in certain developmental anomalies, and in response to local irritants. The radiographic densities of pulp chambers and canals differ because of size, position in the tooth, and radiographic angulation, but not because of vitality. Gradual reduction in the size and shape of the pulp chamber and canal is marked by the deposition of secondary dentin at the walls of the

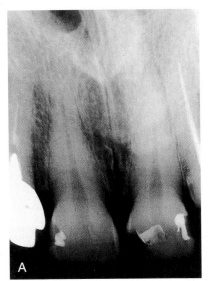

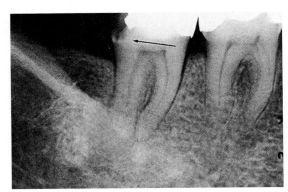

• **Figure 22.3** Secondary dentin formation in second molar *(arrow)* in response to caries and restoration.

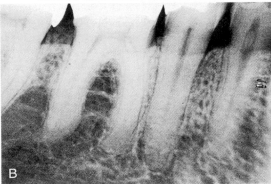

• **Figure 22.1** Normal pulp chambers in anterior **(A)** and posterior teeth **(B).** Note the different shapes and densities and the presence of a pulp denticle in the first premolar.

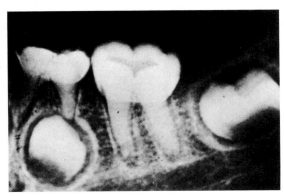

• **Figure 22.4** Dentinogenesis imperfecta. Note the early calcification of the pulp chamber and canals.

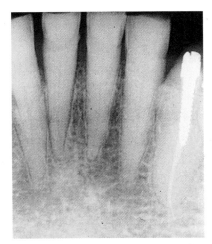

• **Figure 22.2** Pulp chambers receded with age. Secondary dentin formation.

chamber and canals and the appearance on radiographs of a radiopacity to replace the radiolucent area (Fig. 22.2). Radiographically, secondary and regular dentin appear the same and can only be differentiated by the changes in the shape of the chamber and canals that accompany

aging. The formation of secondary dentin with the resulting obliteration or narrowing of the pulp chamber and canals can be caused by different types of irritants. The most common causes are deep caries, pulp capping, deep-seated restorations, attrition, abrasion, and a healed tooth fracture (Fig. 22.3). This decrease in pulp and root chamber size also can be seen in the developmental disturbances dentinogenesis imperfecta and dentinal dysplasia (Fig. 22.4).

Pulp Calcifications
Radiographic Appearance/Characteristics

Pulp denticles or pulp stones are calcifications that appear as well-defined radiopacities within the pulp chamber (Fig. 22.5). A radiolucent line may be seen separating the stone from the pulpal wall and may give the appearance of a "free-floating" denticle, but it is actually attached to the floor or wall of the chamber. The stones, which are composed of either dentin or calcified salts, have the density and appearance of dentin. Other than blocking endodontic access, pulp calcifications have no clinical significance and do not cause pulp strangulation, as was once thought.

Pulpitis
Radiographic Appearance/Characteristics

There are no radiographic signs of pulpitis in the pulp chamber. Normal, inflamed, or necrotic pulp all appear the same, because their densities are the same. The only possible

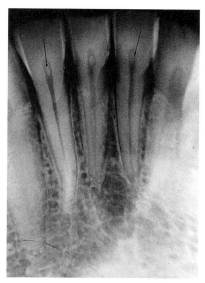

• **Figure 22.5** Pulp stones in lower incisors.

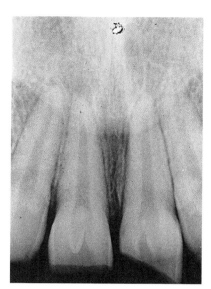

• **Figure 22.7** Fractured crowns of maxillary central incisors. Note the proximity of the fracture lines to the pulp chambers.

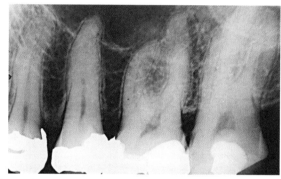

• **Figure 22.6** Pulpitis with no apical changes. The second premolar was acutely sensitive to thermal stimulation and found to be partially nonvital.

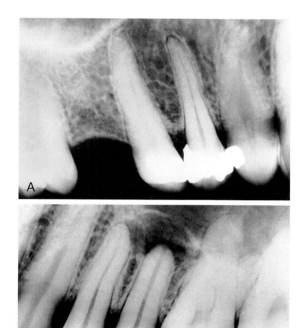

• **Figure 22.8** **A,** Thickened periodontal membrane and early apical bone change on maxillary first bicuspid. **B,** Early apical bone resorption.

radiographic findings related to pulpitis are the causative factors, such as caries, pulp exposure, tooth fracture, previous pulp capping, or deep restorations (Fig. 22.6). The pulps of teeth may appear to vary in radiographic density. This is not because of differences in vitality, but because of the differences in object density of the overlying tooth structure.

Periapical Lesions

Periapical Pathologic Conditions

Radiographic Appearance/Characteristics

Periapical lesions are seen in the apical tissues surrounding the tooth after the pulp has become necrotic. The periodontal membrane, lamina dura, and alveolar bone are the affected tissues. This necrosis, or degeneration of the pulp, may be a result of carious invasion of the pulp, tooth fracture, and physical or chemical trauma (Fig. 22.7). The exudate from the pulp first spills into the periodontal ligament, causing a thickening that can be seen radiographically. The pressure then causes resorption of the lamina dura

and alveolar bone (Fig. 22.8). Depending on certain factors, a cyst, granuloma, or dentoalveolar abscess may develop at this point. If the exudate reacts with some residual epithelial rests, then a periapical cyst will form. The strength and type of bacteria and the tissue resistance determine whether a granuloma or abscess will develop. It is almost impossible to differentiate radiographically between a periapical granuloma and a periapical cyst (Figs. 22.9 and 22.10).

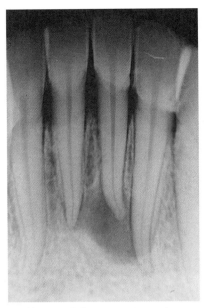

• **Figure 22.9** Periapical granuloma.

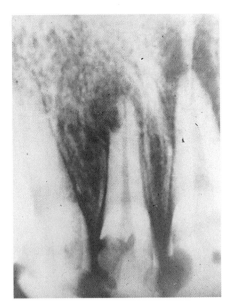

• **Figure 22.11** Dentoalveolar abscess.

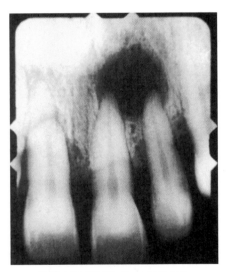

• **Figure 22.10** Periapical cyst.

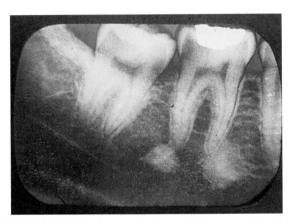

• **Figure 22.12** Periapical condensing osteitis on mesial and distal roots of the first molar.

The **dentoalveolar abscess (dental abscess)** may cause root resorption and a more diffuse radiolucency (Fig. 22.11). If present, a fistulous tract leading from the abscess to the oral cavity is very difficult to see on radiographs because of its tortuous course through the bone. It would only be evident if the fistulous tract and the central ray were in the same cross-sectional plane. Furthermore, clinical evidence of a dental abscess including pain, swelling, and exudate may be present.

Periapical Condensing Osteitis
Radiographic Appearance/Characteristics

Periapical condensing osteitis is recognized by the formation of dense bone around the apex of a tooth in response to low-grade pulpal necrosis. This radiopaque asymptomatic condition is seen most often at, but is not limited to, the mandibular premolar and molar apices (Fig. 22.12). In almost all cases, the teeth are shown to be nonvital through pulp testing. Although the condition may be asymptomatic, it should be considered a radiopaque type of periapical pathologic condition and treated accordingly, with either root canal therapy or extraction.

Residual Periapical Lesions
Radiographic Appearance/Characteristics

Residual periapical lesions are radiolucencies that appear in edentulous areas of either the maxilla or the mandible. They represent pathologic areas that arose from teeth extracted in the area. If a granuloma or cyst that surrounds the apex of a nonvital tooth is not curetted out at the time of extraction, it may remain, grow, and destroy bone or move and possibly devitalize teeth. Such a lesion is considered either a **residual cyst** or **residual granuloma** (Figs. 22.13 and 22.14). Residual periapical lesions are quite common and are always considered in a diagnosis of an infrabony lesion.

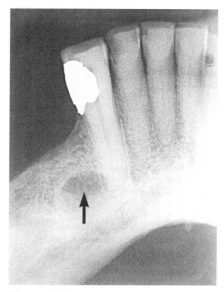

• **Figure 22.13** Residual cyst of the mandible.

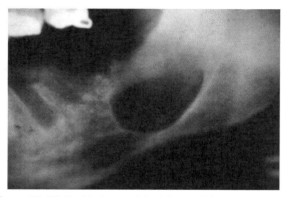

• **Figure 22.14** Residual cyst of the left mandible seen on a portion of a panoramic film.

Root Resorption

Root resorption can be caused by chronic periapical or periodontal infection, trauma, pressure from tumors or cysts, or rapid excessive orthodontic pressure, or it can be idiopathic (i.e., an unknown cause; Figs. 22.15 to 22.18). In a differential diagnosis, it is important to distinguish between smooth (cysts, tumors) and rough (infection, trauma) root resorption.

Internal Resorption
Radiographic Appearance/Characteristics

The cause of the destructive process known as internal resorption (Fig. 22.19) is unknown. The pulpal tissue resorbs the dentin surrounding the pulp chamber or canal and eventually perforates to the periodontal ligament. The radiographic findings of internal resorption are irregularities and widening of the usually smooth, tapered outline of the root chamber. In advanced cases, the irregular outline of the resorption can be seen perforating the root structures and reaching the periodontal ligament.

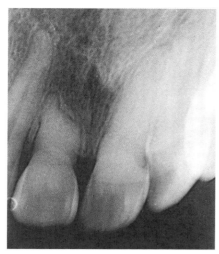

• **Figure 22.15** Root resorption resulting from trauma.

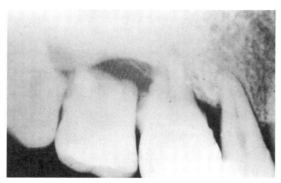

• **Figure 22.16** Root resorption resulting from chronic periodontal infection.

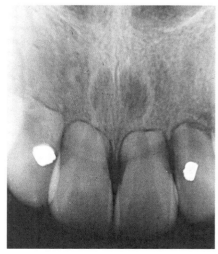

• **Figure 22.17** Root resorption resulting from excessive and rapid orthodontic movement.

External Resorption
Radiographic Appearance/Characteristics

The cause of external resorption is also unknown. In this case (Fig. 22.20), the cells of the periodontal ligament resorb the cementum and dentin of the root or pulp chambers

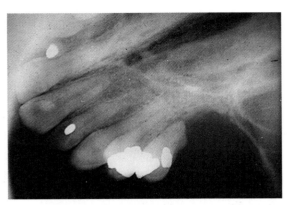

• **Figure 22.18** Root resorption resulting from a malignant tumor.

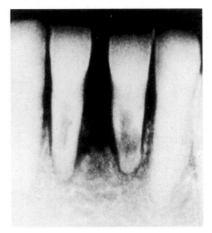

• **Figure 22.19** Internal root resorption.

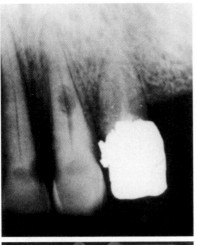

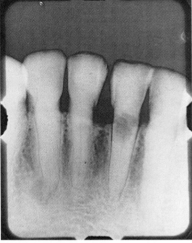

• **Figure 22.20** External root resorption in maxillary and mandibular anterior teeth.

to reach the pulp. Radiographically, teeth with external resorption have a round or oval radiolucency lateral to or superimposed over the pulp canal. If it is superimposed, the outline of the normal canal can be seen through the superimposition. If the radiolucency is lateral to the pulp canal, it can be seen leading from the periodontal ligament. It does not affect the pulp canal in its early stages; however, it perforates into the pulp canal and devitalizes the pulp tissue in its later stages.

Cemento-Osseous Dysplasia

Cemento-osseous dysplasia (COD) is a condition of the jaws that is inherently a benign lesion. It arises from the fibroblasts of the periodontal ligaments.

> **NOTE**
> These conditions frequently affect middle-aged African-American females but are certainly not limited to this demographic group.

There are three types of COD:

1. Periapical cemento-osseous dysplasia (PCOD), which is also known as periapical cemental dysplasia (PCD; Fig. 22.21).

Radiographic appearance/characteristics: PCOD (PCD) is a three-stage lesion that is asymptomatic and self-limiting and for which no treatment is indicated. It is found in the apical region of vital mandibular anterior (canine-to-canine) teeth and originates in the periodontal membrane of the tooth. In its first stage, it is radiolucent and resembles periapical disease. The second stage is mixed (radiolucent and radiopaque), because the radiolucent lesion starts to calcify. In its third stage, it is totally radiopaque. Clinically, the teeth always test vital, and in all cases no treatment is indicated. PCOD (PCD) must be differentiated from periapical pathologic conditions and condensing osteitis by vitality testing.

2. Focal cemento-osseous dysplasia (FCOD) is a condition similar to PCOD but occurs in the posterior mandible, distal to the canines. It usually occurs as a single-site lesion.

3. Florid cemento-osseous dysplasia (FLCOD) is also considered a type of COD but can occur in both maxilla and mandible and in multiple quadrants.

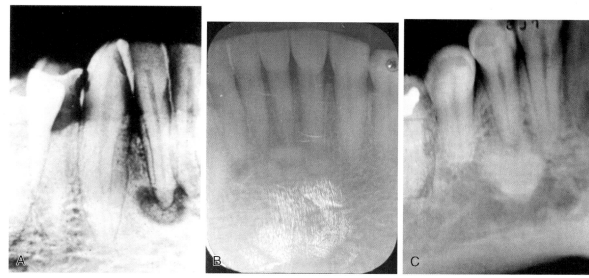

• **Figure 22.21** **A,** First-stage periapical cemento-osseous dysplasia (COD) resembling periapical disease. **B,** Second-stage (mixed) radiolucent lesion starting to calcify. **C,** Third-stage radiopaque area surrounding the tooth apex. All teeth test vital in all stages.

Chapter Summary

- Identification of deviations from the normal appearance of the pulp chamber, pulp canal, and the surrounding periapical supportive structures is an important function of dental radiographic images.
- Pulpal calcifications, such as pulp stones (pulp denticles), are recognized solely by radiographic examination. Clinical examination will not reveal calcifications in the pulp of a tooth. Pulpitis itself cannot be seen radiographically; however, the causative factors of pulpal inflammation, such as caries, can be seen on dental images.
- The differentiation between periapical cysts and granulomas cannot be made radiographically. A dentoalveolar abscess appears differently on radiographs than periapical

cysts and granulomas, and clinical signs and symptoms of an abscess may also be present.
- Periapical lesions on radiographs can appear radiopaque, radiolucent, or they may have a combination of both radiopaque and radiolucent components and thus may be considered "mixed lesions." These periapical lesions include periapical condensing osteitis, residual cysts, residual granulomas, and the three types of CODs.
- External and internal resorptions both appear radiolucent on dental images, because they are resorptive processes that, although both radiolucent, are specifically identified by their radiographic characteristics and location on the teeth that they affect.

Chapter Review Questions

State whether the following pulpal and periapical lesions appear radiolucent (RL), radiopaque (RO), or "mixed" on dental radiographic images. If the lesion does not appear RL, RO, or "mixed" on radiographs, please classify it as not applicable (NA).
1. PCOD stage 2
2. Periapical granuloma
3. Periapical condensing osteitis
4. External root resorption
5. PCOD stage 3
6. Periapical cyst
7. Residual granuloma
8. Pulpitis
9. Dentoalveolar abscess
10. Pulp denticles
11. PCOD stage 1
12. Residual cyst

Critical Thinking Exercise

A 50-year-old female African-American patient presents to a dental facility for a routine dental examination. The patient's radiation history and risk factors for dental diseases are determined, and the appropriate radiographic prescription is advised. The patient does not have any clinical signs or symptoms of any dental-related issues in the mandibular anterior region. Upon viewing the radiographs that were respectively prescribed, the dental professional notices multiple radiolucent lesions in the periapical region of the mandibular central and lateral incisors. Discuss the steps that the dental professional would take in formulating a differential and definitive diagnosis of these radiographic lesions. Please include the following in your discussion:

a. Describe the lesions as being radiolucent (RL), radiopaque (RO), or "mixed."
b. Describe the location of the lesions.
c. State the results of a clinical examination of this area.
d. State whether there was evidence of caries in the area of concern.
e. State the significance of the "positive" vitality test on the four teeth involved.
f. Present your conclusion based on the information given and your knowledge of pulpal and periapical lesions as seen on dental images.

Bibliography

Iannucci JM, Howerton LJ: *Dental radiography: Principles and techniques*, ed 5, St Louis, MO, 2016, Elsevier Saunders.

White SC, Pharoah MJ: *Oral radiology: Principles and interpretation*, ed 5, St Louis, MO, 2004, Mosby.
White SC, Pharoah MJ: *Oral radiology: Principles and interpretation*, ed 7, St Louis, MO, 2013, Mosby.

23

Developmental Disturbances of Teeth and Bone

EDUCATIONAL OBJECTIVES

Upon completing this chapter, the student will be able to:

1. Define the key terms listed at the beginning of the chapter.
2. Understand the formation and radiographic appearance of developmental lesions of the teeth and surrounding bone, as well as recognize developmental lesions of the teeth and bone on dental images and know which radiographic projections are necessary to formulate a diagnosis.

KEY TERMS

amelogenesis imperfecta
anodontia
cleft
concrescence
cyst
deciduous teeth
dens invaginatus (dens en dente)
dental papilla
dentinogenesis imperfecta
dentigerous cyst (follicular cyst)
dilaceration
distodens (distomolar, paramolar, or fourth molar)

enamel pearls (enameloma)
fissural cysts
follicle (dental sac)
fusion
gemination
globulomaxillary cyst
hypercementosis
hypodontia
impaction
malposed
median palatine cyst
mesiodens
mixed dentition

nasopalatine cyst
oligodontia
overretention
primordial cyst
supernumerary teeth (hyperdontia)
taurodontia (taurodontism)
tooth eruption
transposed

Introduction

The recognition of developmental conditions of the teeth and surrounding bone is an important part of the dental professional's diagnostic responsibility. Most of the lesions can be detected radiographically, and their early recognition can prevent further problems. The most common conditions are discussed in this chapter. There are many developmental conditions that are linked to systemic problems; an atlas or textbook discussing these lesions will complement the material presented here.

Tooth Development (Odontogenesis)

The developing tooth can be seen at all stages on radiographs. The tooth germ (Fig. 23.1) before calcification appears as a round or oval radiolucency in the body of the maxilla or mandible. As crown formation progresses, the radiolucent follicle (dental sac) is seen surrounding the crown of the

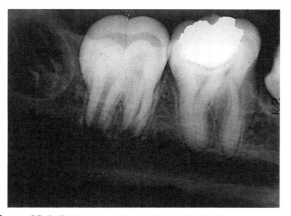

• **Figure 23.1** Tooth germ of mandibular third molar.

tooth (Fig. 23.2). After the tooth erupts, the dental papilla appears at the forming apices (Fig. 23.3).

Radiographic examination by either an intraoral series or panoramic projections (extraoral projections) is essential in determining the progress and pattern of tooth eruption

(Figs. 23.4 and 23.5). In this manner, conditions such as premature loss of primary teeth, anodontia, hypodontia, over-retained teeth, ankylosis, tumors, and supernumerary teeth, which can affect the eruption pattern, can be identified (Figs. 23.6 and 23.7).

Eruption of Teeth

Periapical radiographs of patients, generally up to age 12 years, reveal some evidence of a mixed dentition (both primary and secondary teeth are present). The permanent teeth (secondary teeth) or tooth buds are seen apical to the deciduous teeth (primary teeth) that they will replace (Figs. 23.8 and 23.9). The first, second, and third permanent molars, which have no deciduous predecessors, also can be seen in various stages of formation (Fig. 23.10). The force of the erupting permanent tooth causes resorption of the deciduous roots, with resulting loosening and loss of the tooth (Fig. 23.11). If root formation is not complete, a radiolucent area may appear around the root tip. This radiolucency is the dental root sack and should not be confused with periapical pathologic conditions (Fig. 23.12). There is a range of ±9 months in the normal development and eruption time of the dentition. Systemic diseases, such as hypopituitarism and hypothyroidism, can cause delayed development. Other diseases, such as cleidocranial dysostosis, can cause overretention of the primary teeth and postponed permanent tooth eruption (Fig. 23.13).

Impacted Teeth

The radiograph is the prime diagnostic tool in locating and defining the relative position of the impacted tooth, because most impacted teeth are not visible on intraoral examination. The maxillary and mandibular third molars are the most common impactions. These teeth must be

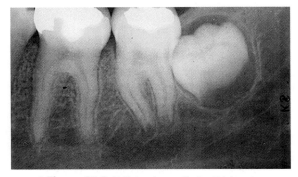

• **Figure 23.2** Follicle of mandibular third molar.

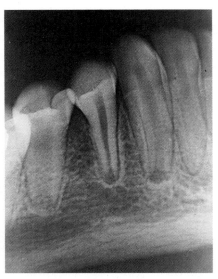

• **Figure 23.3** Dental papilla.

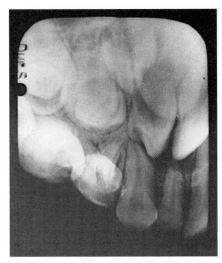

• **Figure 23.4** Mixed dentition in a child.

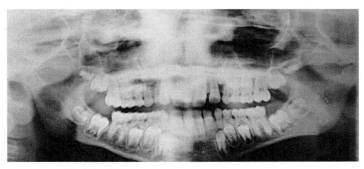

• **Figure 23.5** Mixed dentition on a panoramic image.

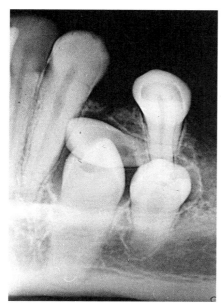

• **Figure 23.6** Supernumerary tooth blocking eruption of the first premolar.

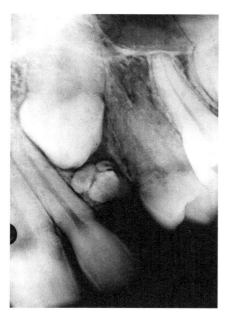

• **Figure 23.7** Odontoma blocking eruption of a permanent canine.

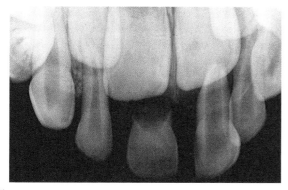

• **Figure 23.8** Maxillary central incisor area in a child. Permanent teeth are seen in bone. Note the root resorption of deciduous central incisor resulting from an eruptive force.

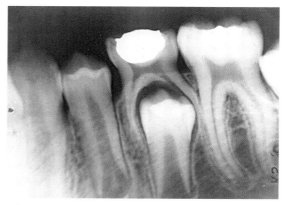

• **Figure 23.9** Mixed dentition in the mandibular molar area.

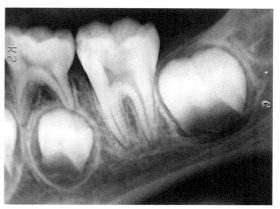

• **Figure 23.10** Mandibular mixed dentition.

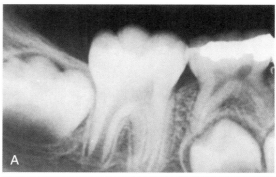

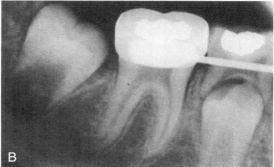

• **Figure 23.11** Root resorption of deciduous second molar. **A,** Early. **B,** Late.

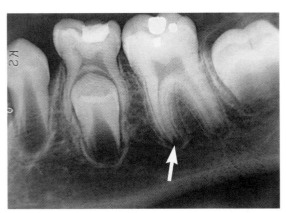

• **Figure 23.12** Root sack *(arrow)* on developing first permanent molar.

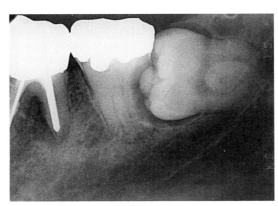

• **Figure 23.14** Bony impaction of the mandibular third molar. Note the relationship of the tooth to the mandibular canal and root resorption of the second molar.

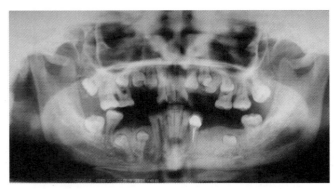

• **Figure 23.13** Overretention of primary teeth as seen in an 18-year-old with cleidocranial dysostosis.

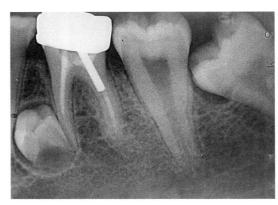

• **Figure 23.15** Soft tissue impaction. Note the supernumerary tooth in the premolar area.

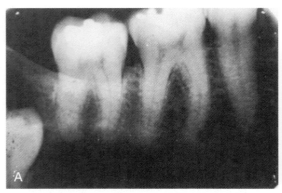

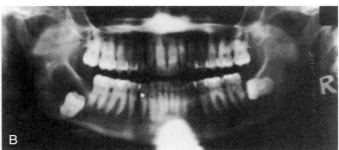

• **Figure 23.16** A, Impacted mandibular third molar, not seen completely. B, Panoramic radiograph shows the extent of the dentigerous cyst.

localized not only in their mesiodistal position by periapical, panoramic, or lateral oblique projections but also in the buccolingual relationship by right-angle (90-degree/cross-sectional) occlusal projections and/or computed tomographic or cone beam computed tomography (CBCT) scanning.

Radiographically, bony impactions may be seen completely or partially covered by bone (Fig. 23.14). A soft tissue impaction is not covered by bone. In some cases, the outline of the covering soft tissue appears on the radiograph (Fig. 23.15).

Periapical radiographs of impacted teeth must show the entire tooth and at least 2 to 3 mm of surrounding bone. If periapical projections cannot accomplish this, a panoramic or another extraoral projection should be used. If the entire tooth is not seen, a lesion (such as, the dentigerous cyst (follicular cyst) seen in Fig. 23.16) might be missed, with negative consequences for the patient.

> **NOTE**
>
> The generalized definition of a cyst is that they are abnormal, closed sac-like structures within a tissue that contain a liquid, gaseous, or semisolid substance. A dentigerous or follicular cyst usually forms around the crown of an unerupted or impacted tooth. The cyst encircles the crown from the cementoenamel junction (CEJ) of one side of the tooth to the other side of the same tooth and represents a retained intact tooth follicle that is usually shed when a tooth erupts into the oral cavity. The term *dentigerous* by definition actually means "containing or bearing teeth."

Supernumerary Teeth (Hyperdontia)

Supernumerary teeth (hyperdontia), or extra teeth and their relative position to other teeth are easily detectable on the proper radiographs. As with impacted teeth, the buccolingual relationship can be established by the use of right-angle occlusal projections. The most common supernumerary teeth are mandibular premolars, maxillary incisors, and fourth molars (Fig. 23.17; see Fig. 23.15). If the supernumerary tooth occurs between the maxillary central incisors, it is called a mesiodens (Fig. 23.18). If it is positioned distal to the third molar, it is referred to as a distodens (distomolar, paramolar, or fourth molar).

Supernumerary teeth may erupt into the mouth or remain impacted. They may delay or prevent the eruption of the normal dentition. Supernumerary roots also can occur on teeth and may or may not be detected radiographically (Fig. 23.19).

Congenitally Missing Teeth

Hypodontia is the failure of teeth to develop. It can occur in either the primary or adult dentition. It can be a single missing tooth, many missing teeth (known as oligodontia), or a complete absence of teeth, known as anodontia). Missing teeth can be detected clinically. However, the diagnosis of hypodontia is made definitively only by radiographic examination of the underlying bone (Fig. 23.20).

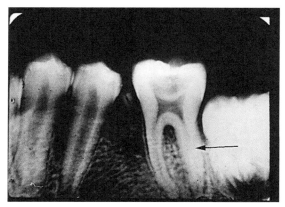

• **Figure 23.19** Supernumerary roots. After extraction, two distal roots were found on the first molar. Note how wide the distal root is *(arrow)*.

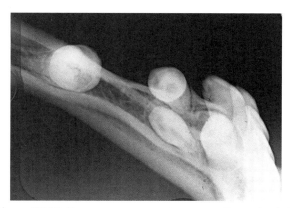

• **Figure 23.17** Supernumerary premolar seen on the occlusal view.

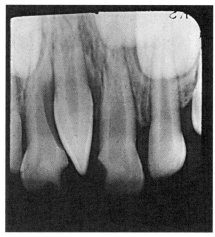

• **Figure 23.18** Mesiodens. Supernumerary tooth between the central incisors.

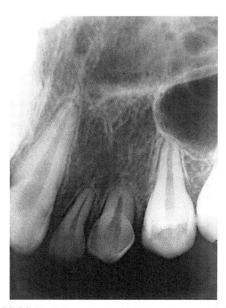

• **Figure 23.20** Partial anodontia. Note the absence of the permanent lateral incisor and canine.

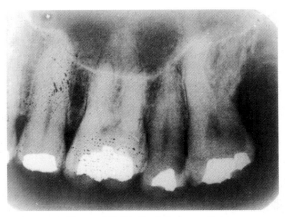

• **Figure 23.21** Tooth transposition.

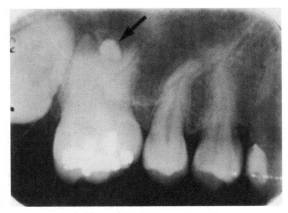

• **Figure 23.23** Enamel pearl.

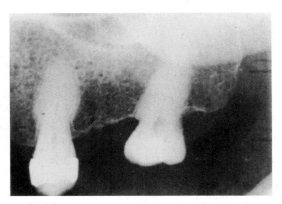

• **Figure 23.22** Hypercementosis. Note the club-shaped root on the second premolar.

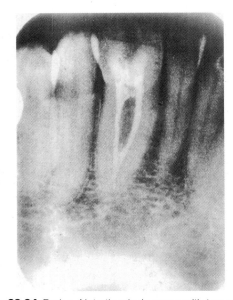

• **Figure 23.24** Fusion. Note the single crown with two root canals.

Malposition of Teeth

Teeth that do not occupy their normal position in the mouth are said to be malposed. Tumors, cysts, supernumerary teeth, or lack of space may keep a tooth from achieving its proper position. If a tooth occupies the normal position of another tooth, it is said to be transposed (Fig. 23.21).

Hypercementosis

Hypercementosis is a condition characterized by the buildup of cementum on the root of the tooth. Normally, it is difficult to distinguish cementum from dentin because of its thin layers and similar densities. The buildup of cementum makes the root appear club-shaped instead of its usual conical appearance (Fig. 23.22). This condition can be seen in patients who have Paget's disease of bone.

Enamel Pearls

Enamel pearls (enameloma) are small, spherical-shaped pieces of enamel attached to the roots of teeth. Enamel pearls usually are seen at the trifurcation of maxillary molars or the bifurcation of mandibular molars. They are asymptomatic and are usually discovered through routine radiographic examination (Fig. 23.23).

Fusion

Fusion is a condition that occurs when two teeth join early in their development. The result is usually a single large crown with two root canals (Fig. 23.24).

Gemination

Gemination occurs when a single tooth germ splits during its development. It usually appears as two crowns with a common root canal (Fig. 23.25).

Concrescence

Concrescence is the joining of two or more teeth by cementum. Although seen radiographically, it may be very difficult to differentiate concrescence from teeth in close contact or those superimposed on one another.

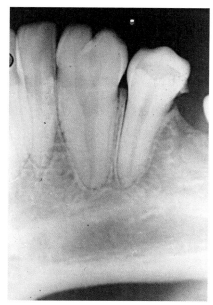

• **Figure 23.25** Gemination. Note two crowns with a common root canal.

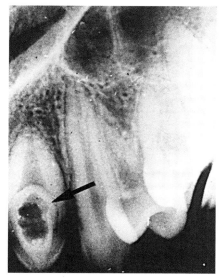

• **Figure 23.26** Dens invaginatus *(arrow)*.

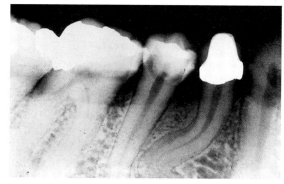

• **Figure 23.27** Dilaceration. Note the curved root on first premolar.

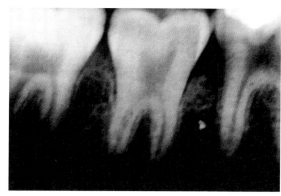

• **Figure 23.28** Taurodontia. Note the longitudinal distortion and short roots.

> **NOTE**
>
> It is important to distinguish between dilaceration and a distorted or bent image caused by overbending of the film packet during film placement. This occurs when film packets, as opposed to digital sensors, are being used as the receptor. To differentiate between dilaceration and an image caused by overmanipulation of a film packet, remember that only one part of the image of the tooth is distorted when the tooth is dilacerated and the rest of the structures are normal. When the manipulation of the film packet is the cause, the whole image, or at least a majority of the image, is distorted.

Dens Invaginatus

Dens invaginatus, or dens in dente, is not a "tooth within a tooth," as it is commonly referred to, but an invagination of the enamel organ within the body of the tooth. The point of invagination of the enamel is usually the cingulum of the tooth (Fig. 23.26).

Dilaceration

Dilaceration is a permanent distortion of the shape and relationship of either the crown or the root of the tooth. This abnormality would present a problem only if the tooth required root canal therapy or extraction. It is thought to be caused by trauma during development of the tooth (Fig. 23.27).

Taurodontia (Taurodontism)

In taurodontia (taurodontism), the body of the tooth is elongated with the extension of the pulp chamber into the elongation; the roots are short, but the size of the crown is normal (Fig. 23.28). It acquired its name because of a likeness to a bull's head. The crown of the tooth is compared to the bull's head, and the horns are represented by the roots of the tooth.

Amelogenesis Imperfecta

Amelogenesis imperfecta is a hereditary disturbance that affects both the primary and secondary dentition. The dentin and root formation are normal. The enamel on the teeth is thin and of poor quality and may fracture away completely. Radiographically, the absence of enamel or thin enamel is apparent (Fig. 23.29).

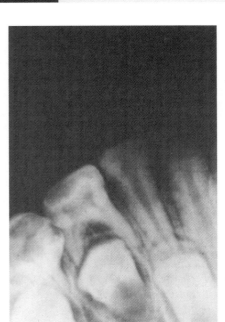

• **Figure 23.29** Amelogenesis imperfecta.

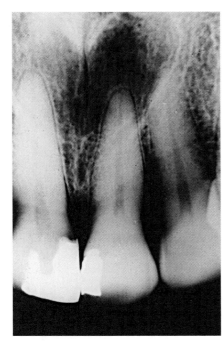

• **Figure 23.31** Nasopalatine cyst.

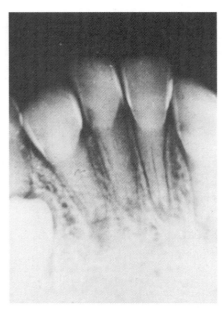

• **Figure 23.30** Dentinogenesis imperfecta.

Dentinogenesis Imperfecta

Dentinogenesis imperfecta is also a hereditary disturbance that affects both the primary and secondary dentition. It is characterized by poor enamel that may wear thin or chip, early calcification of the pulp chambers and canals, and short roots, especially noticeable in the permanent teeth (Fig. 23.30).

Fissural Cysts

Fissural cysts are always found in predictable anatomic locations, because they develop along embryonic suture lines.

The nasopalatine cyst where the teeth are vital appears as a radiolucency in the midline near the apices of the maxillary central incisors and must be differentiated from periapical pathologic processes. It was previously thought that the globulomaxillary cyst is a fissural cyst seen as a pear-shaped radiolucency between the maxillary lateral incisor and canine. However, this entity is now considered controversial as a result of more current research. The median palatine cyst is seen as an oval radiolucency in the midline of the palate. The nasopalatine and globulomaxillary cysts appear on periapical projections of their respective areas; the median palatine cyst is seen best on occlusal projections (Figs. 23.31 to 23.33).

Cleft Palate

The failure of embryonic processes to fuse in development causes clefts. These clefts can occur in the hard palate, soft palate, or both. Clefts can disturb the dental lamina, resulting in anodontia, malposition, or supernumerary teeth. Radiographically, the cleft appears as a radiolucent area in which one would normally expect to find bone (Fig. 23.34).

Dentigerous Cyst

A dentigerous cyst, as previously discussed in this chapter, forms when the developing tooth bud undergoes cystic degeneration. The cyst may surround or be lateral to the developing tooth. It is most commonly seen in association with third molars. A cyst that forms from the dental lamina before the tooth bud forms is called a primordial cyst (Figs. 23.35 and 23.36).

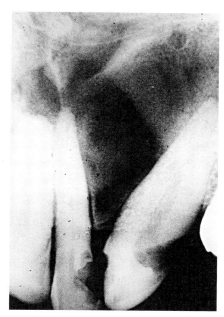

• **Figure 23.32** Globulomaxillary cyst.

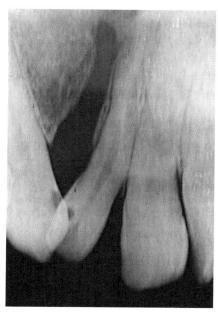

• **Figure 23.34** Cleft palate. Note the radiolucent defect between the lateral incisor and canine.

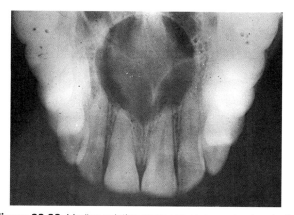

• **Figure 23.33** Median palatine cyst seen on an occlusal projection.

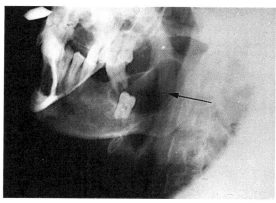

• **Figure 23.35** Dentigerous cyst *(arrow)* seen on a lateral oblique projection.

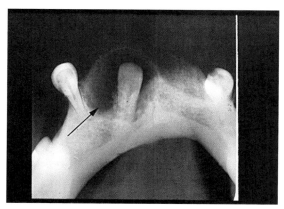

• **Figure 23.36** Dentigerous cyst *(arrow)* seen on a mandibular occlusal projection.

Chapter Summary

- A majority of the developmental disturbances of the teeth and surrounding bone are primarily recognized on a radiographic examination of the dental patient. It is important that dental professionals are able to radiographically identify these conditions and proceed with the patient's diagnosis and treatment accordingly. It is also important to be able to request the appropriate radiographs for proper identification of these disturbances.
- The dental professional is responsible for knowing the radiographic appearance of normal tooth development and eruption patterns. This ability should include being able to recognize the absence of teeth, as well as the presence of supernumerary teeth.
- Changes in the tooth anatomy can also be recognized radiographically, including hypercementosis, fusion, gemination, concrescence, enamel pearls, dens invaginatus, taurodontia, and dilaceration.
- The recognition of various cysts—including fissural cysts, dentigerous cysts, and primordial cysts—are also a valuable skill when interpreting dental images.
- Hereditary disturbances of tooth formation, such as amelogenesis imperfecta and dentinogenesis imperfecta, require both clinical and radiographic identification.

Chapter Review Questions

Matching

Match the term in Column A with the appropriate radiographic appearance in Column B.

Column A

1. Taurodontia
2. Mixed dentition
3. Concrescence
4. Hypercementosis
5. Mesiodens
6. Dentigerous cyst
7. Dens invaginatus
8. Dilaceration
9. Fusion
10. Amelogenesis imperfecta
11. Nasopalatine cyst
12. Dentinogenesis imperfecta
13. Distodens
14. Enamel pearl
15. Gemination

Column B

a. Supernumerary tooth distal to the third molar
b. Two teeth joined: single large crown and two root canals
c. Club-shaped root
d. Spherical-shaped piece of enamel on the tooth's root
e. Split tooth germ forming a tooth with two crowns/one canal
f. Invagination of the enamel organ
g. Permanent distortion of the crown or root
h. Poor enamel, calcified pulp, and short roots
i. Both primary and secondary teeth are present
j. Joining of teeth at the cementum
k. Extra tooth between the upper central incisors
l. Cyst around an unerupted or impacted tooth
m. Hereditary absent or thin enamel
n. Fissural cyst at the apices of teeth #8 and #9
o. Tooth that looks like a bull's head

Critical Thinking Exercise

1. An 18-year-old male patient presents to your dental facility with "missing teeth" as his chief complaint. What steps would appropriately be taken in establishing an explanation for his clinically apparent hypodontia? Please include the following in your discussion:

   a. The appropriate radiographic prescription
   b. A thorough medical history
   c. Classification of anodontia or oligodontia

Bibliography

White SC, Pharoah MJ: *Oral radiology: Principles and interpretation,* ed 7, St Louis, MO, 2013, Mosby.

24

Bone and Other Lesions

EDUCATIONAL OBJECTIVES

Upon completing this chapter, the student will be able to:

1. Define the key terms listed at the beginning of the chapter.
2. Utilize descriptive terminology in providing an interpretation of bone and other oral lesions.
3. Discuss the following related to cysts, tumors, and bone lesions:
   - Recognize cysts, tumors, and bone lesions and differentiate their appearance from normal.

- Understand which radiographic projections are needed to formulate a complete radiographic diagnosis of bone and other oral lesions.
4. Discuss the radiographic appearance of traumatic injuries, foreign bodies and root tips, extraction sockets, salivary stones, exostosis, and enostosis.

KEY TERMS

benign lesion
biopsy
endostosis (dense bone island, idiopathic osteosclerosis)
exostosis (hyperostosis)
extraction socket

fracture
hyperostotic lines
malignancy (cancer)
metabolic condition
mixed lesion
radiolucent (RL) lesion

radiopaque (RO) lesion
salivary stones, sialoliths, or salivary calculi
trabecular pattern

Introduction

This chapter discusses the application of the principles of radiographic interpretation previously included in Chapter 20 to the identification and description of bone and other findings that may be discovered in the oral cavity. It is important for the dental professional to have the skills to properly identify and provide a description of oral lesions (such as, cysts, tumors, metabolic bone lesions, traumatic lesions, foreign bodies, root tips, extraction sockets, and salivary stones) when contributing to a successful diagnostic process.

Description of Lesions

After discovering a lesion radiographically, the diagnostician must know certain facts about its radiographic appearance. In gathering this information, more radiographs may be required to assemble all the information necessary to make the final diagnosis. The following is a repetition of certain diagnostic criteria and categories that illustrate the diagnostic procedures.

Radiolucent versus Radiopaque

In describing or, in some cases, categorizing bone lesions, they are referred to as radiopaque, radiolucent, or mixed. A radiopaque (RO) lesion indicates an increase in the density of the bone or new calcified material being formed (e.g., osteoma), whereas a radiolucent (RL) lesion indicates a decrease in density or destruction of bone (e.g., cyst). Mixed lesions have both processes occurring (e.g., periapical cemental dysplasia).

Location

In making a diagnosis of a pathologic bone condition, location is very important because some lesions have a predilection for certain areas of the mouth (e.g., ameloblastoma in the mandibular third molar region).

Extent of the Lesion

The diagnostician must see the entire lesion and be able to define its borders and extent in three planes before

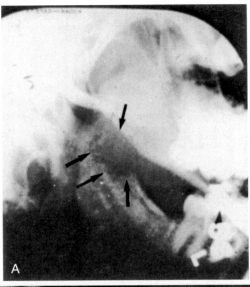

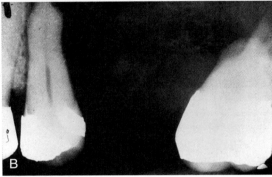

• **Figure 24.1** **A,** Lateral oblique radiograph showing destruction of the coronoid process by a malignant tumor. **B,** Periapical radiograph of the maxillary premolar area showing complete bone destruction as evidenced by the radiolucent (RL) malignant lesion.

any type of treatment is instituted. Large pathologic areas often require the use of panoramic, extraoral, computed tomographic (CT), cone beam computed tomographic (CBCT), or magnetic resonance projections to obtain this information.

Benign versus Malignant

The possibility of malignancy (cancer) must be considered when diagnosing an unknown lesion. In general, malignancies tend to have poorly-defined radiographic borders and destroy normal anatomic structures (Fig. 24.1). Benign tumors and cysts expand slowly, with clearly defined borders referred to on radiographs as **hyperostotic lines**. Their slow growth tends to displace rather than destroy structures. As seen on occlusal projections, **benign lesions** expand the buccal and lingual cortex of bone, whereas malignant lesions perforate and invade neighboring tissue (Fig. 24.2). This effect on the buccal and lingual cortices can be seen best on right-angle occlusal projections of the maxilla and mandible, as well as on CT and CBCT scans.

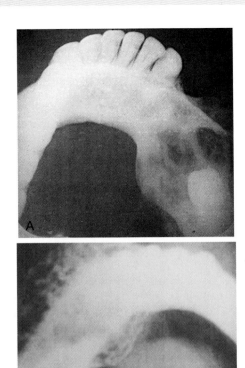

• **Figure 24.2** **A,** Occlusal radiograph showing expansion of the buccal and lingual plates of the mandible caused by a benign tumor. **B,** Occlusal radiograph showing perforation and spread through the buccal and lingual cortices by a malignant tumor.

Cysts and Tumors

All cysts located in bone are seen as RL areas. Tumors can appear RL, RO, or mixed. When the cyst or the tumor appears RL (e.g., ameloblastoma), the lesion has destroyed normal bone and replaced it with less dense cystic or tumor tissue (Fig. 24.3). If the lesion is RO, this signifies that the new tumor tissue being formed has a greater density or size than the tissue it is replacing (Fig. 24.4). The mixed lesion may have a variety of densities. Tumors of bone and cartilage appear RO; all other tumors appear RL. The odontoma has a variety of densities corresponding to the densities of tooth structure (i.e., enamel, dentin, cementum, and pulp; Fig. 24.5).

Metabolic Bone Lesions

Many **metabolic conditions**, which occur when abnormal chemical reactions in the body alter the normal metabolic process, manifest with changes of the trabecular pattern and lamina dura of the bone in the mandible and maxilla. Examples of this type of disease process are Paget's disease (cotton wool bony appearance), hyperparathyroidism, and certain types of anemia. The dental professional's role is not

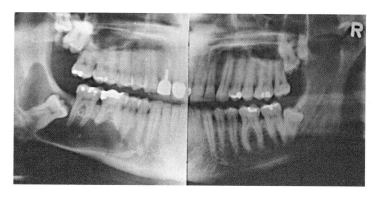

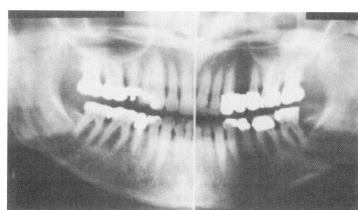

• **Figure 24.3** Radiograph of a tumor (ameloblastoma) enveloping teeth on the right side of the mandible.

• **Figure 24.4** Panoramic radiograph showing a well-defined radiopaque (RO) tumor in the left maxillary sinus. Compare right and left maxillary sinuses.

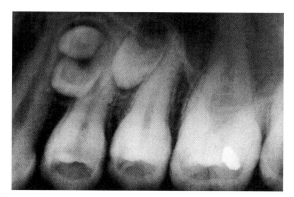

• **Figure 24.5** Radiograph of an odontoma. Note the densities that correspond to tooth structures.

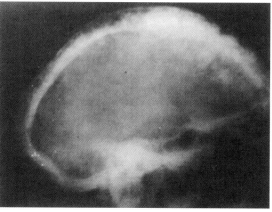

• **Figure 24.6** Paget's disease. Lateral skull projection showing the characteristic "cotton wool" appearance of Paget disease of bone.

NOTE

The following is an exercise in applying the principles of interpretation when identifying an oral lesion: A dental professional described a radiolucent (RL) lesion in the mandibular third molar region as being multilocular and locally invasive on a radiographic image (see Fig. 24.3). Judging by this description, this lesion could be identified as an ameloblastoma, among other possible lesions. An ameloblastoma is a locally aggressive benign tumor, commonly found in the posterior region of the mandible or, less commonly, in the maxilla. This lesion appears RL and could be multilocular or unilocular and can be benign or malignant. Ultimately, the definitive diagnosis would depend on the results of a biopsy (an examination of tissue removed from a lesion to discover the presence, cause, or extent of a disease) performed on the specimen sample.

to diagnose these diseases but rather to recognize the change from normal as seen on the radiographs (Figs. 24.6 to 24.8) and then refer the patient for treatment.

Traumatic Injuries

Fractures of teeth, especially anterior teeth, are very common. Clinically and radiographically, a fracture of the crown of a tooth is easier to detect than a root fracture. The fracture appears on the radiograph as a RL line or the missing part of the tooth is apparent (see Fig. 24.7). A root fracture also is seen as a RL line but is much more difficult to visualize because of superimposition of alveolar

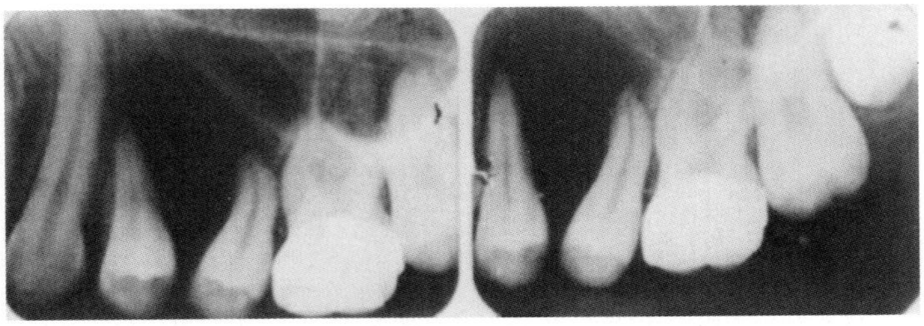

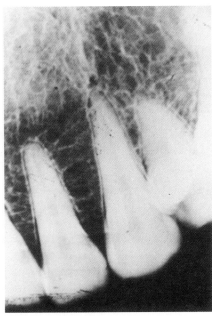

• **Figure 24.7** Radiolucent (RL) lesion of hyperparathyroidism seen between roots of premolars.

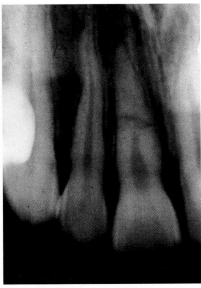

• **Figure 24.10** Root fracture, maxillary central incisor.

• **Figure 24.8** Trabecular bone pattern of anemia. Note the enlarged medullary spaces.

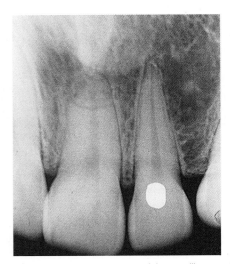

• **Figure 24.9** Root fracture near apex of the maxillary central incisor.

bone trabeculation (Figs. 24.9 and 24.10). Tooth and root fractures can lead to pulp damage and ensuing periapical pathologic conditions. Fractures of the maxilla and mandible may be seen in part on periapical projections, but larger views, such as panoramic or other extraoral films, are needed for complete visualization (Figs. 24.11 and 24.12). The fracture appears as a RL line, and radiographs may show displacement of the fracture segments.

Foreign Bodies and Root Tips

Any sort of foreign body can be embedded in the jawbones. Only those that are RO can be seen radiographically. Metallic foreign bodies are the most common and the easiest to see because of their increased density and appear more RO than bone. These radiopacities may be amalgam, burrs, broken instruments, needles, or metallic fragments from an external source (Fig. 24.13), wires used to reduce fractures, or metallic implants (Figs. 24.14 and 24.15).

Retained root tips have the density of tooth structure (Fig. 24.16); thus, sometimes it is difficult to distinguish between the retained root tip and dense areas of bone. One way to achieve this differentiation is by the appearance of a pulp canal or the conical shape of a root tip. These root tips should be localized radiographically in three dimensions before treatment is attempted.

Extraction Sockets

Extraction sockets may be radiographically evident in the bone up to 6 months after surgery. They initially appear as

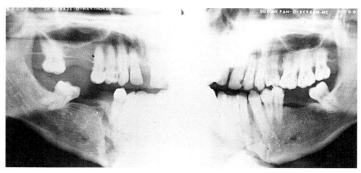

• **Figure 24.11** Panoramic radiograph showing fractured mandible.

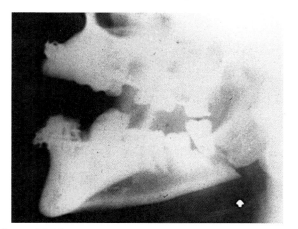

• **Figure 24.12** Fracture of mandible on a lateral oblique projection.

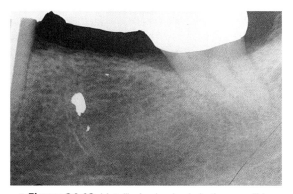

• **Figure 24.13** Metallic foreign body in the mandible.

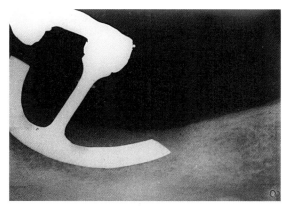

• **Figure 24.14** Metallic implant of the mandible serving as a distal abutment. Note the thinning of bone, indicating start of the rejection process.

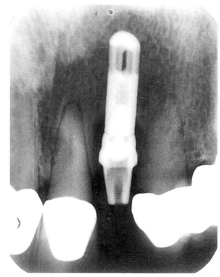

• **Figure 24.15** Osseointegrated (endosseous) implant seen on a periapical radiograph.

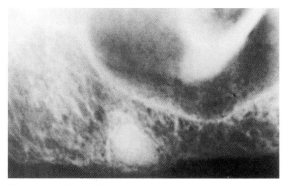

• **Figure 24.16** Retained root tip in the maxillary molar region.

RL areas, and then the area eventually fills in with bone in the normal trabecular pattern (Fig. 24.17).

Salivary Stones (Sialoliths or Salivary Calculi)

Although not a bone lesion, salivary stones are included here because salivary gland disease is often treated by the dentist and can be seen on dental radiographs. Although the salivary glands and ducts are soft tissue, radiographs are still important in the diagnostic workup. Salivary stones, also known as sialoliths or salivary calculi, are a common cause of obstruction, secondary swelling, and infection. Because the sialolith is calcified, it can be seen on radiographs. Stones in the submandibular duct can be seen best on a mandibular right-angle occlusal projection (Fig. 24.18). Stones also can be seen on panoramic radiographs and periapical projections but may appear as superimpositions on the radiograph (Fig. 24.19). Advanced imaging systems, including CBCT and CT scanning images, are also used to locate salivary stones. For the parotid gland, in which stones are not so common, a lateral oblique, posteroanterior, CT scan, or soft tissue projection with the receptor placed in the mucobuccal fold can be employed.

Exostosis and Enostosis

An exostosis (hyperostosis), by definition, is an overgrowth of bone on the surface of the alveolar bone. Both torus palatinus and torus mandibularis are considered to be areas of exostoses but are located in their respective specific locations as discussed in Chapter 19 of this text. Other areas of external bone growth can be present anywhere in the oral cavity but most commonly occur on the buccal surfaces of the maxillary canines and molar regions. An endostosis, also known as a dense bone island or idiopathic osteosclerosis (Fig. 24.20) is an internal growth of bone that is considered to be the internal version of exostoses. Both exostoses and enostoses appear RO on radiographic images and are asymptomatic and within normal limits. Exostoses are identified on clinical and radiographic examination. The identification of endostosis (dense bone island, idiopathic osteosclerosis) is usually made as a result of a radiographic examination only.

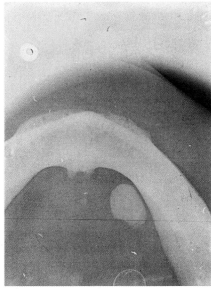

• **Figure 24.18** Occlusal radiograph of an edentulous mandible showing a radiopaque (RO) salivary stone in the submandibular duct in the floor of the mouth.

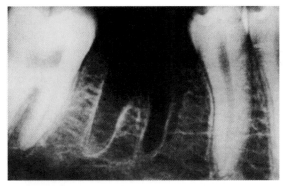

• **Figure 24.17** Extraction socket in the mandible.

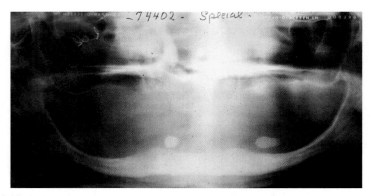

• **Figure 24.19** Salivary stone seen on a panoramic image . The stone is seen twice, as this Panoramic unit produces a redundant image.

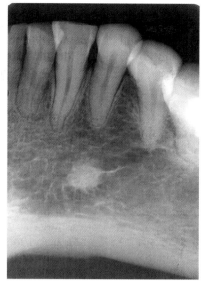

• **Figure 24.20** Endostosis (dense bone island, periapical idiopathic osteosclerosis) in the mandibular premolar region. (From White SC, Pharoah MJ: *Oral radiology: Principles and interpretation,* ed 7, St Louis, 2014.)

Chapter Summary

• When identifying bone and other lesions in the oral cavity, the dental professional should note the radiographic appearance, location, and extent of the lesion.
• The radiographic appearance of the oral lesions discussed in this chapter is dependent on the actual density of the structure.
• The dental professional should choose the type of radiograph that will include the entire lesion on the image.

• The dental professional should know the radiographic appearance and other identifying characteristics of common oral findings, including benign lesions, malignant lesions, various cysts and tumors, metabolic bone lesions, fractures, foreign bodies, retained root tips, extraction sockets, salivary stones, exostoses, and enostoses.

Chapter Review Questions

Matching

Match the term in Column A with the appropriate radiographic appearance in Column B.

Column A	Column B
1. Paget's disease	a. Has poorly defined radiographic borders
2. Odontoma	b. Has the density of root structures
3. Endosseous implant	c. "Cotton wool" appearance
4. Fracture	d. Appears as a RL line
5. Retained root tip	e. Has a hyperostotic border
6. Benign lesion	f. Mixed lesion corresponding to tooth structures
7. Malignant lesion	e. Has the radiopacity of a metallic object

Case-Based Exercises

Identify the oral lesion that the following case descriptions and images are referring to. Provide an answer for items a, b, and c associated with each case.

1. A male patient presents to your dental clinic with pain and swelling in the floor of his mouth. After a clinical examination is performed, a panoramic radiograph is taken of the patient and the lesion plus a ghost image (refer to Chapter 12) of the lesion is seen.

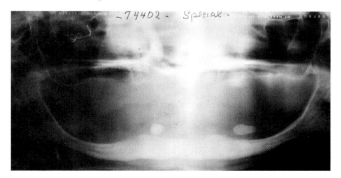

a. Describe the radiographic appearance of the lesion.
b. Discuss the location of the lesion.
c. Comment on whether the radiograph taken is sufficient or if another type of image could be utilized in the case.
d. What do you think this oral lesion could be?

2. A patient presents for a follow-up visit with no complaints or symptoms. A selected periapical radiograph of the area that a recent procedure was performed in is prescribed.

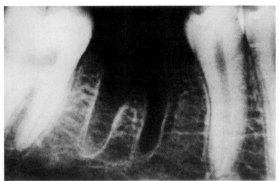

a. Describe the radiographic appearance of the lesion.
b. Discuss the location of the lesion.
c. Comment on whether the radiograph taken is sufficient or if another type of image could be utilized in the case.
d. What do you think this oral lesion could be?

Bibliography

White SC, Pharoah MJ: *Oral radiology: Principles and interpretation*, ed 7, St Louis, MO, 2013, Mosby.

25

Legal Considerations

EDUCATIONAL OBJECTIVES

Upon completing this chapter, the student will be able to:

1. Define the key terms listed at the beginning of the chapter.
2. Describe and be able to differentiate between state and federal regulations as they pertain to dental radiology and licensure.
3. Discuss risk management, including:
   - Understand the concepts of risk management as they apply to patient relations, ownership and retention of radiographs, and the medical and radiation history.
   - Understand the concept of informed consent.
4. Understand the legal status of insurance forms and the dental records.

KEY TERMS

confidentiality
direct supervision
federal regulations
full disclosure
general supervision
Health Insurance Portability and
    Accountability Act (HIPAA)

informed consent
liability
licensure
negligent
radiation inspection
records
res gestae

respondeat superior
risk management
standard of care
statute of limitations

Introduction

It may be a sign of the times, but a discussion of a subject in the health sciences cannot be considered complete today without mentioning the legal aspects that affect the profession. Radiology is no exception; it is probably the most regulated discipline within dentistry, with its registration and certification of x-ray machines, laws, and special testing for operators of the equipment. Therefore, the dental professional must understand the laws and regulations, both local and federal, that govern the use of radiation in this profession.

The legal considerations with which the dental professional should be familiar regarding the use of ionizing radiation in dentistry fall into three major categories: (1) federal and state regulations regarding x-ray equipment and its use, (2) licensure for users of x-ray equipment, and (3) risk management.

Federal and State Regulations

All dental x-ray machines either manufactured or sold in the United States must adhere to federal regulations (federal government's performance standards), which include safety specifications for minimum filtration and accuracy and reproducibility of the milliamperage time and kilovoltage settings. These standards are discussed in Chapters 1 and 3.

Actually, all x-ray equipment, regardless of the date of manufacture, is subject to state, county, or city radiation health codes. It is not unusual for the registration of x-ray machines to be required and a fee charged for such a permit. Many states or other jurisdictions require regular radiation inspections of the x-ray machines in the dental office. Violations of the radiation code can lead to fines or suspension of a dentist's radiation permit. The positive aspect of these inspections is that they serve as a quality assurance (QA) procedure. The inspectors, as they measure for violations, perform recommended QA procedures that dental professionals could not do themselves because of the need for sophisticated radiation-monitoring equipment.

Licensure

Regarding licensure, each state has its own policy for the user of dental radiation. The dentist and dental hygienist, who in all states is a licensed professional, usually do not have to take an additional examination to be certified to perform dental radiography. Generally, the dentist is also responsible for prescribing the appropriate radiographs for the patient and for formulating a diagnosis and treatment plan as a result of a clinical and radiographic examination. However, the dental hygienist may interpret or "read" the radiographs without formulating an actual diagnosis based on their interpretation.

The dental assistant may be required to take a radiology examination other than the national certifying examination to be authorized to perform dental radiography. Some states have exceptions in their radiation rules that allow an uncertified dental assistant to take radiographs under the direct supervision of a dentist. Direct supervision means that the dentist is physically present in the office when the radiographs are taken. Hygienists may take radiographs under the general supervision of a dentist, which means that the hygienist is performing these tasks in a licensed dentist's office or clinic, and the dentist can be reached if necessary. In most states, dental assistants cannot take extraoral projections other than a panoramic image.

Each state deals with dental radiography differently. It is not the purpose of this text to compile lists of these requirements, because they change rapidly. Dental professionals should be knowledgeable about the rules and regulations of the state or jurisdiction in which they are working and should not assume that all state regulations are the same.

Risk Management

By far the most important legal aspect of dental radiology is risk management. Risk management concerns the policies and procedures designed to reduce the likelihood of suits for malpractice against dentists and dental radiographers. All members of the dental staff must be aware of and participate in the risk management efforts of the office if they are to be effective.

First, it must be pointed out that liability, both professionally and legally, rests with the dentist and not the dental hygienist or dental assistant. This is called the doctrine of respondeat superior, or the "captain of the ship" principle; more simply put, the captain of the ship is responsible for the actions of the sailors. The dental professional may be named in a lawsuit, but the liability is ultimately with the employing dentist.

A dental hygienist falls under the doctrine of respondeat superior if the hygienist is an employee. If the hygienist is the one found to be negligent, the dentist's insurance company may decide to subrogate (sue the hygienist's company for a share of the award) the payment of the claim against the hygienist or the hygienist's insurance company. Therefore, the hygienist is well advised to carry professional liability insurance. Hygienists who are independent contractors may be sued alone.

Patient Relations

Avoiding misunderstandings is a critical component of risk management. Dental office staff must communicate in advance to patients about how the office policy deals with financial arrangements, payments, recall procedures, and the filing of insurance claims.

Dental professionals should never say anything negative to a patient about equipment, procedures, staff, or anything else in the office. Remarks such as, "This timer is always off," or "These films weren't processed properly," are unnecessary. These comments are considered "admissions against interest," also known as the theory of res gestae. Statements made by anyone spontaneously at the time of an alleged negligent act are admissible as evidence.

Informed Consent

The dental professional may participate in the process of obtaining informed consent, which entails explaining to the patient the nature and purpose of the procedure. This is called full disclosure. In the case of taking radiographs, full disclosure entails explaining to the patient, in lay terms, the risks and benefits to be derived. Recent legal decisions have noted that it is equally important to inform the patient of the risks of not having a specific procedure. In this case, the patient must be told about the diseases that might go undetected without radiography and the possible consequences. If the patient is a minor, the parent or guardian must consent.

If a patient refuses a recommended radiographic examination, this should be entered into the patient's record to justify why treatment will not be rendered. There are few if any dental procedures that should be done without current and diagnostic radiographs, because their use is now the accepted standard of care. Patient refusal is not a valid reason for treating without radiographs.

Health Questionnaire

The dental professional always should review the patient's health history and questionnaire and update as necessary. The dental professional should call to the dentist's attention any information that might contraindicate or change the number and type of radiographs that are to be taken.

Records

It has been said that the three most important parts of a defense in a malpractice suit are "records, records, records." Dental radiographs are considered part of the patient's dental record and are considered legal documents. The number and quality of the radiographs may be an important issue in any litigation. If the quality is poor and nondiagnostic and the procedures in question are based on the radiographs, this substantially weakens the defense. If the radiographs cannot be found or retrieved (if they are digital images), again, the case for the defense is seriously compromised.

The most common error is the failure to make an entry in the patient's record when radiographs are taken; the date, number, and type of radiograph should always be recorded. There are no exceptions to this rule. Postoperative, working endodontic, or retakes must be recorded or the records will be deemed incomplete. Individual radiographs, a series of radiographs, and panoramic radiographs should be appropriately labeled and dated. The issue of the legal status of digital radiographs and possible alterations of the images is discussed in Chapter 15.

Confidentiality

The patient's records are confidential. The contents or findings in these records should never be discussed or shown to anyone outside the office. Confidentiality also pertains to any radiographs or photographs that are part of the record. Since April 2000, it has also been necessary that all records comply with the Health Insurance Portability and Accountability Act (HIPAA; Box 25.1).

Ownership

The dentist is the guardian and keeper of dental records; these records are the property of the dentist. Patients may request a copy of their radiographs; this request should be written and signed by the patient. A fee may be charged for this duplication. Laws differ from state to state on whether a dental office must give the radiographs to the patient if the fee for this service has not been paid. In some states, the radiographs or copies must be given to the patient even if the fee has not been paid. The dentist may pursue collection but only after giving the radiographs to the patient. This is not true in all states, which underscores that members of the dental team must be familiar with the laws regulating practice in the state in which they work.

The dentist should be informed of this request and an entry made in the record of when and to whom the

---

• BOX 25.1   Health Insurance Portability and Accountability Act of 1996

The Health Insurance Portability and Accountability Act (HIPAA) of 1996 was signed into law by President Bill Clinton on August 21, 1996. Conclusive regulations were issued on August 17, 2000, to be instated by October 16, 2002. HIPAA requires that the transactions of all patient health care information be formatted in a standardized electronic style. In addition to protecting the privacy and security of patient information, HIPAA includes legislation on the formation of medical savings accounts, the authorization of a fraud and abuse control program, the easy transport of health insurance coverage, and the simplification of administrative terms and conditions.

HIPAA encompasses three primary areas, and its privacy requirements can be broken down into three types: privacy standards, patients' rights, and administrative requirements.

1. *Privacy Standards.* A central concern of HIPAA is the careful use and disclosure of protected health information (PHI), which generally is electronically controlled health information that can be distinguished individually. PHI also refers to verbal communication, although the HIPAA Privacy Rule is not intended to hinder necessary verbal communication. The U.S. Department of Health and Human Services (USDHHS) does not require restructuring, such as soundproofing, architectural changes, and so forth, but some caution is necessary when exchanging health information by conversation.

   An Acknowledgment of Receipt Notice of Privacy Practices, which allows patient information to be used or divulged for treatment, payment, or health care operations (TPOs), should be procured from each patient. A detailed and time-sensitive authorization can also be issued, which allows the dentist to release information in special circumstances other than TPOs. A written consent is also an option. Dentists can disclose PHI without acknowledgment, consent, or authorization in very special situations, such as perceived child abuse, public health supervision, fraud investigation, or law enforcement with valid permission (i.e., a warrant). When divulging PHI, a dentist must try to disclose only the minimum necessary information to help safeguard the patient's information as much as possible.

   It is important that dental professionals adhere to HIPAA standards because health care providers (as well as health care clearinghouses and health care plans) who convey

electronically formatted health information via an outside billing service or merchant are considered covered entities. Covered entities may be dealt serious civil and criminal penalties for violation of HIPAA legislation. Failure to comply with HIPAA privacy requirements may result in civil penalties of up to $100 per offense with an annual maximum of $25,000 for repeated failure to comply with the same requirement. Criminal penalties resulting from the illegal mishandling of private health information can range from $50,000 and/or 1 year in prison to $250,000 and/or 10 years in prison.

2. *Patients' Rights.* HIPAA allows patients, authorized representatives, and parents of minors, as well as minors, to become more aware of the health information privacy to which they are entitled. These rights include, but are not limited to, the right to view and copy their health information, the right to dispute alleged breaches of policies and regulations, and the right to request alternative forms of communicating with their dentist. If any health information is released for any reason other than TPO, the patient is entitled to an account of the transaction. Therefore, it is important for dentists to keep accurate records of such information and to provide them when necessary.

   The HIPAA Privacy Rule determines that the parents of a minor have access to their child's health information. This privilege may be overruled, such as in cases in which there is suspected child abuse or the parent consents to a term of confidentiality between the dentist and the minor. The parents' rights to access their child's PHI also may be restricted in situations in which a legal entity, such as a court, intervenes and when a law does not require a parent's consent. For a full list of patient rights provided by HIPAA, be sure to acquire a copy of the law and understand it well.

3. *Administrative Requirements.* Complying with HIPAA legislation may seem like a chore, but it does not have to be so. It is recommended that dental professionals become appropriately familiar with the law, organize the requirements into simpler tasks, begin compliance early, and document their office's progress in compliance. An important first step is to evaluate the current information and practices of the office.

   Dentists need to write a privacy policy for their office, a document for their patients detailing the office's practices

Continued

• BOX 25.1 **Health Insurance Portability and Accountability Act of 1996—cont'd**

concerning PHI. The American Dental Association's HIPAA Privacy Kit includes forms that the dentist can use to customize a privacy policy. It is useful to try to understand the role of health care information for patients and the ways in which they deal with the information while they are visiting the dental office. The dentist should train the staff, making sure they are familiar with the terms of HIPAA and the office's privacy policy and related forms. HIPAA requires that the dentist designate a privacy officer, a person in the office who will be responsible for applying the new policies, fielding complaints, and making choices involving the minimum necessary requirements. Another person with the role of contact person will process complaints. *A Notice of Privacy Practices*—a document detailing the patient's rights and the dental office's obligations concerning PHI—also must be drawn up. Furthermore, any role of a third party with access to PHI must be clearly documented. This third party is known as a business associate (BA) and is defined as any entity who, on behalf of the dentist, takes part in any activity that involves exposure of PHI. The HIPAA Privacy Kit provides a copy of the USDHHS "Business Associate Contract Terms," which provides a concrete format for detailing BA interactions.

The main HIPAA privacy compliance date, including all staff training, was April 14, 2003, although many covered entities who submitted a request and a compliance plan by October 15, 2002, were granted 1-year extensions. The dentist can contact the local branch of the ADA for details. It is recommended that dentists prepare their offices ahead of time for all deadlines, which include preparing privacy policies and forms, business associate contracts, and employee training sessions.

For a comprehensive discussion of all of these terms and requirements, a complete list of HIPAA policies and procedures, and a full collection of HIPAA privacy forms, contact the ADA for a HIPAA Privacy Kit. The relevant ADA website is www.ada.org/goto/hipaa. Other websites that may contain useful information about HIPAA are:

- USDHHS Office of Civil Rights (www.hhs.gov/ocr/hipaa)
- Work Group on Electronic Data Interchange (www.wedi.org/SNIP)
- Phoenix Health (www.hipaadvisory.com)
- USDHHS Office of the Assistant Secretary for Planning and Evaluation (http://aspe.os.dhhs.gov/admnsimp/)

Data from: HIPAA Privacy Kit and http://www.ada.org/prof/prac/issues/topics/hipaa/index.html.
(Reproduced with permission from *Mosby's Dental Dictionary*, St Louis, MO, 2004, Mosby.)

---

duplicate radiographs were sent. In the case that the patient is going to another dental office, it is usually not advised to send dental records, including radiographs, directly to the patient but rather to the new dental practice instead. It is also not recommended to send or give the original radiographs to a patient. There is no defense if there are no radiographs in the possession of the dental office. However, on occasion, the court may request or subpoena the original radiographs. If this happens, the dental professional must comply with the court's request.

Retention

Dental radiographs should be kept for 7 years after the patient ceases to be a patient in the office, depending on the specific state's laws. Ideally, they should be kept for as long as possible. Actions that can be brought against a dentist depend on the statute of limitations. The usual time limitation for an adult is 3 years after the discovery of the injury or when the injury should have been discovered.

For children, it is 3 years after they reach their maturity, which in some states is 21 years. Suits therefore can be brought many years past the mandated 7 years of retention of radiographs.

Insurance Claims

It is the legitimate right of the insurance company to request copies of pretreatment radiographs to evaluate a treatment plan. The original conventional or digital radiographs should never be sent to the insurance company because they may be lost. In either case, the dentist is left without an important part of the patient's record and, in case of litigation, the fact that the originals were lost is not an appropriate defense.

As mentioned in Chapter 6, radiographs should never be taken to prove to the insurance company that the services have been performed. The result of this action would be an administrative radiograph, which is considered unsuitable.

Chapter Summary

- The dental professional should be familiar with the legal considerations concerning the use of ionizing radiation in dentistry. These concerns include the state and federal regulations regarding x-ray equipment, licensure requirements for dental radiographers, and risk management procedures and policies.

- Dentists and dental hygienists have certain specific responsibilities that they are permitted to perform in regard to dental radiography by virtue of their licensing regulations. The rules concerning dental assistants' use of radiation in a dental practice vary from state to state.

- If and when a patient refuses radiographs, the dental professional is advised not to render treatment to that individual as it is not acceptable to treat a patient without the appropriate diagnostically acceptable radiographs available to the respective operator as a result of the patient's refusal.

- Dental professionals are responsible for knowing the legal regulations of the state that they are employed in regarding confidentiality, the ownership of the radiographs, informed consent, and the retention of a patient's dental records, including their dental radiographic images.

Chapter Review Questions

Short Answer Questions

1. Is the insurance company permitted to request pretreatment and posttreatment radiographs? Explain your answer.
2. Who has ownership of the radiographs? What are the patients' rights in requesting their radiographs? Explain your answer.
3. How long is a dental practice required to keep a patient's records, including radiographs, after the patient has left the practice? Explain your answer.
4. What are the licensing and certification requirements for each dental professional regarding the use of radiation in dentistry? Explain your answer.
5. What is the purpose of the HIPAA Act? Explain your answer.
6. What is meant by the terms:
   a. Risk management
   b. Respondeat superior
   c. Res gestae
   d. Informed consent
   e. Full disclosure

Bibliography

Iannucci JM, Howerton LJ: *Dental radiography: Principles and techniques*, ed 5, St Louis, MO, 2016, Elsevier Saunders.

Weissman BJ, Serman NJ: The law and who can expose dental radiographs, *Oral Surg Oral Med Oral Pathol Oral Radiol Endod* 90:663–665, 2000.

Appendix A

Common Error Summaries

TABLE A1 Common Processing Errors

Common Processing Error	Appearance	Cause	Remedy
Fogged film	Overall gray appearance due to diminished contrast.	Darkroom errors: Light leaks, smartphone light exposure, improper safelight, improper film storage, and outdated film.	Check for light leaks. Turn off smartphone before entering a darkroom. Check safelight with "coin test." Store film in cool area and away from sources of scatter radiation. Check expiration date on film box, and use old film first.
Underdeveloped film (thin image)	Light (thin) in appearance.	Insufficient developing time. Cold developing solution. Weak developing solution.	Change solution every 2–3 wks (or more frequently if necessary). Use time–temperature method of developing. Utilize "reference film," step wedge, or dental radiographic normalizing and monitoring device to check solution strength.
Overdeveloped film (dense image)	Dark (dense) in appearance.	Prolonged developing time. Hot developing solution.	Use time–temperature method of developing. Perform daily quality assurance (QA) checks on solution strength.
Developer cutoff	A straight radiopaque border on the upper edge of the top film on the processing rack or was not exposed to developing solution in the automatic processor.	This represents an undeveloped area of the film. When the solutions are allowed to deplete in the processing tanks, the films on the top positions of the racks may not be covered by solution when the racks are placed in the tanks. This error should be differentiated from collimator cutoff, which will give a curved radiopaque border if circular collimation is used and a straight border if rectangular collimation is used. In collimator cutoff, the film portion is unexposed. In developer cutoff, the film portion is undeveloped.	Keep processing tanks full. If the level of solution has dropped, do not add water. Add replenisher solution to maintain the desired levels. This error can also occur in automatic processing.
Clear films	No image is seen. Emulsion is removed completely.	Films remain in the water bath from 24 to 48 hours. Films are in the fixer for prolonged periods of time. Film is unexposed. Films are placed in the fixer before the developer.	Films should be removed from the water bath before the end of the day. Films should not be left in the fixer overnight or for prolonged periods. Keep unexposed and exposed films separated. Remember to plug the machine in and turn it on before exposures are performed. Do not process unexposed films. If processing manually, place the films in the developer solution before the fixer. Make sure the fixer solution is positioned after the developer (from left to right) in the automatic processors.
Stained films	Splotches on the film (dark spots = developer; light spots = fixer.)	Wet or dirty working surface.	Keep all surfaces in the darkroom clean and dry.
Discolored films	Yellowish-brown films.	Inadequate fixation.	Fix film optimally for at least 10 minutes or double the developing time. Return all "wet readings" (which are fixed for 3 minutes) to the fixer tank after the patient has been treated (for at least 7 more minutes to equal an optimal fixing time of 10 minutes).

Continued

TABLE A1   Common Processing Errors—cont'd

Common Processing Error	Appearance	Cause	Remedy
Torn emulsion	Film emulsion is torn off.	If films overlap or touch while drying, they will stick together. In separating the films, the emulsion is usually torn off the base in the overlapped areas.	Check that drying films do not touch. If they are stuck together, separate them by applying water.
Scratched films	Radiopaque line on film.	Not carefully placing a second film rack into a tank already containing one rack. Not discarding racks with broken clips. Fingernails too long.	Be careful not to touch one film rack with another film rack when placing them into the tank. Discard any film racks that have sharp edges or broken clips. Keep fingernails trimmed and avoid scratching films with fingernails. Don gloves when applicable.
Lost films in tank	Missing films/films on the bottom of the tank.	Films not firmly clipped onto rack.	Check that films are firmly clipped onto the rack before placing them into the developer.
Fluoride artifact	Black mark on radiograph.	Some fluorides, especially stannous fluoride, will produce black marks on radiographs.	Operator should wash hands thoroughly before handling films or change gloves when applicable.
Reticulation	Image has a wrinkled or stained-glass appearance.	Film developed at an elevated temperature and then placed in a cold water bath (or vice versa); the sudden change in temperature causes the swollen emulsion to shrink rapidly and gives the image a wrinkled (or stained-glass) appearance.	Avoid a sharp contrast in temperature between processing solutions and the water bath.
Air bubbles	White (unprocessed) spots on radiograph.	If air bubbles are trapped on the film, the chemicals cannot affect the emulsion in that area.	Film hanger should be gently agitated when placed into the solutions.
Static marks	Multiple black linear streaks or spots seen most often on cold, dry days.	Intraoral film packets forcefully opened in the darkroom. Extraoral film not carefully slid out of the box. Extraoral film not carefully loaded and unloaded into and out of the cassette. Dragging feet over carpeting and not grounding yourself before unwrapping the film.	Carefully remove film from packet or extraoral film box. Carefully load and unload extraoral film in cassette. Operators should ground themselves and should avoid friction that will produce static electricity.
Automatic Processing			
Daylight loaders: Light leak	Film fog, a ruined film, or unusual artifacts.	Removing one's hands from the baffles before the film has entered the processor.	Operator must keep hands inside the daylight loader until the film has been completely taken up by the automatic processor. Hand baffles that have lost their elasticity should be repaired or replaced.
Dirty rollers	Radiolucent bands or white chalky smudges appear on finished film.	Rollers are not cleaned properly.	Rollers should be cleaned periodically by soaking them according to the manufacturer's recommendations. A piece of extraoral film should be run through the processor every workday to clean the rollers.
Overlapped films	Image of overlapped film on finished film.	Films are fed into the processor too quickly.	The operator should not feed the film into the processor immediately after placing the previous film. The operator should wait at least 10 seconds before putting another film into the processor.

New York University College of Dentistry Radiology Department.

TABLE A2 Common Exposure Errors

Common Exposure Error	Appearance	Cause	Remedy
***Collimator cutoff (cone cutting)	A curved or straight radiopaque border representing an unexposed area on the image.	The x-ray beam is not centered on the receptor.	The central ray of the x-ray beam should be aligned with the center of the receptor. Utilization of a localizing ring with a receptor-holding device can decrease or eliminate the incidence of collimator cutoff. Make sure the patient does not move after the PID is placed for an exposure.
*Film reversal (formerly known as the "herringbone effect")	A light film with the geometric pattern from the lead foil backing embossed on it.	The receptor is placed backward in the mouth.	Always note the front and the back of the film packet. Place the white side (front) of the film toward the lingual (palatal) aspect of the tooth.
****Improper receptor placement	The entire desired area (tooth or teeth) does not appear on the image.	***The patient does not bite down completely on the bite piece of the receptor-holder (inadequate closure). ***The center of the receptor is not aligned with the center of the appropriate tooth (depending on the specific projection being exposed). **Incorrect placement of the sensor on the adhesive bite piece or *failure to place the film to the base of the slot in the film holder (the incisal edge or occlusal surface is cut off).	***Make sure that the patient bites completely on the bite piece with both opposing maxillary and mandibular teeth. ***Align the center of the receptor with the center of the area (tooth or teeth) being radiographed. **Make sure that the placement of the sensor is on the adhesive bite piece or *the film packet is entirely in the bite piece slot correctly.
***Horizontal overlapping	The interproximal areas of the teeth appear to be overlapped when they are not actually overlapped in the patient's mouth.	The central ray is not directed perpendicular to the receptor in the horizontal plane. The receptor is not placed parallel to the tooth or teeth in the horizontal plane.	Direct the central ray through the contact areas in the horizontal plane. Place the receptor parallel to the tooth or teeth in the horizontal plane.
*Black straight or crescent marks	Black marks (artifacts) appear on the film.	Excessive bending of the film packet that results in a cracked emulsion.	Do not bend or over-manipulate the film while placing it in the film holder or in the patient's mouth.
***Underexposed image (light image) [Conventional and digital radiographic error. However, light images can be adjusted with contrast/density modifications when utilizing a digital radiographic system.]	Light (thin) in appearance.	Inadequate exposure due to improper settings, including size of the patient setting, conventional vs. digital setting, and exposure time setting. Failure to press and hold the exposure button until the indicator light goes off and the sound signal ends. Failure to place the PID as close to the localizing ring and to the patient as possible.	Check that all settings on the control panel are correct for each patient and exposure. Maintain pressure on the exposure button until the indicator light goes off and the sound signal ends. Make sure that the PID is as close to the localizing ring and to the patient as possible.

Continued

TABLE A2   Common Exposure Errors—cont'd

Common Exposure Error	Appearance	Cause	Remedy
***Overexposed image (dense image) [Conventional and digital radiographic errors. However, dark images can be adjusted with contrast/density modifications when utilizing a digital radiographic system.]	Dark (dense) in appearance.	Excessive exposure due to improper settings, including the size of the patient setting, conventional vs. digital setting, and exposure time setting.	Check that all settings on the control panel are correct for each patient and exposure.
*Double exposure	Two images appear on one film.	Using the same film packet for more than one exposure.	Separate the exposed films from the unexposed films. When using a film packet with a barrier envelope, remove the barrier envelope immediately after exposure so that it is easy to distinguish between the exposed and unexposed films.
***Blurred images	Wavy or fuzzy image.	Patient, receptor, or tubehead (PID) movement during exposure.	Adjust the tubehead/arm to prevent vibration and drifting. Always keep an eye on the patient, especially when exiting the operatory. Ask the patient "not to move" before exiting the operatory. **When using a digital sensor with an attached wire, watch the wire for any movement that might indicate that the sensor moved inside the patient's mouth.
***Failure to remove dental appliances and facial jewelry	Radiopaque (metal) images are superimposed on the image.	Failure to ask the patient to remove any metallic objects from the mouth or facial area that may be in the way of the primary beam.	For intraoral radiographs, remove any obstructive intraoral appliances, eyeglasses, and facial jewelry before exposure. For panoramic/extraoral radiographs, remove any obstructive intraoral appliances; facial, intra/extraoral and neck jewelry; hair accessories; and hearing aids before exposure.
*Sensor cable artifact on a digital image	The sensor cable wire is superimposed over the oral structures being imaged.	Failure to move the wire (and its metallic components) out of the way of the primary beam.	Be sure to move the sensor wire out of the way of the primary beam before leaving the x-ray cubicle (or room) to press the exposure button. If the sensor is placed upside-down on the bite piece, the wire will be more difficult to keep out of the way of the primary beam. This could be a warning sign that the sensor is not in the holder correctly.

Error	Description	Correction
***Elongation	Lengthening of the image.	Inadequate vertical angulation. Improper occlusal plane orientation because of patient positioning. Poor receptor placement.	Increase the vertical angulation. The occlusal plane should be parallel to the floor. The receptor should be placed parallel to the tooth in the paralleling technique and as close to the tooth as possible (forming an angle with the tooth) when utilizing the bisecting angle technique.
***Foreshortening	Shortening of the image.	Excessive vertical angulation. Improper occlusal plane orientation because of patient positioning. Poor receptor placement.	Decrease the vertical angulation. The occlusal plane should be parallel to the floor. The receptor should be placed parallel to the tooth in the paralleling technique and as close to the tooth as possible (forming an angle with the tooth) when utilizing the bisecting angle technique.

Bitewing Radiographs

Error	Description	Correction
***Horizontal overlapping	The interproximal areas of the teeth appear to be overlapping when they are not actually overlapped in the patient's mouth.	The central ray is not directed perpendicular to the receptor in the horizontal plane. The receptor is not placed parallel to the tooth or teeth in the horizontal plane.	The beam should be aligned in the horizontal plane so that it is at right angles to the tooth and receptor. The receptor should be placed parallel to the tooth or teeth in the horizontal plane.
***Collimator cutoff (cone cutting)	A curved or straight radiopaque border representing an unexposed area on the image.	The x-ray beam is not directed at the center of the receptor.	Make sure to aim the central ray at the center of the receptor. If a bitewing tab is being used, the bite tab could be kept visible by asking the patient to smile and revealing the tab for better aim. The operator can keep a finger on the tab while positioning the PID and directing the central ray at the tab. A localizing ring can be used to help center the x-ray beam.
***Improper receptor placement	The entire desired area (tooth or teeth) does not appear on the image.	Failure to center the receptor so that all desired structures are seen. The patient fails to close completely on both sides (maxillary and mandibular) of the bite piece (Inadequate Closure).	Place the receptor so that its center is lined up with the recommended central area for that specific bitewing projection (e.g., 2nd premolar for the premolar bitewing). Make sure that the patient closes down on both sides of the bite piece when taking bitewings so that the maxillary and mandibular teeth are represented equally on the image.

*Errors involving conventional (film-based) radiography only
**Errors involving digital radiography only
***Errors involving conventional (film-based) and digital radiography
New York University College of Dentistry Radiology Department.

TABLE A3   Common Errors in Conventional/or Digital Panoramic Radiography

Common Error/Cause	Resultant Image	Panoramic Remedy
Patient positioned too far forward	Upper and lower teeth are blurred and narrow; spinal column is superimposed on the ramus; premolars are overlapped.	Patient's teeth or edentulous ridges must be in proper anterior-posterior position on the bite block.
Patient positioned too far back	Upper and lower teeth are blurred and widened; increased ghosting of the mandible also appears.	Patient's teeth or edentulous ridges must be in proper anterior-posterior position on the bite block.
Patient's head tilted up; forehead too far back; chin is too far forward	Upper incisors out of focus; the radiopaque hard palate is superimposed over the apices of the upper teeth; condyles are off the image.	The reference lines on the patient's face, the Frankfort plane or the ala-tragus line, should be aligned parallel to the floor.
Patient's head tilted down; chin is back; forehead is forward	Lower incisors are blurred; the radiopaque image of the hyoid bone is superimposed on the anterior part of the mandible; the superior portions of the condyles may be cut off the image; premolars are overlapped.	The reference lines on the patient's face, the Frankfort horizontal plane or the ala-tragus line, should be aligned parallel to the floor.
Patient moved during exposure	The part of the receptor being exposed at the time of movement appears blurred.	Talk to patients prior to and, if possible, during exposure to remind them not to move.
Patient failed to place the tongue on the roof of the mouth	An airspace is created that produces a radiolucent band below the palate and superimposed over the apices of the maxillary teeth.	Remind patients to keep their tongue against the roof of their mouth during exposure.
Patient does not sit or stand erect (patient is slouching)	The spinal column causes a triangular radiopacity to be superimposed on the anterior teeth.	Keep patient's spine erect during positioning.
Failure to remove metallic objects, such as dentures, jewelry (including facial jewelry), hair accessories, hearing aids, and eyeglasses from the face, head, neck, and mouth	Radiopaque ghosting will appear on the opposite side and higher than the actual image with less detail and definition than the actual image and may obscure desired structures.	Remove all metallic objects from the face, head, neck, and mouth regions before exposure.
Lead apron placed above the level of the clavicles	A large radiopacity will appear on the image.	Keep the lead apron low on the patient (below the level of the clavicles); never use a thyroid collar.
Film cassette slowing down because of patient contact	Black vertical band will appear on the image due to localized overexposure. Exposing the patient to unnecessary radiation.	Position the patient carefully; make sure that the receptor will not contact the patient before actually exposing the projection (especially patients with large frames).
Static electricity (conventional panoramic radiography only)	Electrostatic artifact; black linear streaks resembling bare tree branches without leaves.	Be careful not to pull film quickly and forcefully out of box and not to rub film on film screens during film loading, especially on cold/dry days. The operators should ground themselves and avoid friction that will produce static electricity.

New York University College of Dentistry Radiology Department.

Glossary

A

abrasion The wearing away of tooth structure by mechanical means (e.g., toothbrush).

absorption A process in which the intensity of a beam of radiation is reduced as a result of the interactions involved in passing through matter.

acquired immunodeficiency syndrome (AIDS) The group of disease entities caused by the human immunodeficiency virus (HIV).

actual focal area The true representation of the area of the anode of an x-ray tube that the electrons actually strike.

acute (short-term) effects The effects of radiation that manifest themselves within minutes, days, or weeks after exposure.

administrative radiograph A radiograph taken for other than diagnostic purposes, such as a radiograph taken for verification of third-party payment.

advanced caries Caries that has penetrated through the dentin and is about to reach the pulp chamber.

ALARA principle (concept) The acronym for *as low as reasonably achievable*. This term refers to reducing radiation exposure to patients as much as possible within the dental office without excessive cost or inconvenience to the patient.

ala-tragus line An imaginary line between the ala of the nose and the tragus of the ear that is kept parallel to the floor particularly for panoramic radiographs.

alpha particle A positively charged particle emitted from an atomic nucleus.

alternating current (AC) Current that flows in one direction and then in the opposite direction in the circuit.

alveolar bone The bone of the mandible and maxilla that supports and surrounds the roots of the teeth.

alveolar crest The most coronal portion of the alveolar bone found between the teeth.

amelogenesis imperfecta The hereditary developmental defect of enamel seen in both the primary and secondary dentition.

American Academy of Oral and Maxillofacial Radiology (AAOMR) An organization established to promote and advance the art and science of radiology in dentistry and to provide a forum for communication among and professional advancement of its members.

American National Standards Institute (ANSI) Institute that designates film speed (sensitivity) by using the letters A through F (A for the slowest film and F for the fastest).

Amperage (ampere) (A) The unit of measurement of the amount of current flowing in an electric circuit. The unit milliampere (mA) is one-thousandth of an ampere and is the important unit of current measurement pertaining to an x-ray tube.

analog Relating to a mechanism in which data are represented by continuously variable physical quantities.

angstrom unit (Å) A unit of measurement equal to one-millionth of a centimeter; x-ray wavelengths are expressed in angstrom units.

angulation The direction of the primary x-ray beam in relation to the tooth and receptor.

anode The positively charged side of the dental x-ray tube. It contains the tungsten target at which the electrons are aimed and from which x-rays are emitted.

anodontia The developmental absence of teeth. It can be complete or partial.

ANSI See *American National Standards Institute.*

anterior nasal spine The radiopacity seen in the midline of the maxilla at the inferior termination of the nasal septum.

anterior palatine foramen The opening in the midline of the palate just posterior to the central incisors through which vessels and nerves emerge.

anteroposterior projection An extraoral radiograph of the skull seen in the coronal plane.

antibiotic prophylaxis The antimicrobial drugs prescribed before dental treatment for patients whose medical conditions can be affected by a bacteremia resulting from dental treatment.

antiseptic A substance that inhibits the growth of bacteria.

antral or inverted "Y" The radiopaque "Y" formed by the anterior and inferior border of the maxillary sinus as the arms and the floor of the nasal cavity as the stem which is useful in the mounting orientation of maxillary canine projections.

arch The formation of teeth seen in the axial plane.

arthrography Modality for radiographic evaluation of a bone joint after injection of a radiopaque contrast medium.

atom The basic unit of matter, composed of a positively charged nucleus around which negatively charged electrons revolve.

atomic mass The total number of protons and neutrons in the nucleus of an atom and is designated by the letter A.

atomic number The number of protons in the nucleus of an atom. The symbol is Z, and it is written as the subscript, for example, 3Li.

attenuation Absorbing or weakening of an x-ray beam because of passage through a material.

attrition The wearing away of teeth by occlusal forces.

autoclaving The sterilizing of instruments by steam.

automatic processing The processing of radiographs by machine, eliminating the need for human interaction to move the films through the processing solutions. This technique employs a standardized procedure for processing films as it is basically an automated time-temperature method.

autotransformer A transformer that has only one coil and a series of taps that allow it to increase or reduce voltage.

axial plane The plane of the head that is parallel to the floor.

B

background radiation The ever-present manmade or naturally occurring ionizing radiation in the environment. Its sources include cosmic rays, radon, radioactive materials, industrial waste, and nuclear fallout.

barrier A radiation-absorbing material such as lead, concrete, or plaster used to protect an area from radiation. The term also refers to protection used against microorganisms, such as the use of gloves, masks, glasses, and surface coverings.

barrier envelope A plastic bag that the x-ray film packet is placed in to prevent contamination by saliva.

becquerel (Bq) The Système International (SI) unit of radioactivity produced by the disintegration of unstable elements. It replaces the curie.

bedridden A term used to describe a patient who cannot leave his or her bed; such patients cannot travel to a dental office to have radiographs exposed on them or receive dental treatment.

benign lesion A term applied to tumors that may be harmful but not life-threatening.

beta particles Electrons emitted from the nuclei of radioactive atoms.

bilateral lesion A lesion that is on both sides of the oral cavity. Most bilateral findings are normal anatomic landmarks.

binding energy The energy (expressed in electron volts) that binds the orbiting electrons around the nucleus of an atom.

biopsy An examination of tissue removed from a living body to discover the presence, cause, or extent of a disease.

bisecting-angle technique (bisecting the angle) A technique for intraoral periapical radiography in which the receptor is positioned as close to the tooth as possible and the central x-ray is directed vertically perpendicular to an imaginary line that bisects the angle formed by the long axis of the tooth and the receptor .

bite block A device used to support and position dental receptors in the patient's mouth.

bitewing projections (radiographs) Intraoral images that show only the crown portions of opposing teeth in the biting position primarily utilized to view interproximal areas.

blurred image An image showing decreased detail and definition as a result of patient, film, or x-ray source movement during an exposure.

bone marrow The soft inner portion of bone.

bone window The density range in computed tomography in which bone images are seen without superimposition of soft tissue.

bremsstrahlung (general) radiation Literally *braking radiation*, the release of a photon of energy by a bombarding electron slowed and bent off course by an atom.

buccal caries Demineralization of the hard tissue structure present on the outside surface of the tooth that is difficult to detect radiographically.

buccal-object rule In localization, if an object on a second radiograph moves in the opposite direction of the horizontal tube shift, then the object is buccally positioned.

buccinator shadow The radiopaque area seen mostly in the maxillary premolar area that represents the soft tissue density of the muscle in the cheek (buccinator muscle).

C

calibration procedure When dental x-ray machines are adjusted for accuracy at regular intervals. X-ray machine calibration is performed by a competent technician to confirm that the radiographic equipment is functioning properly in producing consistently diagnostically acceptable radiographic images.

calcification Hardening of a structure caused by calcium deposition.

calcium tungstate The fluorescent material used to coat intensifying screens, emitting a blue light.

calculus The radiopaque calcification concretion that adheres to the teeth.

cancellous bone Bone that is composed mainly of marrow.

caries Demineralization of the hard tooth structure with subsequent destruction. Appears radiolucent on radiographs.

cassette A wrapping or container for x-ray film that is light-tight yet permits penetration of x-rays. Cassettes may be plastic, cardboard, or metal.

cathode The negatively charged side of the dental x-ray tube. It contains the tungsten filament and the molybdenum focusing cup.

cathode ray The stream of electrons in the x-ray tube traveling from filament to target.

cell recovery The process by which cells heal themselves from the effects of radiation.

cementoenamel junction That place on the tooth where the enamel ends and the cementum begins.

cemento-osseous dysplasia (COD) Is a condition of the jaws that is inherently a benign lesion. It arises from the fibroblasts of the periodontal ligaments.

cementum The calcified tissue that surrounds the root and helps to support the tooth.

centers of roatation In tomography, the point around which the source of radiation rotates. The center of rotation changes as the receptor and x-ray source rotate which allows the image layer (focal trough) to conform to the shape of the dental arches.

Centers for Disease Control and Prevention (CDC) The U.S. governmental agency based in Atlanta, Georgia, that is responsible for tracking and responding to outbreaks of infectious disease.

central ray That x-ray located in the center of the x-ray beam as it leaves the tube head.

cephalometric radiography The modality for measuring the skull by means of radiography.

cephalostat The head-holding device used in cephalometric radiography.

Certified Radiation Equipment Safety Officer (CRESO) Those who perform the inspection and calibration of x-ray equipment. Their responsibilities include performing checks on the kilovoltage, milliamperage, output, timer accuracy, tube head stability, and x-ray beam alignment of the dental x-ray unit.

cervical burnout The shadow seen interproximally on radiographs that is caused by the concavity in the root surface at that area. It may resemble caries.

chair position The position of the chair and its head rest and back rest during radiographic procedures.

characteristic radiation X-rays produced when orbiting electrons in an atom fall from outer shells to inner shells after an orbiting electron is knocked out of one of the inner shells by bombarding electrons.

charge-coupled device (CCD) A type of electronic sensor used in direct digital radiography.

chromosomes One of a definite number of rodlike bodies, containing genes, found in the nucleus of a cell. At the time of cell division, they duplicate, divide, and distribute evenly in the resulting cells.

chronic effects See *long-term effects.*

clear film A film that after processing does not show an image.

cleft palate The developmental condition in which embryonic fusion of the palate fails to occur.

clusters The high incidence of cancers in certain geographic areas.

coherent scatter An interaction of x-rays with matter in which the path of the x-ray is deviated without a loss of energy.

coin test A test carried out in the darkroom to test the effectiveness of the safelight.

collimation The process of restricting the size and shape of the x-ray beam.

collimator A device that limits the size and shape of the x-ray beam.

collimator cutoff (cone cutting) A curved or straight radiopaque border representing an unexposed area on the image caused by not centering the x-ray beam on the receptor while using a circular- (cylindrical) or rectangular-shaped PID

complementary metal oxide semiconductor (CMOS) A type of electronic sensor used in direct digital radiography.

composite Synthetic restoration primarily used in anterior regions.

Compton effect An interaction between x-rays and matter whereby the x-ray photon is deflected from its path after dislodging a loosely bound electron from an atom. This interaction takes place about 62% of the time in dental radiography.

computed tomography (CT) scanning Tomographic process in which x-ray scanning produces digital data that measure the extent of the energy transmission through an object. This information is stored and transformed by a computer into a density scale that is used to generate an image.

concavity A depression.

concha The radiopaque outgrowth of tissue from the lateral walls of the nasal cavity.

concrescence The condition in which two or more teeth are joined by their cementum.

condensing osteitis A condition characterized by the formation of dense bone around the apex of a tooth in response to low-grade pulpal necrosis.

cone The pointed position-indicating device on the dental x-ray machine through which the x-rays travel after leaving the tube.

cone beam computed tomography (CBCT) A more recent means to acquire a CT image for dental purposes and is also known as cone beam volumetric tomography (CBVT). This technique involves use of a round or rectangular cone-shaped x-ray beam on a two-dimensional x-ray sensor.

cone cutting The error produced by not centering the x-ray beam on the receptor, producing unexposed areas on the image while using a cone-shaped PID .

confidentiality The state of being free from unauthorized disclosure. For example, material in a dental chart is confidential information.

congenital A condition that is present at birth.

contrast The difference in densities between adjacent areas on the radiograph.

coronal plane An orientation plane that divides the head into front and back portions.

coronoid process of the mandible The mesial superior radiopaque part of the ascending ramus of the mandible that is seen in the distal inferior portions of maxillary molar periapical radiographs.

cortical bone The dense outer layer of the mandible and maxilla.

cosmic ray Radiation that has its origin outside of the Earth's atmosphere (e.g., radiation from the sun).

coulombs/kg The unit for expressing x-ray exposure in the SI system.

CRESO See *Certified Radiation Equipment Safety Officer.*

crest The height of an energy (i.e. x-ray) wave.

critical organ An organ that if damaged by radiation will seriously affect a patient's quality of life.

cross-contamination The spreading of microorganisms from one instrument or patient to another.

crown-root ratio The relationship between the length of the tooth that is embedded in bone and the part that is not.

CT number A number indicating the density of a tissue on a CT scan.

Cummulaive effective dose (CUMEfd) The accumulated lifetime dose of radiation that dental personnel should not exceed.

cumulative effects These are effects that are additive, as repetitive exposure can damage cells that are not repaired and can lead to health problems.

cupping The change of shape seen radiographically in the crest of the interseptal bone that is cup-shaped.

curie (Ci) The unit of measurement of the number of nuclear disintegrations of a radioactive element. The curie was superseded by the becquerel in 1985.

cut A tomographic plane.

cycle (of electric current) The sine wave plot of the change in polarity of an alternating current circuit in which the current travels first in the positive direction and then in the negative direction.

cyst A pathologic radiolucent lesion in which a bone cavity is lined by epithelium.

D

dark (dense) image A dense or black image.

darkroom A room with controlled lighting where x-ray film is handled and processed.

darkroom maintenance Steps taken to ensure quality assurance in the darkroom.

daylight loader The device attached to an automatic processor that allows the operator to develop film in ambient light.

Deciduous teeth The primary dentition.

definition (detail) The degree of clarity on a radiograph.

definitive diagnosis A final diagnosis that is made after getting the results of all performed diagnostic examinations (i.e. prescribed radiographs).

dens invaginatus A developmental disturbance whereby the enamel organ invaginates into the pulp of the tooth.

Dense (dark) image A dark or black image.

density (receptor) The degree of blackness on a radiograph.

density (object) The relative mass of an object through which an x-ray beam passes, causing it to appear radiopaque or radiolucent.

dental papilla Appears at the root apex as the newly erupted tooth progresses into the oral cavity.

deterministic or nonstochastic effects These effects have a clear relationship between the exposure and the effect. In addition, the magnitude of the effect is directly proportional to the size of the dose.

dentigerous cyst (follicular cyst) A cyst that develops from the enamel organ of a tooth. It may contain the tooth or be adjacent to it.

dentin Comprises the major part of the tooth structure and is seen in both the crown and the root portions of the tooth. Dentin is radiopaque on radiographs.

dentinogenesis imperfecta A hereditary disturbance that affects both the primary and secondary dentition. It is characterized by poor enamel that may wear thin or chip, early calcification of the pulp chambers and canals, and short roots, especially noticeable in the permanent teeth.

dentoalveolar abscess An abscess in bone resulting from a necrotic pulp.

detail See *definition.*

detector The digital electronic sensor (receptor) that is used in digital radiographic techniques to produce an image of the oral structures after it is exposed to x-radiation and is connected to a computer in some manner.

developer The solution used in the processing of exposed x-ray film that softens the emulsion and precipitates silver from the silver bromide crystals of the film emulsion that have been energized by x-rays.

developer cutoff The blank area on processed radiographs that results from an insufficient level of solution in the darkroom developer tank.

developmental disability Patients who are mentally disabled or have other physical conditions, such as cerebral palsy or autism, and are afflicted before the age of 22.

diaphragm The lead-collimating device found in the dental x-ray machine that limits the beam size.

DICOM images The digital receptor receives the information generated by the radiation exposure. This raw data is three-dimensional, goes through reconstruction, and forms a pile of images known as DICOM images. These images are transferred to the software that allows the dental professional to view the area of interest (FOV) in the axial, coronal, and sagittal planes.

differential diagnosis The process that the diagnostician goes through with the use of radiographs, clinical examination, and patient history to formulate a diagnosis.

digital image An image formed by a computer after the conversion of analog penetration data to digital expression.

digitize Convert to numbers.

dilaceration A developmental disturbance that results in an abnormally curved root or crown.

dimensional accuracy The accurate dimensional relationship of one part of a tooth to another on a radiographic image.

dimensional distortion The distortion seen primarily with the bisecting-angle technique in which parts of the object farther from the receptor are foreshortened in relation to parts of the object that are closer to the receptor (e.g., the buccal roots of maxillary molars versus the palatal root).

direct current (DC) Electric current that flows in one direction and does not reverse itself.

direct digital radiography Digital modality that involves use of a (wired or wireless) sensor that has a direct relationship to the computer, with the sensor being either a charge-coupled device or a complementary metal oxide semiconductor.

direct effects of radiation Radiation effects that are the results of the x-radiation striking the affected cell.

direct supervision Referring to the physical presence of the dentist during a staff member's performance of duties.

disability A physical or mental condition that limits or impairs a person's life activities.

disclosure The process of informing the patient about the risks and benefits of a procedure.

disinfection The process of destroying disease-causing microorganisms by physical or chemical means.

distodens (distomolar, paramolar, or fourth molar) A supernumerary tooth seen distal to the third molar.

distortion A change in the size or shape of an object seen on a radiograph.

divergent beam The primary beam of x-radiation that spreads as it leaves the tube.

dose The amount of radiation energy absorbed per unit mass of tissue at a particular site.

dose equivalent A concept that allows for the fact that not all radiations are identical in biologic effects. The dose equivalent is expressed in rems or sieverts.

dose rate The dose in rads or grays absorbed per unit of time.

dose-response curve The plot of the effect of radiation as a function of the dose given.

double exposure An error in which the same film packet is used twice, producing superimposed images.

double film packet A dental film packet in which there are two pieces of film.

drying A step in the processing of radiographs where any residual water is removed.

duplicating film A reversal film used to replicate original images.

duty cycle The portion of every minute that the dental x-ray machine can be used without overheating.

duty rating The number of consecutive seconds in a minute that a dental x-ray machine can be operated without overheating.

E

effective dose A calculation that considers the difference in tissue sensitivity. It is the preferred method for comparing effective tissue sensitivity.

effective focal area The apparent size and shape of the focal spot when viewed from a position in the primary beam.

electric current The flow of electricity through a circuit.

electromagnetic radiation A grouping of energy waves that have the weightlessness of the waves and the speed of which they travel (the speed of light-86,000 miles per second) in common.

electromagnetic spectrum The spectrum of energy-bearing waves whose properties are determined by their wavelength, frequency and penetrating ability.

electron A negatively charged particle, which is a constituent of every neutral atom.

electron cloud The electrons at the cathode surrounding the tungsten filament.

electronic timers Timers that are used with the newer dental x-ray units. The use of electronic timers, as opposed to mechanical timers, is imperative as short exposure times are employed with digital sensors and faster, more sensitive contemporary x-ray films.

electrostatic artifact Black linear streaks or black spots on the radiograph caused by static electricity.

elongation The distortion on a radiograph that results in lengthening of the image particularly caused by insufficient vertical angulation.

emulsion The silver halide suspension in gelatin that is coated on the x-ray film base.

enamel The radiopaque covering of the crown of the tooth.

enamel hypoplasia A defect associated with a reduced thickness of enamel that is formed during the developing stages of the enamel.

enamel pearls (enameloma) Small, rounded, hyperplastic area of enamel seen on the roots of the teeth.

endostosis (dense bone island, idiopathic osteosclerosis) An internal growth of bone that is considered to be the internal version of exostoses that appears radiopaque on radiographic images and are asymptomatic and within normal limits.

enlargement An increase in the size of the image.

erosion A condition of the teeth that results from a chemical action not involving bacteria on the tooth surface. Areas of erosion appear as radiolucent defects on the tooth and can be mistaken for caries radiographically.

eruption The emergence of teeth into the oral cavity.

exostosis (hyperostosis) An overgrowth of bone on the surface of the alveolar bone.

exposure A measure of the ionization in air produced by x-ray or gamma radiation.

exposure routine The order in which exposures are taken.

exposure technique The technique used by the operator to exposure radiographic images. The goal of the dental professional is to perfect their technique, reduce radiographic retakes and produce diagnostically acceptable radiographs with the least amount of radiation exposure to the patient and to themselves.

exposure time The amount of time, expressed in fractions of seconds or impulses, that x-rays are generated.

extension paralleling technique A technique for intraoral radiography that uses a 16-in target-receptor distance, receptor placement parallel to the long axis of the teeth, and a central ray direction perpendicular to both the object and the receptor.

external oblique ridge A radiopaque line seen in mandibular posterior periapical radiographs that appears higher and shorter than the internal oblique or mylohyoid ridge.

external resorption The idiopathic condition seen radiographically where the tissue from the periodontal ligament causes resorption of the dentin.

extraction socket The radiolucent area on a radiograph that has not filled with bone after a tooth is removed from that area.

extraoral projections Radiographs that are taken with the receptor and source of radiation outside of the patient's mouth.

F

fallout A form of background radiation produced by a nuclear explosion.

federal regulations A set of regulations promulgated by the U.S. government governing the manufacture and performance of dental x-ray machines.

field of view (FOV) The patient's maxillofacial area that is of interest when taking a CBCT (CBVT) image.

filament The tungsten wire found at the cathode in the x-ray tube that when heated boils off electrons.

filling overhang Poorly contoured filling that allows accumulation of debris.

film A transparent sheet of cellulose acetate or a similar material that is coated on both sides with an emulsion sensitive to radiation and light.

film badge A recording device worn to record one's exposure to ionizing radiation.

film base The cellulose acetate sheet on which the emulsion is coated.

film contrast The difference in the degrees of density.

film fog An overall gray appearance due to diminished contrast.

film hanger The device that carries the film through the manual processing procedure.

film-holding device The device used to hold a film in place for intraoral radiography.

film mount A cardboard or plastic holder for finished radiographs.

film packet The film receptor used in conventional (film-based) radiography consisting of the an outer vinyl package wrapper, a black paper film wrapper, an x-ray film, and a lead foil backing.

film reversal The improper placement of the film packet in the patient's mouth that results in an underexposed film with a geometric pattern (i.e. herringbone pattern), caused by the useful beam striking the lead foil backing before the film.

film roller That part of an automatic processor that moves the film along from one step to another in the automatic processing sequence.

film-screen system The imaging system used in conventional extraoral radiography in which the film is used in combination with intensifying screens.

film speed (sensitivity) An expression of how much radiation for a given period of time is necessary to produce an image on film.

film viewing The positioning of the finished radiographs on an illuminating device for reading and interpretation.

filter An aluminum disk placed in the path of the useful beam that absorbs the softer, less penetrating radiations.

filtration The removal of long (soft), nonpenetrating x-ray photons from the x-ray beam.

fissural cysts Cysts that are always found in predictable anatomic locations because they develop along embryonic suture lines.

fixation The localization of an object in three planes.

fixer The solution used in the processing of exposed x-ray film that removes the unaffected silver bromide crystals from the emulsion and hardens (preserves) the image.

flexible cassette A cassette that can be wound around a drum for panoramic radiography.

floor of maxillary sinus The radiopaque horizontal line seen above the apices of the maxillary premolars and molars on periapical films.

floor of the nasal cavity The horizontal radiopaque line seen in the maxillary incisor maxillary incisor, canine and posterior regions.

florid cemento-osseous dysplasia (FLCOD) Is considered a type of COD (cemento-osseous dysplasia) but can occur in both maxilla and mandible and in multiple quadrants.

fluorescence The property of emitting visible light when struck by radiation.

focal-film distance (FFD) The distance from the focal spot (target) at the anode of the dental x-ray tube to the receptor . It is usually expressed in inches (e.g., an 8-in FFD). Currently known as the target-receptor distance.

Focal-object distance The distance from the focal spot (target) at the anode of the dental x-ray tube to the object (i.e. tooth) being radiographed.

focal cemento-osseous dysplasia (FCOD) Is a condition similar to PCOD (periapical cemento-osseous dysplasia) but occurs in the posterior mandible, distal to the canines. It usually occurs as a single-site lesion.

focal spot (area) See *target.*

focal trough That plane of an object that is seen clearly on a tomogram also known as the *plane of acceptable detail.*

fog A detrimental density imparted to a radiographic image by the film base and chemical action on unexposed silver grains. An overall gray appearance due to diminished contrast. Fog is increased by inadvertent exposure to white light.

follicle (dental sac) As crown formation progresses, the radiolucent follicle (dental sac) is seen surrounding the crown of the tooth. This is a sac containing the developing tooth and its odontogenic organ.

foramen A normal radiolucent opening in bone.

foreshortening The distortion on a radiograph that results in shortening of the image primarily caused by excessive vertical angulation.

fossa A radiolucent depression in bone.

fracture The breaking of a part of an oral structure, usually resulting in a radiolucency.

Frankfort plane The imaginary line connecting the floor of the orbit and the superior border of the external auditory meatus.

free radical An uncharged molecule that exists with a single unpaired electron in its outer shell.

frequency The number of oscillations that an energy wave makes per second.

full-mouth series (full-mouth survey) A series of intraoral radiographs that gives diagnostic information for all teeth and desired bony areas. It is usually composed of periapical and bitewing projections.

furcation The area between the roots of a multi-rooted tooth.

fusion The developmental disturbance in which two teeth are joined, resulting in a large crown and two root canals.

G

gag reflex The retching or coughing, caused by contact of the receptor, or holding device with the patient's palate or other intraoral tissues.

gamma rays Electromagnetic radiation of short wavelengths that emanate from radioactive materials.

gelatin The material coating the cellulose acetate base of film in which the halide crystals are suspended.

gemination The developmental disturbance of teeth whereby a tooth has one root canal but two crowns.

gene The basic unit of inheritance, located in the chromosome, which determines hereditary characteristics.

general supervision Referring to the fact that the dentist need not be directly present during a licensed staff member's performance of duties.

genetic effects The changes produced in an individual's genes and chromosomes; usually refers to those changes in reproductive cells.

genial tubercle The radiopacity seen apical to the teeth on mandibular central incisor periapical radiographs at the midline of the mandible.

ghost image The objects that have the greatest density (e.g., bone or metal objects) and are out of the plane of acceptable detail (focal trough) are shown in two places on the panoramic image. One place is the intended image or the usable image, and the other is referred to as the ghost image. The ghost image is always reversed, has less sharpness and is seen at a point higher on the projection than the desired image.

gray (Gy) The Système International (SI) unit for absorbed dose. One gray equals 100 rads.

gray level The density seen on a digital image.

grid A device used to prevent object scatter from affecting the receptor.

group D film An ANSI rating for intermediate-speed film.

group E film An ANSI rating for fast film.

group F film An ANSI rating for the fastest film available.

H

H & D curve The H & D (Hunter and Driffield) curve is a plot that shows the relationship between film exposure and its resultant density.

half-value layer The thickness of a specific material that attenuates the x-ray beam intensity to one half. It is an expression of beam quality.

half-wave rectified The blocking of the reversal of current across the dental x-ray tube.

halide Compound of metal with the halogen element bromine, chlorine, or iodine.

hamular notch The radiolucent anatomic landmark that is located distal to the maxillary tuberosity.

hamular process (hamulus) The radiopaque bone that is located distal to the hamular notch.

hard copy The printout of a digital image.

headrest position Proper position of the patient's head for radiographic exposure.

Health Insurance Portability and Accountability Act (HIPAA) Enacted in April 2000 to ensure patient confidentiality in healthcare delivery.

hearing-impaired Physical disability that affects a person's ability to hear efficiently.

hemostat An instrument that can serve as an intraoral receptor holder.

hepatitis Infectious disease categorized by inflammation of the liver caused by the hepatitis virus. Dental personnel should be immunized (vaccinated) for the hepatitis B virus (HBV).

high contrast High contrast images appear mainly black and white with very few gray tones, and the densities (black and white) seen are easy to distinguish from each other. They also are referred to as short-scale contrast images and are produced by a lower kilovoltage range.

horizontal angulation The aiming of the x-ray beam in the horizontal plane.

horizontal bone loss Interproximal periodontal bone loss in the horizontal plane.

Hounsfield unit A unit used in computed tomographic scanning to express the density of a specific area of the image.

human immunodeficiency virus (HIV) The virus that compromises the immune system, leading to acquired immunodeficiency syndrome (AIDS).

hypercementosis A condition that results in formation of excess cementum on the root of a tooth.

hyperdontia (supernumerary teeth) Supernumerary, or extra, teeth. The most common supernumerary teeth are mandibular premolars, maxillary incisors, and fourth molars.

hyperostotic lines Clearly defined radiopaque borders of slow-growing benign lesions.

hypodontia Is the failure of teeth to develop. It can occur in either the primary or adult dentition.

I

illuminator See *viewbox.*

image A picture or representation of an object.

image acquisition Acquisition of a computerized image in computed tomographic scanning and digital radiography.

image density The degree of blackness on an image.

image layer See *focal trough.*

image manipulation The changing or modification of a digital image.

image receptor The component of an imaging system that the x-ray photons strike.

imaginary bisecting line The line that bisects the angle formed by the long axis of the tooth and the receptor.

imaging The visual representation of an object.

imaging plate Reusable plastic storage phosphor sensor that is employed in indirect digital radiography and is not wired to the computer but uses a laser scanner to produce an image.

imaging system The film, digital sensor, or film-screen combination that the x-rays strike to produce the visible image.

immunization Protection of an individual from a communicable disease achieved by giving the patient a modified or weakened form of the causative microorganism.

impaction The condition of a tooth not being able to erupt by its expected time.

implant fixture The radiopaque metallic device that is placed in the maxilla or mandible to replace a missing tooth.

impulse The radiation generated during a half cycle of an alternating current.

incipient caries Caries that radiographically is only in the enamel.

incisive canal The radiolucent anatomic landmark in the maxillary anterior region that can be seen leading to the incisive foramen.

incisive foramen See *nasopalatine foramen.*

indirect digital radiography A kind of digital radiography in which the finished radiograph is scanned to produce a digital image.

indirect effects Cell damage caused when the cells hit directly by radiation produce toxins that affect cells not in the radiation beam.

infection Contamination caused by disease-producing microorganisms.

infectious waste Waste that is contaminated with blood, saliva, or other body fluids.

inferior alveolar canal (mandibular canal) The radiolucent band seen on mandibular molar and premolar radiographs. It originates at the mandibular foramen and runs downward and forward to end at the mental foramen.

inferior border of the mandible A broad radiopaque band that represents the thick cortical bone of the inferior portion of the mandible. The inferior border of the mandible can be seen in all of the intraoral mandibular projections.

inferior nasal concha (turbinate) The radiopacity that sometimes projects into the nasal fossa from its lateral wall and can be seen on maxillary anterior radiographs.

informed consent The permission granted or implied by the patient to allow treatment to be rendered after a full explanation of the treatment has been made.

infrabony pocket The area created and seen on radiographs as the result of crestal bone loss.

intensifying screen A coating of fluorescent material on a suitable base that intensifies the radiation, thus permitting a decrease in exposure time.

intensity The product of the quantity and the quality of the x-ray beam per unit of area per time of exposure.

interaction The result of radiation reacting with any form of matter.

internal oblique ridge (mylohyoid ridge) The radiopaque line that is seen running anteriorly on radiographs from the ascending ramus to the genial tubercles of the mandible that appears longer and lower than the external oblique ridge.

internal resorption The process in which pulpal cells resorb the walls of the pulp chamber or canal to form a communication to the periodontal ligament.

interpretation An explanation of radiographic findings.

interproximal caries Caries on the mesial or distal surfaces of teeth that are best viewed on bitewing radiographs.

intraoffice peer review The evaluation mechanism for maintaining superior levels of chairside technique between personnel within a dental office.

inverse square law An expression of the relationship between the exposure time and focal-film distance (target-receptor distance). This law states that the intensity of radiation is inversely proportional to the square of the distance between a point source and the irradiated surface.

ion An electrically charged (+ or −) particle of matter.

ionization The process by which an electrically stable or neutral atom or molecule gains or loses electrons and thereby acquires a positive or negative charge.

ionizing radiation The property of radiation that produces ions when interacting with matter.

isotope An atom whose nucleus has the same number of protons but a different number of neutrons.

K

kilovoltage (kilovolt) (kV) An electric potential difference as measured in kilovolts (a unit of measurement equal to 1000 V). Controls the quality of the x-ray beam in the dental x-ray tube.

kilovolt peak (kVp) A unit of measurement used in dental radiology to express the kilovoltage setting on the control panel. It implies that not all the x-rays generated are of the penetrating power called for; rather, the numerical setting is the peak and is usually employed with x-ray machines that operate on an alternating current.

L

labial mounting A means of mounting and viewing processed radiographs so that the observer's point of view is looking into the patient's mouth with the patient's right side on the viewer's left.

lamina dura A radiopaque line of cortical bone that surrounds the periodontal ligament surrounding the tooth's root.

laminogram (tomogram) A radiograph of a three-dimensional object that shows a predetermined plane clearly while blurring out all other superimposed structures.

latent image The term used to describe the x-ray film after it has been exposed. The film contains the latent image that will be made visible by film processing.

latent period The delay between exposure of an organism to radiation and manifestation of change produced by that radiation.

lateral fossa A depression in the labial plate in the maxillary lateral incisor region. It appears as a radiolucency between the maxillary lateral incisor and canine.

lateral oblique projection of the mandible Projection used for surveying one side of the mandible.

lateral skull projection (cephalometric projection) An extraoral radiograph that shows the entire skull in the sagittal plane.

lead apron The flexible lead or lead-equivalent drape placed over the patient's torso to shield from secondary radiation.

lead foil backing One of the components of the intraoral film packet that prevents backscatter.

lead-lined boxes Shielded boxes used in the past, for unprotected film that over time may contaminate the film with an oxidized leaded white powder.

liability The responsibility for a deed or decision.

licensure The permission granted by a governmental body that allows one to work in his or her profession.

light leak The area where unwanted white light is entering a darkroom.

light-tight A term used in radiography to indicate that there is no white light exposure.

line pairs per millimeter A measure of contrast discrimination (gray levels) in an image.

lingual caries Demineralization of the hard tooth structure on the lingual surface of a tooth.

lingual foramen A radiolucent opening in the lingual surface of the mandibular anterior bony structure and appears at the center of the genial tubercles on a radiograph.

lingual mounting A means of mounting and viewing processed radiographs so that the observer's point of view is looking at the teeth from within the patient's mouth with the patient's right side on the viewer's right and the patient's left side on the viewer's left.

litigious Tending to bring legal action.

localization Locating radiographic structures, particularly in the buccolingual plane.

localized exposure The measurement of radiation to the area of the body that is in the path of the direct beam of radiation.

localizing ring The extraoral part of an intraoral paralleling receptor-holding device that aligns the x-ray beam with the film or sensor (receptor).

long axis The imaginary line that divides the tooth vertically in two halves.

long cone Used to refer to position-indicating devices on x-ray machines where the target-receptor (focal-film) distance is 16 in or greater.

long-scale contrast Film contrast in which the gray tone is predominant.

long-term effects Effects of radiation that appear years or decades after exposure to radiation.

low contrast See *long-scale contrast.*

M

magnetic field The field used in MRI that changes the alignment and orientation of the protons in the patient's body.

magnetic resonance imaging (MRI) An imaging modality that uses magnetic fields and radio frequencies to view pathologic lesions in the soft tissues of the body.

magnification The proportional enlargement of a radiographic image.

malignant growth (malignancy or malignant lesion) A type of tumor that can be locally destructive or metastasize and can result in a fatality.

malposed A tooth that is out of line with the dental arch.

mandibular canal (inferior alveolar canal) See *inferior alveolar canal.*

mandibular foramen Appears radiolucent on radiographs and is where the mandibular (inferior alveolar) canal originates. The mandibular foramen cannot be seen on intraoral radiographs.

mandibular tori (torus mandibularis) A specifically placed exostosis that is bilateral, appears radiopaque, and is located in the mandibular premolar region on dental radiographs.

manual processing The process of developing radiographs where the film hangers are manually placed in the processing solutions.

marking grid The device used to superimpose either radiopaque or radiolucent lines in 1-mm vertical and horizontal increments.

mass number The number of nucleons (protons and neutrons) in the nucleus of an atom.

maxillary sinus The radiolucent area seen apical to the maxillary posterior teeth.

maxillary torus (torus palatinus) A specifically placed exostosis at the midline of the palate that appears radiopaque on dental radiographs.

maxillary tuberosity The distal portion of the maxillary alveolar ridge.

maxillofacial radiology That specialty of dentistry concerned with exposure and interpretation of diagnostic imaging used for examining the craniofacial, dental, and adjacent structures.

maximum permissible dose (MPD) The amount of whole-body radiation to which an occupationally exposed person (or the general public) can be exposed to without any harm during a specific period of time (i.e. yearly).

median palatal suture The radiolucent line seen running vertically between the roots of the maxillary central incisors.

medullary spaces Radiolucent areas seen in bone representing the bone marrow.

mental foramen The round radiolucent area seen near the apices of the mandibular premolars.

mental ridge The V-shaped radiopacity seen in mandibular anterior radiographs.

mesiodens A supernumerary tooth found in the midline of the maxillary arch.

metabolic lesion A radiographic finding caused by a generalized pathologic condition.

microorganism An organism, such as bacteria, of microscopic or ultramicroscopic size.

midsagittal plane The imaginary line that divides the skull in equal parts in the sagittal plane.

milliamperage (mA) Current strength expressed in milliamperes (one thousandth of an ampere). The mA setting controls the quantity of the x-ray beam in the dental x-ray tube.

milliroentgen (mR) One thousandth of a roentgen.

mixed dentition Both primary and secondary teeth are present in the oral cavity.

mixed lesion A radiographic lesion that has both radiolucent and radiopaque components.

molecule The smallest particle of a substance that retains the properties of the substance.

monitor Computer image screen used in digital radiography.

monitoring device The instrument that measures radiation exposure.

mounts The cardboard or plastic sheets used to hold and view a finished radiograph.

Multiplanar reconstructed images (MPR images) When these axial, coronal, and sagittal CBCT images are viewed simultaneously.

mutation The chemical effect of a change in a gene or a chromosomal aberration.

mylohyoid ridge See *internal oblique ridge.*

N

nasal cavity The bilateral radiolucent areas seen superior to the maxillary central incisors.

nasal septum The radiopaque vertical line separating the right and left nasal cavities.

nasolabial fold A radiolucent area seen distal to the canine.

nasopalatine (incisive) foramen The oval radiolucent landmark located between the roots of the maxillary central incisors.

negligent Failure to exercise the care that a prudent person would usually exercise in the same situation.

neutron A particle that has no charge but has mass. It is found in the nucleus of an atom.

nucleus The positively charged, relatively heavy inner core of an atom.

normalizing device The device utilized in the procedure for testing the strength of the processing solutions. This procedure involves placing the processed film in a slot and moving the measured densities until a visual match of densities is achieved. If the test densities are too light, the solutions are too weak or too cold. If the densities are too dark, the solutions are too concentrated or too warm.

nutrient canals Pathways for blood vessels and nerves that appear as radiolucent vertical lines in alveolar bone.

O

object The structure being radiographed, such as tooth or bone.

object density The density (thickness) of the teeth, bone, and soft tissue being radiographed, which is determined by the structure of the object being radiographed, and the image density, which is the degree of blackness on an image.

object-film distance The distance between the object and the x-ray film. Currently known as the *object-receptor distance.*

object-receptor distance See *object-film distance.*

occlusal caries Caries that are found on the biting surfaces of teeth and are usually not seen well on radiographs.

occlusal receptor A large intraoral receptor (#4) placed on the occlusal surfaces of either the upper or lower teeth and used to portray objects in the buccolingual dimension.

occlusal plane The imaginary plane formed by the occlusal contact of upper and lower teeth.

occlusal projection A radiographic projection of the mandible or maxilla that shows either a larger area or a right-angle (axial) relationship of the objects being radiographed.

Occupational Safety and Health Administration (OSHA) The federal agency that oversees health and safety in the workplace.

oligodontia The absence of many teeth (many missing teeth).

open contact When the interproximal surfaces of teeth or restorations do not touch.

operator concern Radiation concerns that lie with the operator.

Optically scanned digital radiography The process in indirect digital imaging whereby a finished conventional radiograph is scanned and then digitized and the information is sent to the computer.

orbit A prescribed path or ring in which electrons travel around the nucleus of an atom.

orientation dot This is a small, convex-concave area that indicates which side of the film was facing the tooth and the source of radiation and helps to orient the developed film in mounting.

osteoradionecrosis An area of bone does not heal from the high levels of radiation used in radiation therapy.

output The amount of radiation produced by the x-ray machine (measured in roentgens per second).

overdeveloped The condition of a radiograph being too dark because of the film's having been left in the developer solution too long.

overexposure A dark or dense image due to improper settings (kV, mA, exposure time) causing excessive exposure due to overpenetration of the x-ray beam.

overlapping The interproximal surfaces of adjoining teeth are superimposed on each other because of improper horizontal angulation or improper placement of the receptor in the horizontal plane.

overretention The state of the deciduous teeth not being shed at the expected time.

P

packet A wrapping or container for intraoral x-ray film that is light-tight and permits penetration of x-rays. Packets are usually made of plastic, paper or cardboard.

panoramic image An extraoral radiograph that shows both the mandible and the maxilla and other structures out of the realm of intraoral radiographs in their entirety on a single image.

Panorex The commercial name for one of the earliest panoramic units.

pantomogram A panoramic radiograph produced by curved surface tomography.

paperless office A dental office where all records, including radiographs and photographs, are produced and stored in digital form on a computer.

parallel Moving or lying in the same plane, equidistant, and never intersecting.

paralleling technique A technique for intraoral periapical radiography in which the receptor is positioned parallel to the long axis of the tooth and the central ray is directed perpendicular to both the tooth and the receptor.

pathogen A disease-causing microorganism.

patient concern Radiation concerns that lie with the patient.

patient movement When a patient moves during an exposure causing a blurred radiographic image.

penetration The ability of x-rays to pass through an object and reach the receptor.

penumbra The vague or blurred area that surrounds the edge of the radiographic image.

periapical abscess A type of periapical pathologic process whereby an abscess forms at the apex of a tooth.

periapical cemento-osseous dysplasia (PCOD) (periapical cemental dysplasia - PCD) A three-stage asymptomatic lesion seen on mandibular anterior periapical radiographs.

periapical condensing osteitis The apical bony response to low-level infection that appears radiopaque on dental radiographs.

periapical cyst A cyst formed at the apex of a tooth.

periapical projection Intraoral image representing the entire tooth from the incisal or occlusal surface to the apex of the root and 2-3 mm of surrounding bone.

periapical granuloma A granuloma formed at the apex of a tooth.

periapical lesions Radiolucent or radiopaque lesions appearing at the apex of the tooth.

periapical pathologic condition The infectious condition that arises at the apex of a tooth as the sequela of pulpal necrosis.

periapical radiograph An intraoral image that shows the entire tooth and surrounding bony structures.

period of injury This period occurs after radiation exposure and the latent period, and can include changes in the cell's or tissue's function.

periodontal abscess A soft tissue abscess of the gingiva that is seen as a radiolucency interproximally on radiographs.

periodontal disease Disease of the supportive structures of the teeth.

periodontal ligament Radiolucent area around the root of the tooth between the cementum and the lamina dura.

permissible dose The amount of radiation that one can receive without suffering any clinical effects.

personal protective equipment (PPE) Personal barriers to the transmission of infective microorganisms including gloves, masks, protective eyewear, and protective clothing that must be worn in the dental environment.

perpendicular Intersecting or meeting at a 90-degree angle.

phosphor A substance that when struck by radiation will emit light.

photoelectric effect An interaction of an x-ray photon with an atom in which an inner shell electron is released and the total energy of the photon is absorbed.

photon A discrete unit of energy.

photostimulable phosphor plate An electronic sensor used in indirect digital radiography that is read by a laser beam scanner.

physical disability A condition that limits the patient's ability to perform certain movements.

pixel A discrete point of information utilized in digital radiography to produce the digital image.

pocket dosimeters Small ionization chambers that the operator wears to measure radiation occupational exposure.

point of entry Anatomic location on the patient's face at which the central x-ray is aimed so that the x-rays strike the center of the receptor in the patient's mouth.

point of rotation A point in a tomographic unit around which the sensor and source of energy rotate.

position-indicating device (PID) That part of the x-ray machine (cone, rectangle, or cylinder) that aligns the useful beam to the object and receptor.

posteroanterior projection The companion projection to the lateral skull used to survey the skull in the anteroposterior plane, which provides a means of localizing changes in a mediolateral direction.

pregnancy The condition in which a woman is carrying a fetus in her womb.

primary dentition The first (deciduous) set of teeth.

primary radiation X-rays coming directly from the target of the x-ray tube.

primordial cyst A cyst seen in the jaws that forms instead of a tooth.

progeny The descendants of an individual.

proton A positively charged particle that has mass. It is found in the nucleus of an atom.

pterygomaxillary fissure It is a radiopaque outlined triangular interval, formed by the divergence of the maxilla from the pterygoid process of the sphenoid bone. It appears as an inverted teardrop on extraoral radiographs.

pulp calcifications The condition in which the pulp canals and chambers are completely filled with dentin.

pulp canal and chamber The space within the crown and root of the teeth where the soft tissue of the pulp is found.

pulp denticle (pulp stone) A calcification formed in either the pulp chamber or the pulp canal.

pulp horns An extension of the pulp extending toward the cusp of a tooth.

Q

quality assurance (QA) program A series of tests and procedures to ensure that all components of the radiographic system are functioning at an acceptable level of quality so as to ensure the best radiograph for the radiation exposure.

quality factor An expression of the different types of effects that radiation produces in human tissue (for x-rays, Q = 1).

R

radiation The emission and propagation of energy in the form of waves or particles.

radiation absorbed dose (rad) A unit of absorbed radiation equal to 100 ergs per gram. In dental radiology, 1 rad is equal to approximately 1 roentgen.

radiation caries The type of caries caused by a decrease and changes in saliva secondary to radiation therapy of the head and neck.

radiation exposure The process of being struck by radiation, either primary or secondary.

radiation history The record of a patient's exposure to radiation for diagnostic and therapeutic needs.

radiation inspection The monitoring of x-ray equipment and procedures by some governmental body or CRESO (certified radiation equipment safety officer).

radiation risk The likelihood of ill effects from radiation.

radioactive process The process whereby certain unstable elements undergo spontaneous degeneration and produce high-energy waves called gamma and particulate radiations.

radiobiology Is the study of the effects of ionizing radiation on biologic tissue.

radiofrequency The frequency in the electromagnetic spectrum at which radio waves are found.

radiograph The visual image produced by chemically processing the effects of x-rays on film or the dental image that appears on a computer monitor as a result of digital radiography.

radiolucent (RL) Refers to areas on the radiograph that appear dark. These objects have little or no density.

radiolucent lesion A pathologic lesion that is dark on radiographs.

radionuclide A radioactive substance.

radiopaque (RO) Refers to areas on the radiograph that appear light. These are objects that are dense.

radiopaque lesion A pathologic lesion that is light on radiographs.

radiopaque medium A liquid that is injected into body vessels or spaces whose outline is radiopaque on the radiograph for diagnostic pruposes.

radioresistant cell A cell that is relatively unaffected by radiation.

radiosensitive cell A cell that is sensitive to radiation.

rapid processing The processing of radiographs by either elevated solution temperature or concentration, which markedly shortens the time needed to produce an image. This technique is used when the time it takes to process the film is shortened and is more important than the exacting of the image.

rare earth elements A group of metallic elements that contain oxides classified as rare earths. Such elements are used in intensifying screens to produce light.

receptor The material (film, film screen, or digital sensor) that is affected by the x-ray beam and from which the visible image is formed.

receptor holder The device that holds and positions the receptor (e.g., film) in the patient's mouth.

receptor (film or sensor) plane The plane (axial, sagittal, or coronal) in which the receptor (film or sensor) is held for radiographic exposure.

receptor (film or sensor) position The description of the relationship between the receptor (film or sensor) and the teeth to be radiographed.

recessed target The design of a dental x-ray machine in which the tube is positioned at the back of the tube head that allows for a 12-in to 16-in target-receptor (focal-film) distance and a short position-indicating device (PID).

recessed tube An x-ray tube that is placed in the rear part of the tube head, with the rest of the components placed on both sides of the beam. This design extends the focal distance without increasing the length of the position-indicating device.

record keeping Keeping accurate records of films processed, mounted, and filed as an important part of a QA program in a dental facility.

records The written or electronic description and images of treatment given to a patient.

rectangular collimation Limiting the shape of an x-ray beam to a rectangle instead of the conventional circle.

rectification Blocking of the flow of current in one direction in an alternating current circuit.

reference film An ideally processed film, which is kept on the darkroom viewbox, to which densities and contrasts can be compared to check the strength of the processing solutions.

reformatting In computed tomography, changing the plane of orientation in which the image is portrayed.

replenisher A concentrated form of either the developer or fixer solutions that is used to maintain the volume and concentration of the solutions.

res gestae "Admissions against interest" – These are statements made by anyone spontaneously at the time of an alleged negligent act that are then considered admissible as evidence.

residual cyst A cyst that was not removed with the extraction of the tooth and continues to grow.

residual granuloma A granuloma that was not removed with the extraction of the tooth and continues to grow.

resolution The discernible separation of closely adjacent image details.

resonance The transition from one energy level to another.

respondeat superior The legal doctrine that states that liability, both professionally and legally, rests with the dentist and not the hygienist or dental assistant.

retake The repeating of a non-diagnostic exposure.

reticulation An unsatisfactory image caused by a sudden change in temperature from one processing solution to another.

reverse bitewing A variation of a bitewing whereby the receptor is placed in the buccal sulcus and the central ray directed at the receptor from the other side of the jaw as in a lateral oblique projection.

ridge A radiopaque line representing extra bone seen on radiographs.

right-angle occlusal projection This technique (also known as the 90-degree or cross-sectional projection) employs directing the central ray at an angle of 90 degrees to the receptor. This technique is used for locating an oral finding in the buccolingual or *the third dimension*.

right-angle technique (projection) Another name for the paralleling technique. See *paralleling technique*.

risk estimate The comparing of the presence of a finding between irradiated and nonirradiated populations.

risk factors Are expressed as the number of cases or deaths from a specific disease per million persons.

risk management Office procedures and policies that reduce the likelihood of litigation.

roentgen (R) The basic unit for measuring x-ray (ionizing radiation) exposure in air. It is the amount of radiation needed to produce one electrostatic charge in 1 cm3 of air. The milliroentgen (mR) is one thousandth of a roentgen.

roentgen equivalent man (rem) The expression of dose equivalent; the dose of radiation that produces the same biologic effects in humans as are produced by 1 roentgen of x-radiation. For x-rays the rem equals the roentgen.

root resorption The destruction of the root structure caused by chronic periapical or periodontal infection, trauma, pressure from tumors or cysts, or rapid excessive orthodontic pressure, or it can be idiopathic.

root sack The radiolucent ball seen at the apices of developing teeth.

RVG system One of the earliest dental digital units to be put on the market.

S

safelight Illumination used in the darkroom that does not affect the film emulsion.

sagittal plane (of the head) A vertical longitudinal plane that divides the head into right and left sections.

salivary stones (sialoliths or salivary calculi) Calcifications in the salivary gland or duct that causes an obstruction and possible consequential swelling and infection.

scale of contrast Refers to the range of densities seen in a dental radiographic image.

scanner A device that senses the grayscales of a radiograph and records it in the digital form for a printout or computer storage.

scatter radiation Radiation that during its passage through a substance has been deviated in other directions. It also may have been modified by an increase in wavelength. It is one form of secondary radiation.

secondary dentin Dentin produced by the pulp in response to an irritation or aging.

secondary radiation Radiation that comes from any matter being struck by primary radiation (i.e. scatter radiation). Secondary x-rays are less penetrating than primary x-rays.

selection criteria Those factors that dictate whether radiographs are necessary and useful in a specific clinical situation.

self- or half-wave-rectified The blocking of the reversal of a current (rectification) that the dental x-ray tube operating on an alternating current is designed to produce.

sensor An electronic detector plate that is placed in the patient's mouth to record the penetrating x-ray photons in digital radiography.

septa Radiopaque lines seen dividing bony spaces.

sharpness The visual quality or clarity of a radiograph (conventional or digital), which depends on the resolution, detail, or definition of a radiographic image.

shell See *orbit.*

shielding Preventing or reducing the passage of radiation.

short cone A position-indicating device on dental x-ray machines for which the target-receptor (focal-film) distance is 8 in.

short-scale contrast A reduced range of grays on a radiograph (i.e., high contrast).

sialography A modality for radiographic visualization of salivary glands following the injection of a contrast medium into the salivary ducts for diagnostic purposes.

sialolith A salivary calcification (stone).

sievert (Sv) The Système International (SI) unit for the dose equivalent. One sievert equals 100 rem.

sight development A film-processing technique in which the time the film stays in the developer is subjectively determined by periodically looking at the developing image under safelight conditions.

signal intensity The strength of the radiofrequency wave that comes from the patient back to the detector in magnetic resonance imaging.

silver bromides (a type of silver halide) The x-ray-sensitive crystals used in the film emulsion.

sinus A radiolucent cavity in bone.

slit beam tomogram A tomographic image produced by an extremely narrow, rectangular x-ray beam.

SLOB rule The acronym used to interpret the results of using the tube shift method (Clark's rule, or the buccal-object rule) to determine the relative buccolingual relationship between two structures that appear radiographically superimposed. SLOB stands for *same lingual, opposite buccal* which means that if after the tube shift the object moves in the opposite direction of the tube shift it is said to be buccally positioned and if it stays the same, it is said to be more lingually positioned.

soft tissue window A density range seen in computed tomographic scans that portrays mainly soft tissue.

soft x-rays X-rays of longer wavelengths and low penetration.

software A computer program and other operating information used by a computer.

somatic effects Effects of radiation on all cells except the reproductive cells.

standard of care The quality of care that is provided by dental practitioners in a similar location under the same or similar conditions.

statute of limitations The period of time in which a patient can bring suit against a dentist or dental health professional.

step-down transformer A transformer designed to decrease the voltage.

step-up transformer A transformer designed to increase the voltage.

step wedge The device used to measure the penetration of a dental x-ray beam.

sterilization The process used to destroy all pathogens, including highly resistant bacteria and spores.

stochastic effects The effects of radiation exposure that occur by chance and by changes in the DNA of body cells. In the context of radiation protection, the main stochastic effect is radiation-induced cancer.

stop bath The solution (water in x-ray processing) in which films are placed after the developer.

storage phosphor A type of indirect digital radiography that uses photostimulable phosphor plate technology.

submandibular fossa The broad radiolucent band seen apical to the mandibular molars that represents a medial bone depression.

submentovertex projection An extraoral projection whereby jaws are seen from an inferior view. This projection is used to detect fractures of the zygomatic arch and visualize the sphenoid and ethmoid sinuses as well as the lateral wall of the maxillary sinus. It is also used in tomography as a scout film to determine the positions of the condyles in imaging evaluation of the TMJ.

Système International (SI) units The units of radiation measurement that standardize measurement to the metric system.

T

target That part of the anode that the high-speed electrons strike and that produces x-rays and heat. In dental x-ray tubes, the target is usually made of tungsten.

target-object distance See *focal-object distance.*

target-receptor distance See *focal-film distance.*

taurodontia (taurodontism) A developmental defect of teeth in which the crowns have longitudinally enlarged pulp chambers with short roots.

temporomandibular joint (TMJ) The joint formed by the articulation of the mandibular condyle and the temporal bone of the maxilla.

tesla (T) The unit of measurement for the strength of the magnetic field in an MRI unit.

thermionic emission effect Production of free electrons by the passing of an electric current through a tungsten filament with resultant heating of the filament.

thermometer The device found in the developer solution used to measure the temperature of the solution.

thermostatic valve A device used to control the temperature of the incoming water in the manual developing tanks.

thin image A light image, lacking in density.

threshold erythema dose (TED) The minimal dose of radiation to the skin that will produce a reddening of the skin on the most sensitive patient's skin.

thyroid collar The lead drape put around the patient's neck to shield the thyroid gland during intraoral radiographic procedures.

timer The parameter on the x-ray unit control panel that regulates the exposure time.

time-temperature development A technique used to process x-ray films in which the time the film stays in the developer is calibrated to the temperature of the solution within a stated acceptable range.

tissue sensitivity That scale of sensitivity of various tissues in the body to radiation. Some tissues (e.g., epithelium) are very radiosensitive, whereas others (e.g., bone) are relatively radioresistant.

tomogram A radiograph of a three-dimensional object that shows a predetermined plane with blurring of all other superimposed structures.

tomography A radiographic modality that allows imaging in one plane of an object while blurring or eliminating images from structures in other planes.

tooth eruption The growth and migration of teeth into the oral cavity.

Topographic occlusal projection A type of occlusal radiographic technique that shows a large area, utilizing extreme vertical angulations which are necessary to compensate for the lack of parallelism between the object and the receptor. This projection is a modification of the bisecting-angle technique.

torn emulsion Film-processing error that occurs when the emulsion is removed from the acetate base in a finished radiograph.

total body exposure The radiation dosage that reflects the effects on the whole body of the person exposed.

trabecula Radiopaque line separating marrow spaces in bone.

trabecular pattern The expression of the radiographic appearance of alveolar bone.

transcranial projection An extraoral projection used to visualize the temporomandibular joint.

transformer An electric device that can either increase (step up) or decrease (step down) voltage.

transposed Tooth development in another position in the dental arch.

triangulation A description of the shape of interproximal bone loss when the periodontal ligament separates from the tooth and has a triangular shape with the base of the triangle toward the crown and the point of the triangle toward the root of the tooth.

trismus The state of being unable to open one's mouth.

trough The depth of an energy (i.e. x-ray) wave.

tube head drift Drift of the x-ray tube head from its set position.

tube head leakage Leakage of x-rays from an area in the tube head other than the port.

tube shift A technique used to localize objects in the buccolingual plane by shifting the tube for a comparative radiograph.

tuberosity A normal anatomic bony protrusion.

tuberosity pad The fibrous buildup of soft tissue above the maxillary tuberosity causing a slightly radiopaque shadow on the radiograph in the maxillary posterior region.

tungsten filament Component of the cathode in the dental x-ray tube that heats up and produces the thermionic emission effect resulting in the formation of the electron cloud.

U

ultrasound Mechanical radiant energy above the audible range that can be used in diagnostic imaging.

umbra The sharp area that surrounds the edge of the radiographic image.

underdevelopment A thin (light) film that is the result of weak solutions or incorrect developing time.

underexposure The condition of an image that is light or thin as a result of insufficient exposure time, inadequate kV or mA, or excessive FFD.

unilateral lesion A lesion seen only on one side of a patient.

universal precautions An infection control protocol that is followed for all patients regardless of history and clinical findings.

useful beam The part of the primary radiation that passes through the diaphragm aperture and filter and exits through the position-indicating device.

V

vaccination The introduction of vaccine (i.e., a weakened, dead, or genetically altered form of a microorganism) for the purpose of inducing immunity.

vertical angulation The angle made between the x-ray beam and a line parallel to the floor.

vertical bitewing Bitewing projection in which the receptor is placed in the patient's mouth with its long dimension running vertically.

vertical bone loss Interproximal bone loss in periodontal disease in the vertical plane.

viewbox An illuminated device used to view radiographs.

visible image The image present on a radiograph after the film has been processed.

visually impaired A person who has lost all or part of the ability to see.

vitality testing The technique that uses either thermal or electrical stimulation to determine whether a tooth is vital or nonvital.

voltage The difference in potential in an electric circuit. It is this difference that causes the current to flow.

W

water bath The second and fourth solutions (water) in the manual processing of dental radiographs.

Waters' view The type of posteroanterior extraoral projection that enlarges the middle third of the skull to prevent superimposition, usually used for viewing the maxillary sinus.

wavelength The distance from the crest of one wave to the crest of the next wave. In radiology, wavelength is a measure of energy.

wet reading Interpretation of a radiograph approximately 3 minutes after its initial fixation.

wheelchair access The design of an office that permits unrestricted access and placement of all patients.

X

x-rays Penetrating electromagnetic radiations having wavelengths shorter than those of visible light and that are produced by bombarding a metal target with high-speed electrons.

Z

zygoma (malar bone) The radiopaque bone seen apical to the maxillary molars.

zygomatic arch The cranial bone that runs from the maxilla distally to the temporal bone.

zygomatic process of the maxilla A radiopaque "U"-shaped bone seen on maxillary posterior radiographic projections.

Index

Page numbers followed by "*f*" indicate figures, "*t*" indicate tables, and "*b*" indicate boxes.